The Heritage of NUCLEAR MEDICINE

Editorial Panel:
Marshall Brucer, MD
C. Craig Harris, MS
William J. MacIntyre, PhD
George V. Taplin, MD

Book Coordinator:
James A. Sorenson, PhD

Commemorating the 25th Anniversary of the Society of Nuclear Medicine, 1954–1979

ISBN-O-932004-02-4

Library of Congress Number 79-65338

Published 1979 by the Society of Nuclear Medicine, Inc., 475 Park Avenue South. New York, NY 10016.

Foreword

This volume commemorates the 25th anniversary of two important historical events for the Society of Nuclear Medicine: the first organizational meeting of the Society, which took place in Spokane, Washington, on January 19, 1954, and the Society's first annual meeting in Seattle, May 29–30, 1954.

The papers reprinted in this volume trace the history of the development of basic principles underlying the practice of nuclear medicine, beginning with the fundamental discoveries in physics and radiochemistry of the late 19th and early 20th centuries, and leading to the first descriptions in the 1950's of now commonplace techniques and instrumentation. The papers were selected by a distinguished editorial panel, who themselves have made significant contributions to the develoment of nuclear medicine: Marshall Brucer, Craig Harris, Jim MacIntyre, and George Taplin. The papers are arranged in chronological order, following an introductory article by Dr. Brucer. In Dr. Brucer's article, an asterisk is used to indicate that a particular paper or work is included in the selection of reprinted papers.

It was, of course, impossible to include in this volume all of the important works that led to the development of nuclear medicine. For reasons of space, it was necessary to omit many otherwise worthwhile papers. It was also felt that the sheer volume of papers published since 1960 made the selection of papers from this period an impossible task. The reader should be aware, then, that the papers included are representative but by no means all-inclusive of historically important work. In spite of these shortcomings, however, it is hoped that the selection will prove to be interesting, informative, and rewarding to the reader.

In addition to the editorial panel, who took on the most difficult task of identifying those papers to be included, many other individuals are deserving of special thanks for assistance in the production of this volume: Mr. Julian Maack and the staff of the University of Utah Medical Illustrations Service accomplished the very challenging task of obtaining photographic copies from the original papers. From the Society's central office, Mr. David Kellner provided valuable editorial assistance, Mr. Rodney Hough was responsible for typesetting, and the graphic design was done by Mr. Paul Greenwald with Ms. Laura Chalfin's assistance. The cover photograph, showing Dr. Saul Hertz injecting a rabbit being held by Dr. Arthur Roberts, was taken about 1937, and was kindly provided by Dr. Robley Evans. Dr. William Myers and Dr. Gerry Hine provided translations of papers from foreign languages (papers by Villard [p. 21], and Geiger and Müller [p. 67], respectively). Finally, I offer special thanks to the Society President, Dr. Doug Maynard, and to the Society Publications Committee under the chairmanship of Dr. Rita Hays for their encouragement and support for this project.

James A. Sorenson, Ph.D.
Book Coordinator
Society of Nuclear Medicine

Nuclear Medicine Begins with a Boa Constrictor

Marshall Brucer

In the beginning, a boa constrictor defecated in London and the subsequent development of nuclear medicine was inevitable. It took a little time, but the 139-yr chain of cause and effect that followed was inexorable (*1*).

One June week in 1815 an exotic animal exhibition was held on the Strand in London. A young "animal chemist" named William Prout (we would now call him a clinical pathologist) attended this scientific event of the year. While he was viewing a boa constrictor recently captured in South America, the animal defecated and Prout was amazed by what he saw. The physiological incident was commonplace, but he was the only person alive who could recognize the material. Just a year earlier he had isolated the first pure sample of urea—but from the urine of patients with gout!

Upon seeing the unusual feces, Prout sought out the animal caretaker and requested a sample. Grave robbers were an ongoing scandal in London in those days, but coprophilia was a new twist. The incredulous animal caretaker crossed himself twice and cleaned out the cage. Prout hurried back to his surgery (the British use of the term) with his unusual prize.

In 1815 it was not unusual for a clinical pathologist to practice medicine from his own surgery. It couldn't have been unusual because Prout was the first and only existing clinical pathologist. After getting his M.D. from the University of Edinburgh, Prout walked the wards of the United Hospitals of St. Thomas's and Guy's until licensed by the Royal College of Physicians on December 22, 1812. In addition to seeing patients, he analyzed urine and blood for other physicians, using methods and laboratory equipment of his own design.

Prout dissolved the snake's feces in muriatic acid and then analyzed the insoluble precipitate. Just as he suspected, it was almost pure (90.16%) uric acid. As a thorough scientist he also determined the "proportional number" of 37.5 for urea. ("Proportional" or "equivalent" weight was the current terminology for what we now call "atomic weight.") This 37.5 would be used by Friedrich Woehler in his famous 1828 paper on the synthesis of urea. Thus Prout, already the father of clinical pathology, became the grandfather of organic chemistry.

[Prout was also the first man to use iodine (2 yr after its discovery in 1814) in the treatment of thyroid goiter. He considered his greatest success the discovery of muriatic acid, inorganic HCl, in human gastric juice. He was first to divide the aliments into three classes: sanguinous (carbohydrate), oligenous (fat), and albuminous (protein). He designed and supervised construction of the Royal Society's first

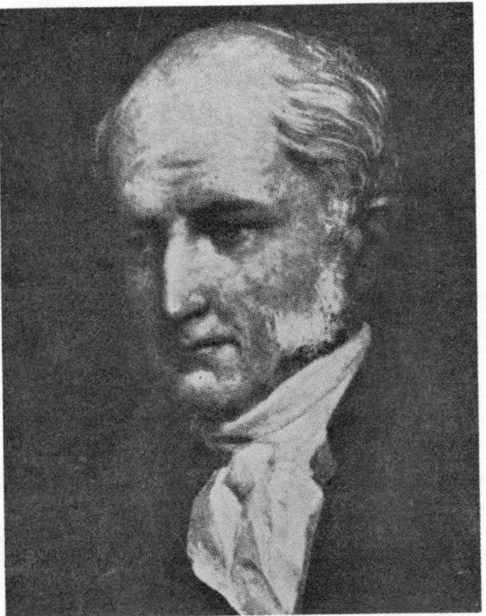

FIG. 1. William Prout MD, FRS, FRCP (1785–1850).

official barometer. From the weather patterns over London he was led by rigid epidemiological reasoning to the cause of London's devastating cholera outbreak; (wrong, of course, but so logical that it puts him in line as grandfather of our modern crusades against cancer).]

In order to determine the proportional weight for urea Prout had to use the "atomic" weights of the involved elements. There were 40–45 chemical elements in 1815 depending upon how many of Davy and Dalton's discoveries you believed. Humphery Davy and John Dalton were sloppy chemists. Thirty-five years later his obituarist would point out that Prout had "a taste for extreme exactitude and unrivaled manual expertness never achieved by John Dalton" (*2*). Prout remeasured the proportional weights of the elements and noted a remarkable consistency. All of the weights were whole numbers —or very nearly so. He argued that with greater accuracy they would all be multiples of the atomic weight of hydrogen. Published in an anonymous paper (*3*) this whole number rule, soon known as Prout's hypothesis, was so highly praised that he quickly acknowledged authorship. But eventually chlorine was its undoing. In 1828 Berzelius proved the atomic weight of chlorine to be midway between 35 and 36. The supposition that half a hydrogen atom entered into the composition of chlorine did violence to Newton's unsplittable atom.

In 1832 the Chemistry Committee of the British Association awarded John Dalton and William Prout 50 pounds to investigate atomic weights and specifically to test the whole number hypothesis. They never did turn in a report because they got involved in an even bigger hassle on chemical nomenclature and formulae. The question of atomic weights was lost in the argument and wasn't "settled" until 1860 when the Belgium chemist, J. S. Stas, measured the weights with great accuracy. He said that the law of Prout was "une pure illusion."

With the Stas measurements, Prout's hypothesis was dead. However, in 1888, William Crookes, a generation more advanced than Stas, arrived at a new conclusion based upon the rapidly developing new technique of spectroscopy. "Probably our atomic weights merely represent a 'mean' value around which the actual atomic weight of the atoms vary within certain narrow limits. . . . when we say the atomic weight of, for instance, calcium is 40, we really express the fact that while the majority of atoms have a weight of 40 . . . a few have 39 or 41, a less number 38 or 42, and so on..." (*4*).*

In 1901 Lord Rayleigh voiced a new scientific consensus "...the atomic weights tend to approximate to whole numbers far more closely than can reasonably be accounted for by any accidental coincidence . . ." (*5*) And then in 1913 H. G. Moseley, using crystal defraction, demonstrated that ". . . as we pass from one element to the next using the chemical order of the elements in the periodic system . . . the number of charges is the same as the number of the place occupied by the element in the periodic system . . ." (*6*). Atomic number, not atomic weight, was critical. The first element, number one at the bottom of the periodic table, was hydrogen. After 98 years, Prout's hypothesis was no longer a hypothesis. But Berzelius and Stas were not false prophets; they could not possibly have foreseen the relationship until a new observation was made at the very top of the periodic table. And this required an observation on uranium that couldn't be made until Spiritualism was revealed in Massachusetts.

THROUGH SPIRITUALISM THE TRUE PATH TO NUCLEAR MEDICINE IS REVEALED

In 1867 Phillip, the youngest brother of William Crookes, died of yellow fever while on a cable-laying expedition in Havana. The circumstances were somewhat confused, and William felt a deep personal tragedy—almost a responsibility. He wanted to know how his brother had contracted this deadly disease (remember, mosquitoes were 30 years in the future). If he could only talk with his brother. Spiritualism, a recent import from Massachusetts, was all the rage in England at the time, and it offered a means.

Although a religious agnostic, Crookes, along with quite a few of England's top scientists, became intrigued by the "physical phenomena" behind the "psychic force." Table rappings, levitations, and apparitions could be investigated by scientific methods. Crookes made some observations and became hooked on the paranormal. He came dangerously close to capturing the Royal Society as an agent for the propagation of Spiritualism. But the cult's scientific dishonesty disgusted many scientists. Faraday commented that "many dogs have come to more logical conclusions" (*7*). But on the surface, Faraday's "fields-of-force" were just as aethereal as Crookes' "psychic-force" and nowhere near as practical—if you wanted to talk to your dead brother. Crookes was almost read out of scientific society. He was deeply hurt by the bitterness of his scientific peers. In his despondency he turned to a piece of scientific scutwork that would saturate his mind.

In 1861 Crookes had discovered the element thallium, but its atomic weight had never been properly measured. If Prout could be called an "exacting chemist" and Stas a "specialist in precision,"

**asterisks indicate papers appearing elsewhere in this volume.*

Crookes became a fanatic. He constructed a new balance enclosed in a specially prepared vacuum case. The expansibility of the weighing arms, knife edges, and weighing pans were all measured. The weights were made of a specially purified platinum. The friction of the forceps against the weights during transfer was obviated with especially made platinum hooks. The thallium sample to be weighed and all of the glass and reagents were prepared from multiple purifications.

Crookes used the Tl_2NO_3 method and arrived at an atomic weight of 203.642. The 1961 accepted value is 204.37. If it can be called an error, he made one error. He had used the Stas values for the atomic weights of nitrogen and oxygen. If he had used 1961 values, his atomic weight would have been 204.02.

The important point, historically, is that Crookes knew that he had committed an error—not in his impeccable chemical technique but in the physical concept of "mass." When daylight was shining on his balance the excursions of the balance needle seemed greater than in the dark. There was too much mass in his platinum balance to check this, and so he suspended pithballs from a straw and balanced these in a vacuum. Different colored rays of light were directed against one ball. It was repulsed by the beam of light, and more by red light than any other color. His demonstration before the Royal Society on April 22, 1874 provoked controversy. Shying away from the controversy, he improved on the unstable pithballs-on-a-straw and on April 22, 1875, demonstrated an instrument he called the "radiometer." Four discs of pith—black on one side, white on the other—were attached to four arms suspended on a steel needle so as to revolve horizontally. The whole was enclosed in a glass globe evacuated to the highest obtainable vacuum. The arms revolved when exposed to visible light. The rate of revolution was proportional to the intensity of the incident radiation. Upon demonstration before the Royal Society the radiometer caused a sensation. To many scientists the first question was, "How did he get that thing into the bottle?"

Maxwell's electromagnetic theory provides for light to exert a pressure. A light particle falling on the black surface would be absorbed and give up its momentum to the vane. Falling on the white surface the light particles would be reflected; the vane would recoil with a momentum equal and opposite to the reflected ray, thus doubling the momentum of an absorbed ray on the black side. Thus, the white side is repelled more than the black side, and Crookes' radiometer will rotate clockwise . . .

But it didn't—it rotated counterclockwise!

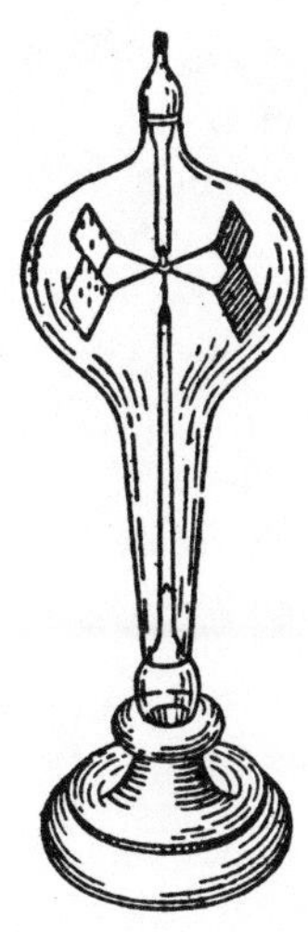

FIG. 2. Drawing of the Crookes Radiometer (c. 1875).

Mathematical physicists quivered when they saw the radiometer rotating in the wrong direction. Arthur Schuster (professor of mathematics at Owens College) had another explanation. The few gaseous molecules left in the vacuum globe impinged on both black and white surfaces of the vanes according to the kinetic theory of gases. When light impinges on the black surface it gets hotter, repels the molecules with greater speed, and their recoil rotates the vanes counterclockwise. A colleague suggested that Schuster set up a proof. If the vanes rotated by pressure from light, the globe itself would not be affected. But if the recoil were of molecules inside the globe, it too should rotate but in the opposite direction. At Owens College a radiometer was suspended by a fine thread so that it could rotate as freely as the vanes.

Maxwell's theory was hanging on a fine thread in Owens College. J. J. Thomson described the anxiety of physicists throughout England on the morning of the experiment:

"I can still remember the excitement and anxiety with which I waited for the verdict. And the relief on hearing that the case had rotated in the opposite direction to the vanes" (*8*).

Crookes had severely shaken but he hadn't cracked the foundations of science.

But making the toy for demonstration was no small task. A laboratory notebook entry by Crookes' lab assistant on March 7, 1876 marks the first rumble of an earthquake that eventually would crumble the foundations:

"Making radiometer for exhibition . . . all went well until putting in bulb when all came to grief . . . had to be taken out, unsoldered, put in another, when the cup took a piece out of the disk . . . I have tried hard to finish it, but find it impossible today" (*9*).

Crookes wrote in the notebook under this entry: "Cheer up!" And then he sketched in a tube with platinum anode and cathode embedded into the ends to modify the radiometer. This new tube was the protoype of the "Crookes tubes" that puzzled Roentgen 19 years later.

J. J. THOMSON CRACKS THE FOUNDATION OF 19TH CENTURY SCIENCE

In Germany a number of physicists had been passing electric currents through evacuated glass tubes that caused the glass to fluoresce. Electricity bore an obscure relationship to light and Crookes thought he could improve upon Johan Hittorf's famous shadow experiment of 1869. In a highly evacuated tube he placed an anode asymmetric so as to leave the path of the cathode ray beam free to strike the glass wall. He also placed a hinged mica maltese cross between the cathode and the glass wall. Upon activation of the cathode a shadow cast by the maltese cross was surrounded by fluorescing glass. After a while the fluorescence began to fade, presumably from fatigue in the glass. A flick of the wrist knocked the cross down and now the shadow itself fluoresced, but the fatigued glass remained dark.

Did this straight-line beam of light (or electricity, in this case) have sufficient mass to rotate his radiometer? He built another modification. In the glass tube he put a pair of glass rails. On the rails a paddlewheel could roll freely from end to end of the evacuated tube. Mica vanes attached to the paddlewheel interrupted the pathway from cathode to anode. He sent a current into the cathode. The paddlewheel rolled toward the anode. He reversed the current. The paddlewheel rolled back. Hence, the cathode rays were particles with mass. J. J. Thomson agreed that they might have mass, but a quick calculation showed that the mass was inadequate to move Crookes' paddlewheel—but he couldn't prove it.

In Germany, Johan Hittorf, a specialist in the transport of ions—atom-sized pieces of matter—should have agreed with Crookes. But he didn't. In 1869 he had put a point cathode into a vacuum bottle, interposed a solid body between it and the glass wall, and produced a sharp shadow in the fluorescence. In 1876 E. Goldstein substituted a very large cathode. It cast a shadow that was not sharp but had an umbra and a penumbra. He introduced the word "Kathodenstrahlen" because these cathode rays cast shadows; hence, like light, they were waves in ether.

This wave-versus-particles controversy lasted until 1895 when Jean Perrin, in France, made another Crookes tube, but this one with a small bucket to collect the ions. He proved that something, and it couldn't be ether waves, accumulated in his collector.

J. J. Thomson, who now agreed with Crookes, modified Perrin's tube and made a long series of measurements to estimate the weights of these "particles of matter." At a Friday evening discourse on April 29, 1897, at the Royal Institution, he disclosed his results. By indirect measurement the negatively charged particles in the cathode ray beam (he called them "corpuscles," we now call them "electrons") had about 1/1837 the mass of a hydrogen ion. A howl of laughter shook bells as far away as the tower of London. J. J. Thomson was "pulling their legs." It had taken over a century to convince scientists that the atom was the smallest piece of matter. Even Thomson didn't believe his own measurements. He reluctantly conceded error. Upon repetition of the experiment, he found there was error. He had made his corpuscles slightly too large!

Particles of matter smaller than an atom? It was hard to believe, and its significance was not appreciated at the time because every physicist was preoccupied with an even more astounding discovery: the invisible rays of Dr. Roentgen that came out of the Crookes tube.

BECQUEREL BREAKS THE LAW

On Monday, January 20, 1896, the regular meeting of the French Academy of Science featured a demonstration of Roentgen's new photography by Henri Poincaré. The Roentgen story had been leaked to the press 2 weeks earlier. (Roentgen didn't give his first paper until January 23, 1896.) But the newspaper article had been well written, and most physicists had a Crookes tube available for a quick check. Poincaré had verified the news story immediately.

Henri Becquerel, as always, attended the meeting. At the end of Poincaré's demonstration, Becquerel asked a question:

"From where do these remarkable rays originate?"

"Undoubtedly," answered Poincaré, "from the spot on the glass wall of the discharge tube rendered fluorescent by the impingement of the cathode rays" (*10*).

Poincaré's answer was technically correct, but Becquerel jumped to the wrong conclusion. Poincaré had not said that fluorescence caused X-rays, but Becquerel's confusion was understandable. His grandfather, Antoine, and his father, Edmund, had been world authorities on light from phosphorescence. As a demonstrator for his father, Henri had prepared a double sulphate of uranium and potassium that was remarkably phosphorescent after exposure to sunlight. If X-rays came from fluorescence on the glass wall of the Crookes tube, obviously they must also come from the intense phosphorescence of the double sulphate of uranium and potassium. Becquerel hurried back to his laboratory to test his misinterpretation.

The story of Becquerel's discovery is well known; the story of the confusion in his mind is not appreciated (*11*).*

The rays from uranium obviously represented the emission of energy. But what was the source of this energy? He proved that it could not come from air surrounding the uranium. It could not come from a chemical reaction. It was a permanent property of all uranium. After hundreds of experiments his interest waned until one of his graduate students, Marie Curie, and her husband Pierre proved that another substance they called polonium gave off, weight for weight, seven hundred times more radiation than uranium. And then, within 6 months, another substance, radium, was found to give off a million times more radiation than uranium.

By this time, December 1898, Becquerel's break with the conservation of energy law was under severe challenge. He was nibbling away at an explanation for each criticism (including his own disbelief). The Curies gave him a pinhead portion of their first radium sample in a glass vial. He carried the vial in his vest pocket to demonstrate to disbelievers that it gave off light, produced heat, and its radiation did not diminish in time. Soon there were no disbelievers, but there was still no imaginable source for the energy. The law of conservation of energy was dead.

WILLIAM CROOKES OPENS THE 20TH CENTURY IN PHYSICS

When the Curies announced polonium on July 18, 1898, there was considerable criticism: the spectroscope said "Bismuth." The criticism stopped when the master spectroscopist, William Crookes, showed that the only thing wrong with the Curies' discovery was that those French kids didn't know how to do spectroscopy. He made up his own sample of polonium and showed that in between the characteristic bismuth lines were a number of new lines never seen before. Polonium was an element.

Crookes used spectroscopy like we use a pencil. He had been the first to adapt photographic recording and was the recognized world authority on spectrum analysis. But it was only a tool; he was more interested in the impossible dilemma his old friend Becquerel had got himself into: energy coming out of uranium with no possible source for the energy.

In 1900 Crookes prepared a solution of uranium and a ferric salt. He added an excess of ammonium hydroxide and ammonium carbonate. The ferric hydroxide precipitate was intensely radioactive. (Remember, he was using Becquerel's photographic method.) "For the sake of lucidity," Crookes reported, "the new body must have a name. Until it is more tractable I will call it provisionally uranium X—the unknown substance Ex-Uranium" (*12*). (We now call it Th-234.) He sent off a letter to Becquerel who immediately confirmed the discovery. Crookes had made one slip. He hadn't run a spectrum of the new substance. He *always* did spectroscopy on every material he worked with. He would have fired an assistant who did not verify an analysis with the spectroscope. Uranium X was thorium. William Crookes's first chemical discovery 40 years earlier had been with the spectroscope, and he was very aware of its insensitivity in highly dilute samples. The distinctive thorium lines could have been obvious to Crookes with only about 15 minutes additional work. But just this once he forgot, and so he missed the greatest scientific discovery of the 20th century: that the elements were naturally transmuted during radioactive decay. But he made up for this horrible mistake by starting off the process whereby transmutation would be discovered.

If he could wash some radioactivity out of uranium, maybe Becquerel was wrong. Maybe all of the radioactivity could be washed out. He made some crystals of uranyl nitrate, did multiple ether separations, evaporated the ether for multiple fractional distillations. After many repetitions he was satisfied and tested his "pure" uranium on a photographic plate—the exposure was a total blank. He put the mother solution on a photographic plate, all the radioactivity was in the solution. With straightforward chemistry Becquerel's "always active" uranium had been washed clean of radioactivity. He immediately wrote to Becquerel:

"I've washed the radioactivity out of your uranium," and told him how to do it.

Upon opening the envelope, Becquerel exploded, "Impossible," and immediately repeated the experiment. He confirmed Crookes . . . but not quite. By this time Becquerel was using the electroscope in addition to the photographic method; the precipitate was very weak but not totally inactive. The mother solution, as Crookes had written, contained almost all the activity.

Becquerel was puzzled. What could he have done wrong to make such a mistake 4 years earlier when he proved that all uranium was "always" radioactive? A few months later he was still worried. He wasn't one to make that kind of mistake. So he dug out the 4-month-old samples and measured them again. On this repeat measurement the uranium was again hot, but now the mother solution was cold. He dashed off a note to Crookes, "Measure your samples again!" Then he began all over from scratch. Crookes broke his daily routine to check Becquerel. His 4-month-old cold uranium sample was now hot. The hot mother solution was now cold. After making some new uranium crystals, he too began all over from scratch.

When Crookes received the note from Becquerel, he had been writing to Rutherford telling him where to buy pure thorium nitrate. After checking Becquerel's finding, he added a paragraph describing the disappearance of radioactivity in UX and its regrowth in the parent uranium. Upon receiving Crookes' letter, Rutherford immediately checked all of his old thorium X samples: washout and regrowth were also true for thorium X.

But what was this thorium X? No such thing had ever been announced as a radioactive element.

THE 3RD SACRED COW OF 19TH CENTURY SCIENCE IS KILLED

It would be historically interesting to read the first draft of the Rutherford-Soddy paper on the radioactivity of thorium compounds. The published second draft gives the first hint of "transmutation" (*13*). But how, in the first draft, could they have explained the concentrations of short-lived (55 sec) radioactivity growing out from the extremely long-lived (14Gy) thorium? Rutherford admits that it can't be explained, and in the middle of a paragraph ThX suddenly creeps in as the explanation. (ThX is a 3.6 day isotope of radium.) Rutherford contradicts himself in mid-paper and proves that thorium X is different from thorium. While writing the paper, undoubtedly stretching his imagination for an explanation, Crookes' uranium X had been announced. Rutherford immediately did the same type of experiment with thorium and discovered thorium X, but he never announced it. The new element just crept into the corrected draft of the paper he was already writing.

Upon receiving this note from Crookes on the regrowth of uranium and the decay of uranium X, he immediately checked his old thorium X samples. All of his cold thorium precipitates were hot again and all the hot thorium X samples were now cold.

[Forget that you know of the existence of isotopes and then look at today's chart of nuclides (Fig. 3). You will then understand the impossible position that Rutherford was in. Uranium decays to thorium, which decays back to uranium, which decays back to thorium. Then look at thorium (Fig. 4). It decays to radium, which decays back to thorium, which decays back to radium. A more perfect system of concealment (without isotopes) is hard to imagine.]

Rutherford had originally said, "There can be no question ThX and [Crookes'] UX are distinct types of matter with definite chemical properties." The thorium manuscript was in press before Christmas (*14*). Upon opening Crookes' letter, Rutherford was astonished to see confirmation of his article which hadn't even been printed yet, and by no less than Crookes and Becquerel. He immediately wrote another article (*15*).* This time he included the forbidden words he had been thinking: ". . . the radioactive elements must be undergoing spontaneous transformation."

In 1897 J. J. Thomson's electron showed there were pieces of matter smaller than the atom, which was hard to swallow. By 1899 radium proved that Becquerel had broken the law of conservation of energy; it had to be believed, whether or not it was hard to swallow—you could see the radium glow. In 1902 Rutherford's "transmutation" was not a public sensation, it was a scientific obscenity—not mentioned in polite conversation. His senior colleagues at McGill begged Rutherford not to publish the second thorium article because it would bring disgrace upon McGill (*16*).

WHO PUT THE OVERALLS IN MRS. MURPHY'S CHOWDER?

Only a few physicists and a handful of chemists really believed in atomic transmutation. Completion of the Periodic Table was the big picture in chemistry. Rutherford's "transmutation" would eventually answer the chemical problem, but in 1902 it was all graphs of electrical measurements. Sir William Crookes, now the foremost chemist in the world, didn't like ionization chambers – too far from reality. He wanted to see, feel, smell, and weigh alpha particles. "How can I demonstrate the luminosity of radium in permanent fashion?" He wrote to a friend, an industrial chemist in Germany (who was selling dilute radium @ £2500/oz).

"Try Zinc Blende," his friend answered.

Crookes exposed some ZnS crystals and found they glowed when exposed to radium – essentially Roentgen's old discovery. He wanted to see what

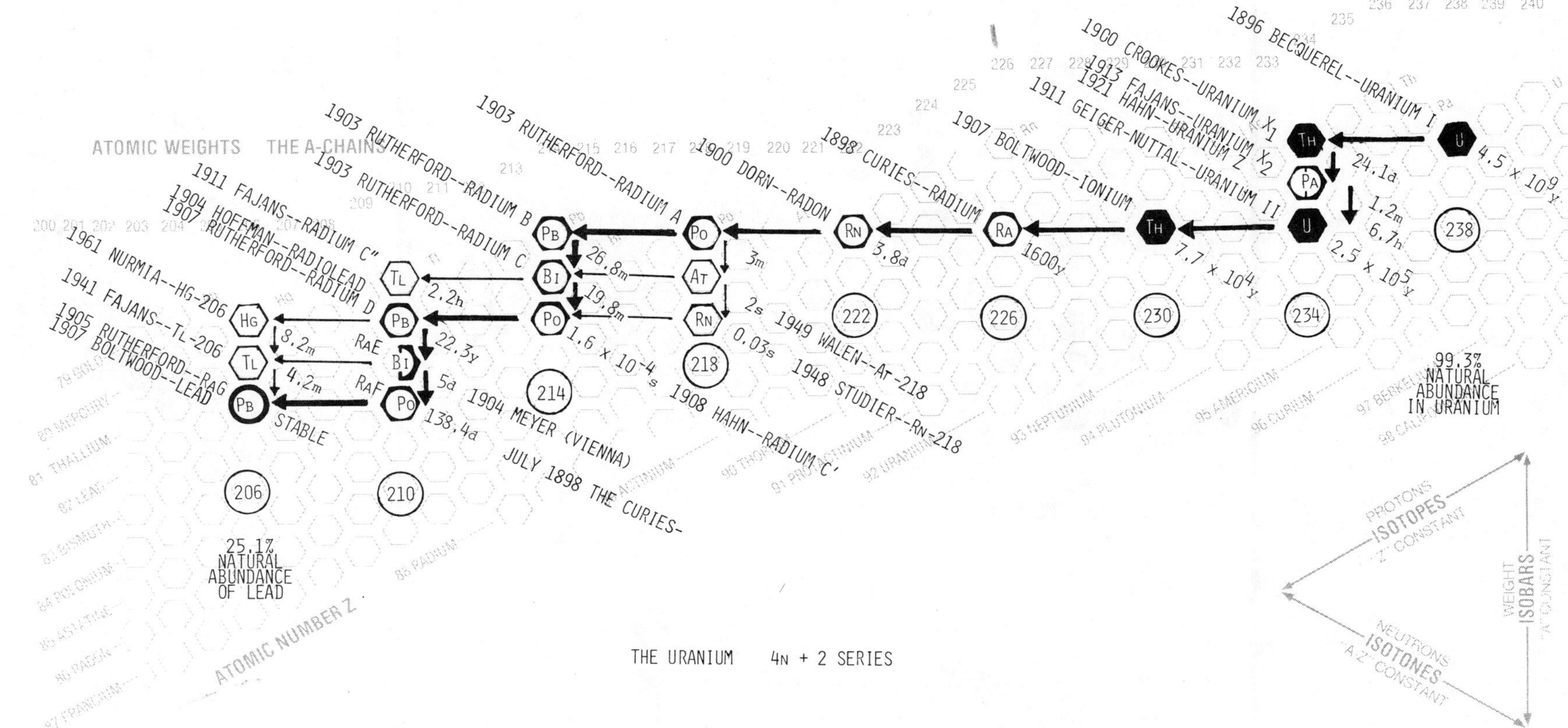

FIG. 3. Uranium Natural Decay Series.

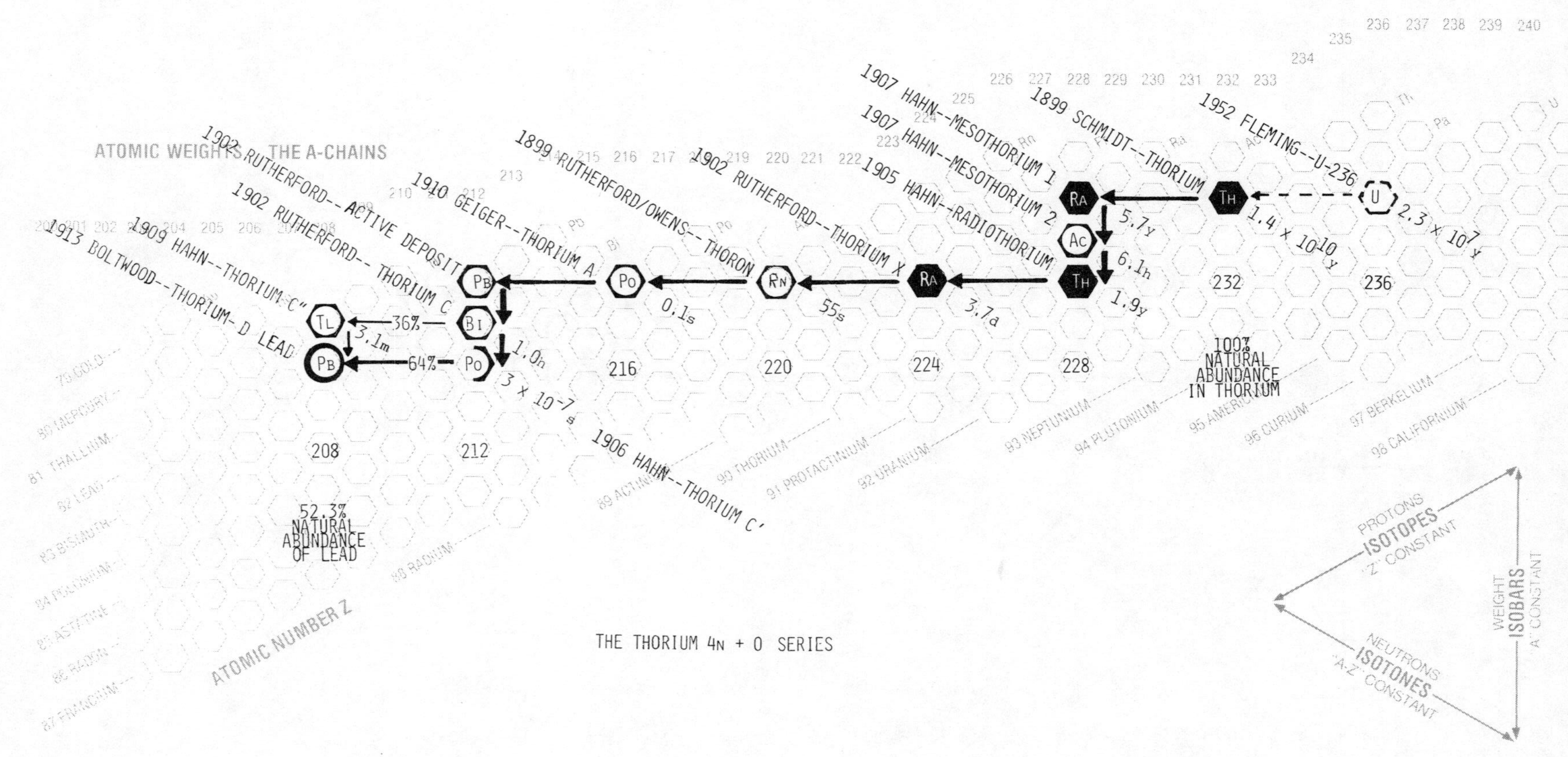

FIG. 4. Thorium Natural Decay.

happened when a single alpha hit a single crystal. He painted the bottom of a short metal tube with ZnS, put in a thumbscrew to regulate the distance of a needle from this ZnS screen and then plugged the other end of the tube with a microscope eyepiece. He dipped the needlepoint in a weak radium solution and positioned it as far from the zinc sulphide crystals as possible. Watching through the eyepiece he could see a faint glow of the ZnS. As he moved the radium on the needlepoint closer to the crystals, suddenly he began to see sparks, and then a cloud of sparks "resembling a swarm of fireflies on a dark night."(*7*)* He called the toy a spinthariscope (from the Greek spintharis = spark) and soon was demonstrating to all his friends that each spark was the interaction of a single alpha particle. Rutherford's curves on graph paper had suddenly become very lively members of scientific society.

When Rutherford arrived at Owens College in Manchester in 1906, he inherited Hans Geiger as his senior laboratory assistant; it proved to be an invaluable inheritance. They teamed up in a remarkable exploitation of Crookes' toy. They could count the number of sparks per minute and then, by replacing the ZnS screen with an electrical collector, they could measure the total charge per minute. By a simple division they had the average charge on each alpha particle and from this they could calculate its mass. Each alpha particle had twice the charge of the electron and four times the mass of a hydrogen atom. On 18 June 1908 they announced: "The alpha particle after it has lost its positive charge, is a helium atom." (*30*)

By 1908 transmutation was no longer a scientific obscenity. It was believable in the natural chains of radioactive decay because Rutherford had furnished a mechanism: transmuted elements were displaced in steps of four mass units with the emission of an alpha particle. Frederic Soddy at Glasgow preached the new chemistry with the fervor of an evangelist. But something was wrong. Not all decays released alpha particles.

Rutherford, Geiger, and a growing group of students kept on modifying the spinthariscope to measure alpha scattering from atoms until Rutherford envisioned something he called "the nuclear atom."* Geiger and the students were furnishing evidence that it was a valid picture – but not a theoretically satisfying picture.

One of Rutherford's transient students, a young theoretical physicist from Denmark, Neils Bohr, was worried about this unsatisfactory picture. Still another student, a physical chemist from Germany, Kasimer Fajans, teamed up with still another student from Oxford, H.G.J. Moseley, to measure the first true transmutation by a change in charge rather than in mass. Fajans went back to Germany to discover the beta displacement law.

Moseley followed his teammate in getting away from alpha particles; instead he looked at the emission of X-rays from elements bombarded with electrons. Still another student, George Hevesy, from Berlin (originally from Hungary), was being tortured by his failure to accomplish a simple task that Rutherford had assigned him: separating the valuable radiolead from a pile of ordinary lead ore, a recent gift from the Austrian government.

The Manchester Lab by 1911 had become a sizeable international gathering of advanced students, and all of them were required to take Geiger's introductory laboratory course in handling radioactive substances. (To Rutherford you weren't a scientist, or even a person, unless you did laboratory work.) Rutherford assigned each student a problem upon completion of the required course; suddenly many of these problems bloomed during the first *annus mirabilis* of nuclear science, 1913.

To start the year Kasimer Fajans announced the alpha and beta displacement laws to explain natural decay with "Pleiades." Then J.J. Thompson (Rutherford's old professor at the Cavendish Lab) demonstrated two neon lines with his new positive ray spectrometer but announced there was no room on the Periodic Table for Ne-22. Then Geiger and E. Marsden (another student) proved the atomic nucleus experimentally. Then Geiger invented a beta counter (the immediate parent of the GM tube). Then Neils Bohr justified the nuclear atom on theoretical grounds. Then F.W. Aston (a Thompson student) demonstrated that his boss was wrong, there was a Ne-22 whether or not the Periodic Table had room for it. Then Frederic Soddy devised theoretical justification and renamed Fajans' pleiades "isotopes" and showed that the Periodic Table had room for expansion.* Then H.G.J. Moseley proved that the fault in the Periodic Table had been the chemist's preoccupation with atomic weight: it was the atomic number that lined up the atoms. Fajans had already sent a student to T.W. Richardson's Lab at Harvard to remeasure the atomic weights of lead and the results were coming in: there were at least two different atomic weights for lead.

George Hevesy decided to turn his failure into a triumph. If you can't separate radiolead from lead, then use the radiolead to trace the kinetic behavior of lead in lead. He became the first convert to isotopes at least a year before isotopes existed. Hevesy had devised a use for radioactive tracers while still a student in Geiger's introductory course in Manchester. You won't find the experiment described in nuclear physics literature because it was an experiment in the field of Home Economics.

George Hevesy, while in Berlin, had been trying to answer a question on energy transfer in gases. The answer might be a problem of electron transfer but nobody in Berlin was acquainted with the new techniques of measuring electrons; he decided to learn them at Manchester. Upon arrival in Manchester he followed the usual custom of boarding in one of the homes close to Owens College. Although Hevesy was well satisfied with the meals served by his landlady, from long experience in boarding houses he suspected that the remains of the Sunday meat course was served later in the week – tastily, of course, but still leftovers. This, his landlady denied fervently so Hevesy conducted the first experiment with tracer methodology:

> "The coming Sunday in an unguarded moment I added some active deposit to the freshly prepared pie and on the following Wednesday, with the aid of an electroscope I demonstrated to the landlady the presence of the active material in the souffle."(*31*)

Thus the first radioactive tracer experiment, strictly speaking, was in humans. But radioactive tracers were limited to a few naturally radioactive heavy elements. Potassium, a biologically significant element, was known to be radioactive but its activity could not be separated. When Urey discovered heavy water in 1932, for the first time a biologically significant isotope (but in highly dilute concentration) became available and Hevesy jumped at the opportunity. He studied its distribution in goldfish, proved it safe, and then swallowed the first human dose himself to demonstrate the first truly biological half-time.* (He was wrong on that safety business; in 18 more years his similar goldfish experiment would teach him that extreme dilution, not deuterium, was biologically safe.)

But stable isotope measurements limited biological studies to large and very slow sampling techniques; nothing approaching the fast kinetics of biochemical behavior. Hevesy needed radioisotopes of biologically significant light elements and there weren't any. Then, suddenly, within the first three months of 1934, such isotopes did exist.

IRENE CURIE COMPENSATES FOR DELAYING THE DISCOVERY OF POLONIUM

Marie Curie was awfully pregnant in 1897. Two embryos were developing. One was the idea of getting her doctor's degree. Mathematics? Physics? Chemistry? Equally proficient in all three, she inclined towards chemistry, and the subject would be an extension of Becquerel's interesting new uranium rays. After 9 months delay waiting for Irene to be born, plus another 9 months gestation, in July 1898 polonium was discovered. Although overshadowed by the radium discovery 6 months later, polonium had a higher energy alpha emission than radium, and it decayed to a clean stability. Irene, the first embryo, felt a kinship to polonium and used it (not the same chunk, but a very similar piece) to bombard aluminum foil 36 years later.

It was already known in 1933 that some light elements when exposed to alpha particles would emit neutrons and positrons. Irene and her husband Frederick Joliot were working on the possibility that high energy gamma rays could produce positron-electron pairs. A thin metal foil was exposed to a polonium source until a burst of radiation was detected. This radiation, of course, ceased immediately upon removal of the polonium and the experiment was over. On 31 December 1933 the Joliot-Curies finished a routine set of cloud chamber measurements. They gave instructions for cleanup and left for home to celebrate New Year's Eve. Their assistant, a German student scientist named W.W. Gentner, began to dismantle the equipment – but something was wrong. After removing the polonium source, the cloud chamber tracks continued. Gentner immediately called the Joliot-Curies back to the laboratory. Upon repeating the student's dismantling procedure they discovered that their experiment was not over:

"Our latest experiments have shown a very striking fact; when an aluminum foil is irradiated the emission of positrons does not cease immediately. . . . The foil remains radioactive and the emission of radiation decays exponentially as for an ordinary [naturally occurring] radioelement. We observed the same phenomenon with boron and magnesium. . . . the transmutation of boron, magnesium, and aluminum by alpha particles has given birth to new radioelements emitting positrons" (*17*).*

The new radiation must be, they thought, from an isotope of phosphorous. Irene's long gestation in chemistry with Marie now paid off; she quickly dissolved the aluminum foil in HCl and separated out a pure phosphate which continued to give off radiation with a half-life of 2.5 minutes. This chemical conversion proved that a new, artificially radioactive isotope had been produced. Joliot suggested adding the prefix "radio-" to distinguish these unstable from stable isotopes.

Upon reading the Joliot and Curie note in *Nature*, Enrico Fermi in the Royal University at Rome saw an easier way to produce these new species without the severe limitations of the alpha source. He obtained some radon (630 mCi) from a medical radium cow and sealed it with berryllium in a glass vial to produce neutrons. He put the vial in a can of paraffin to slow down the neutrons. With this enormous (at least it was the biggest so far), slow neutron source, Fermi irradiated every pure element he could find (eventually 60 in all). Three months later in a letter to the editor of *Nature* (*18*)*, he reported 14 radio-elements. The 11th item was interesting: "Iodine—Intense Effect. Period about 30 Minutes." (Robley Evans in Boston read this note and 2½ years later remembered those seven words.)

Although the Joliot-Curies discovered isotopes, they were not the first to produce them. For over a year the cyclotron at Berkeley had been producing them in great quantities. F. N. E. Kurie told the story at the dedication of the new U.S. Navy Radiation Laboratory at San Francisco in 1955:

"Ernest Lawrence invited Dr. Cooksey and me to come out to Berkeley in the summer of 1932 and see if we couldn't repeat the Cockroft-Walton transmutations. We came out with boxes of Geiger counters which at that time were not very common. The ones Cooksey and I brought out were designed for a particular job, and when it was done they were thrown away. An all-purpose Geiger counter was not known in most laboratories with the result that even though we were simply crawling with artificial radioactivity, we were not the first to discover it."

"We learned about radioactivity one morning in 1934 when a cable came from the Curie-Joliots telling us about their experiment. We verified it. This should have been a lesson, but several months later we got a cable from Fermi telling us that he had discovered that neutrons could make things radioactive. These great discoveries, which really set nuclear physics on the way, were followed by a period of relative stability in which we all found that an easier way to make a living was simply to bombard something new and find new radioactivity. A paper could always be written, and papers were the things that counted. So, literally, for years people would take things and bombard them; then they'd take the neighboring elements of the periodic table and try to figure out what the activities really were."‡

From three radioisotopes in February to 14 three months later—and the number was growing; by the end of 1934 at least 40 radioisotopes had been re-

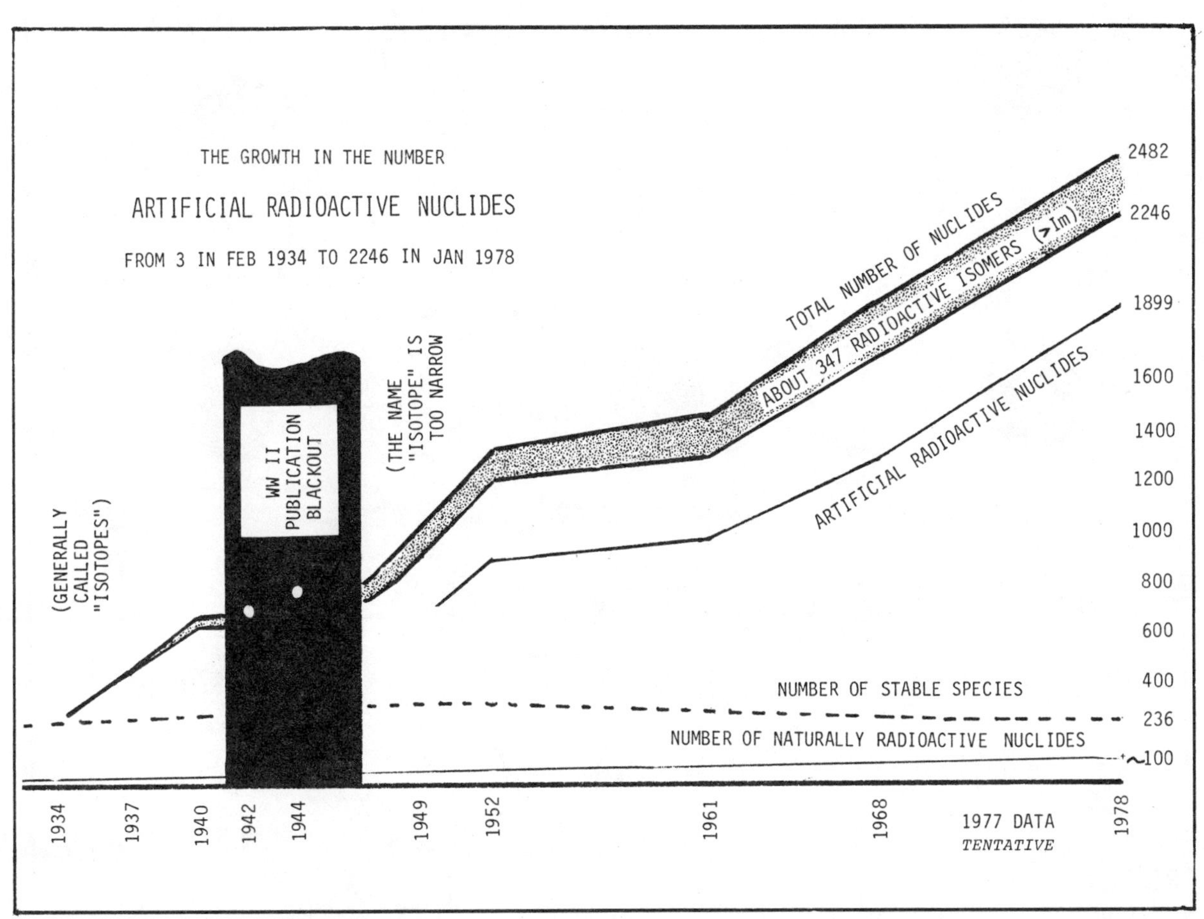

FIG. 5. Number of nuclides, 1934–1978.

ported. Upon receipt of Fermi's cable, the Berkeley group—a rare combination of chemists and physicists—focused a new look at the constitution of matter. The periodic table with stable isotopes was almost complete. (A few numbers, 43 (Tc), 61 (Pm), 85 (At), and 87 (Fr) were still missing.) But now the table was growing again. In his review of the changing table (of December 2, 1936), the University of Chicago chemist, Aristid Grosse (who had envisaged the possibility of artificial radioactive isotopes in 1932), pointed out that "It may be now safe to assume that the little over 400 isotopes [263 stable and 141 radioactive] represent the largest bulk of possible atomic species" (*19*). Grosse was grossly wrong; by 1942 Robley Evans listed 656 isotopes, by 1944 Glenn Seaborg listed 746 and updated his list to 1,314 in 1952.

SULLIVAN CHARTS THE SPECIES

During the last days of 1912 Kasimir Fajans had announced that more than one of the naturally occurring radioactive nuclear species could occupy the same place on the periodic table. By the end of 1913, Frederick Soddy had generalized this to all elements and had adopted the term "isotope".* By this time F. W. Aston had diffused neon through clay pipe to prove that the two lines J. J. Thomson had detected in his 1912 parabolic spectroscopy of neon were not a contamination; the two lines were separate and distinct components. This was the first proof of the existence of isotopes for physicists.

At the spring 1914 meeting of the Bunsen-Gesellschaft in Leipzig, Max Lembert, who Fajans had sent to work with T. W. Richards at Harvard, reported on the different atomic weights of lead from different mineral sources. Chemists were now convinced of the existence of isotopes and the officers of the Bunsen-Gesellschaft gave a special toast to Fajans—he had explained the difference without violating the periodic system.

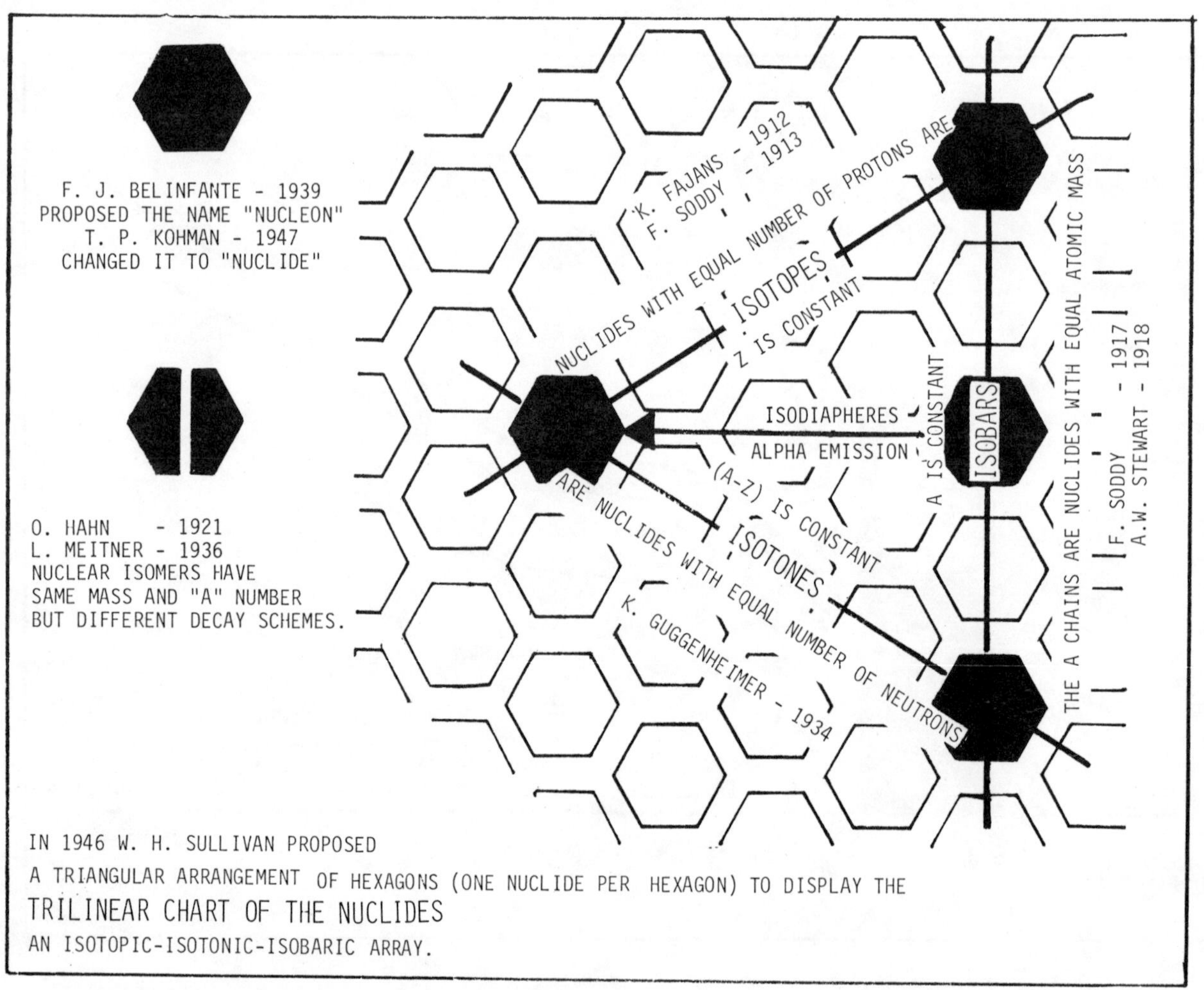

FIG. 6. Nomenclature of nuclides. It took a half century to coin the word "nuclide" to signify a specific nuclear species of atom in a chemically elementary form of matter.

By 1917 more stable isotopes had been found, and Soddy pointed out that if there were isotopes with "the same atomic number but different atomic weight" there must also be species with "the same atomic weight but different atomic number." The British chemist, A. W. Stewart, in 1918 called such species "isobares" (the final "e" was later dropped and the A-chains became "isobars").

When the neutron was discovered a decade later* the definition of "isotope" was changed from atomic weights and numbers to the structural relationship of protons and neutrons. Isotopes were nuclear species with an equal number of protons (their chemical identity is implied). Isobars were nuclear species with an equal number of protons-plus-neutrons (identity of atomic mass is implied). In 1934 the German physicist K. Guggenheimer pointed out that there must be a third set—nuclear species with an equal number of neutrons. Replacing the "p" (for protons) with an "n" (for neutrons), the name "isotones" was coined.

All of these words are plural. The single species in series can be part of either an isotopic or an isobaric or an isotonic chain. In 1939 the Dutch physicist, J. Belinfante, proposed the term "nuclon" (changed to "nucleon" by C. Møller in 1941). It, however, became associated with specific "mass number," and the word "nuclide" was slowly substituted.

Way back in 1921 Otto Hahn had found that uranium Z (Pa-234) had the same atomic number and the same atomic weight as uranium X_2 (Pa-234m), but had a different half-life. By 1935 quite a few of these freak isobaric-isotopic-isotones were detected. Lisa Meitner in 1936 saw an analogy with chemical isomers and called them "nuclear isomers."

During World War II at the Manhattan District's Clinton Laboratories (about to become AEC's Oak Ridge National Laboratory), a great number of unreported nuclides were being worked with. Analytic chemists on the project were finding so many possible reactions in one irradiation that identification required immediate access to long tables that did not give a picture of what might have occurred. Most nuclides decayed by isobaric transition towards stability; the isobars had to be visualized as related. Since chemical identification was required, the isotopes had to be listed in sequence. In Oak Ridge, where neutron bombardment was the prime method, a sequence of nuclides by neutron number was also required.

William H. Sullivan, a chemist at Clinton Labs, tried to organize the rapidly changing nuclear data into an immediately visible form. Since the three important axes, neutron number—proton number—and atomic mass number, were equally important he tried trilinear coordinate paper. A hexagon has three axes and so he placed each nucleon in a hexagon (Fig. 6). When placed on a beehive array, a chart of the elements in nuclear structure was formed. His first chart in four colors (*20*) was 16 ft long unfolded. It contained 935 hexagons, each with up to 13 items of nuclear data. It was out of date before the chart was printed.

For the second edition (*21*), the words "Nuclear Species" had already been replaced by the more popular "Nuclides." The new chart was 17 ft long unfolded, but it did not go out of date because gummed hexagonal stamps were issued periodically to keep the data up to date. By 1961, after nine issues of gummed stamps had been distributed, the chart contained 1,349 hexagons with many double or even triple isomers. But the data by now was becoming so complex that a Nuclear Data Group (first at National Academy of Science—NRC, then at Oak Ridge) had to go back to the tabular form, and thick volumes of Nuclear Data Sheets are still being revised and published periodically (*22*). After Sullivan's death a further simplification of the chart, showing only half-life and decay data, was published by Mallinckrodt. Its revision in 1979 will have 2396 hexagons, including 252 for stable nuclides and 55 for nuclides with $t_{1/2}$ over a million years. I haven't counted the isomers yet. The rapid expansion seems to have slowed down. (I am not as certain of this as Groose was in 1937.)

ROBLEY EVANS MAKES IT MEDICAL

Even before the concept of isotopes had been announced George Hevesy, then with Rutherford in Manchester, had used naturally occurring radioactive lead as a "tag" to study the dispersion of radioactivity in stable lead.* This tag concept required that the chemistry of two disparate nuclear species be identical. In 1927 Hermann Blumgart used a dilute solution of radon as a "tracer" during the first few seconds after injection into the blood stream.* The "tracer" required that there be no physiologic recognition of the foreign nuclide. A "tag" could be a "tracer" but the "tracer" need not necessarily be a "tag." By the time artificial radionuclides were discovered both concepts had already found a use in biological and medical research but not in the practice of medicine.

On November 12, 1936, Karl Compton, president of the Massachusetts Institute of Technology (MIT), was scheduled to address a luncheon in Vanderbilt Hall at Harvard Medical School. His subject: "What Physics Can Do For Biology and Medicine." Robley Evans, on his physics faculty, had slipped him some juicy, physico-biologic tidbits about Hevesy's indi-

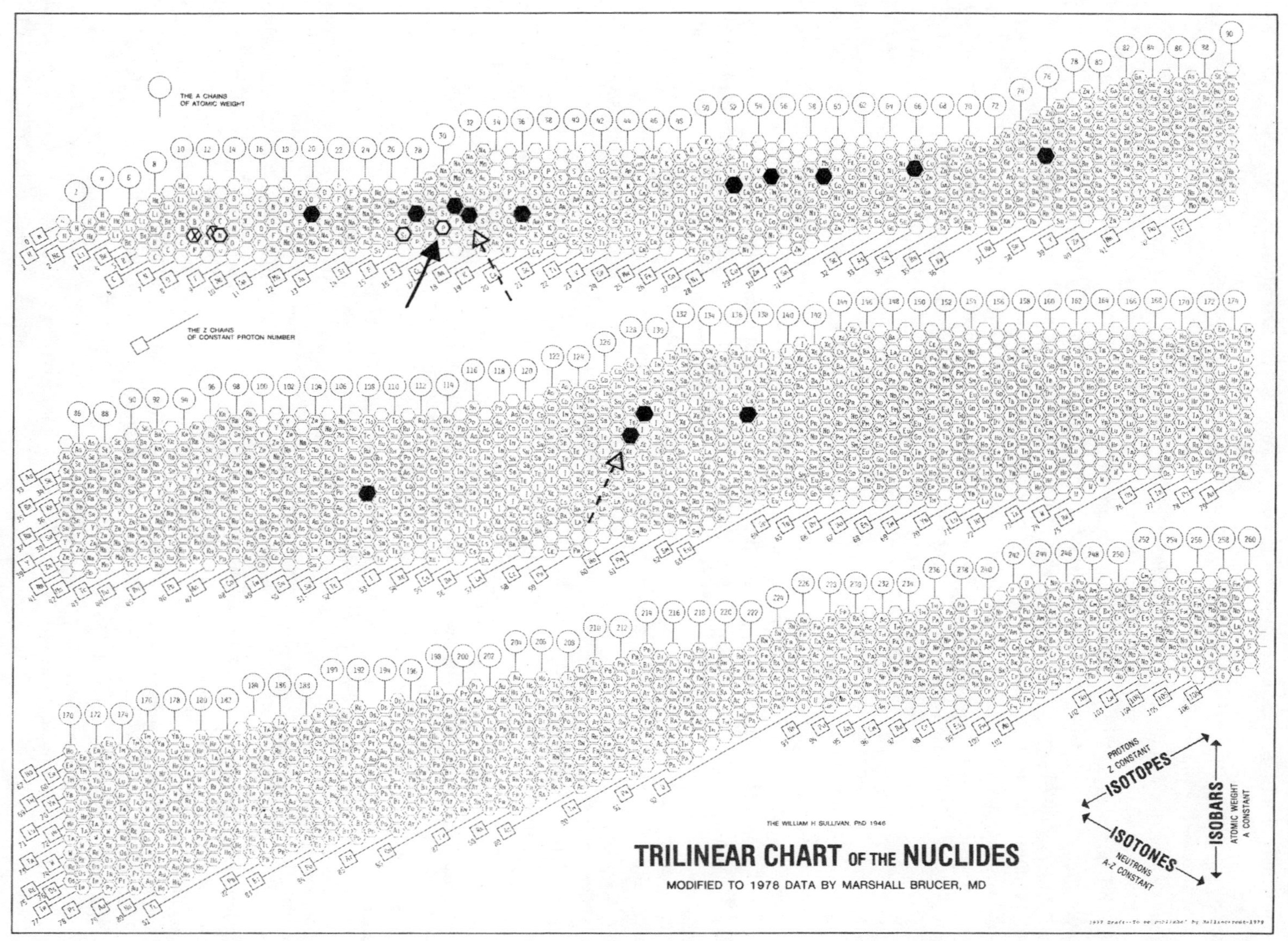

FIG. 7. The first radioactive nuclides: —February 10, 1934. Joliot F. Curie I (Paris): Radionitrogen, radiosilicon, and radiophosphorus produced by the action of α-particles. *Nature* 133: 201, Feb. 10, 1934. —March 14, 1934. Crane HB, Lauritsen CC (Cal Tech); "Induced Radioactivity" in C-11 and N-13 by proton bombardment. *Phys Rev* 45: 497, April 1, 1934. —April 10, 1934. Fermi E (Rome): Fourteen "Unstable Products" of neutron bombardment. *Nature* 133: 757, May 19, 1934.

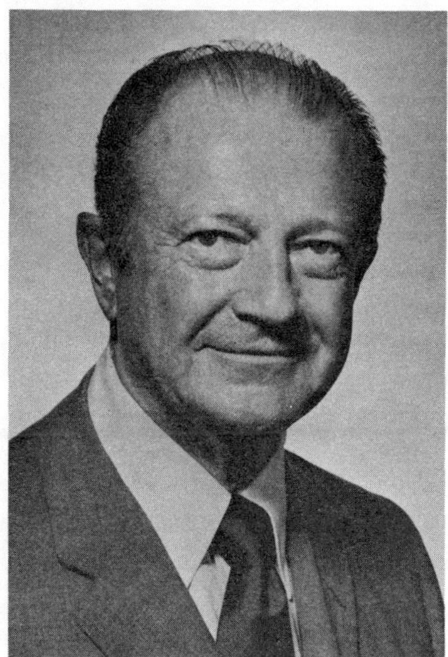

FIG. 8. Robley Evans, Ph.D. Nuclear "medicine" begins on Nov 12, 1936. In Vanderbilt Hall at Harvard Medical School.
J. H. Means, M.D. (Thyroid Clinic, Mass. Gen. Hosp.): *"Is there a radioisotope of iodine?"*
Robley Evans, Ph.D. (Physics, Mass. Inst. Tech.): *"We can make some."*

cator-dilution studies in animals using radioactive tags. Attending the lecture was James H. Means, whose thyroid clinic at Massachusetts General Hospital (MGH) was already world-famous, accompanied by two of his henchmen, Earle Chapman and Saul Hertz. Hevesy's P-32 work was considered very interesting, with possible clinical application, but, asked Means in the post-lecture discussion, "Is there a radioactive isotope of iodine?" (*23*) At this point Robley Evans remembered the seven words he had read in Fermi's article 2½ years earlier. He explained that there was a radioiodine, and it could be made the same way Hevesy made P-32.

During the next 6 months Compton and Means set up a joint MIT-MGH committee to study the feasibility of Evans' interesting idea. Evans knew that MIT could not afford the fantastically expensive 600 mg radium-beryllium neutron source that Hevesy had used. But he knew how Fermi had made his neutron source with medical radon. Huntington Hospital in Boston used many radon needles milked from their radium cow, and discarded them after a short decay. For no cost at all he could gather the discards, mix their remnant activity into beryllium and make a baby brother to Hevesy's neutron source. He put his gadget together, and within a few months proudly showed Compton a few nanocuries of I-128. The thyroid project was feasible; Compton and Means raised $3,000 to start a joint MGH-MIT thyroid-radioiodine research program. Evans persuaded a versatile physicist, Arthur Roberts, to join the full time staff and concentrate on radioiodine production. In late 1937 he and Saul Hertz injected some I-128 into the ear of a rabbit.

After hours of neutron bombardment they hadn't made enough I-128 for more than a teaser. Fortunately a retired physician donated his collection of radium plaques and needles; this new permanent 110 mg Ra-Be neutron howitzer could produce an enormous yield of about 1/20 microcuries of I-128 every day. Now they could really study thyroid metabolism. Hertz, Roberts, and Evans published the first paper on thyroid-radioiodine in May 1938 (*24*).*

Meanwhile, they had encouraged Joe Hamilton, a young neurologist working in Berkeley's Medical Group, to also study I-128 metabolism in animals. He was giving enormous (a new definition of enormous) doses produced by the cyclotron. Anything Berkeley could do, MIT could do better. Compton and Evans went to the Markle Foundation in New York for $30,000 to build a cyclotron.

Joe Hamilton was dissatisfied with the limitations imposed by the 25 minute half-life of I-128 in studying metabolism. One day in the spring of 1938, he ran into Glenn Seaborg on the steps of LeConte Hall at Berkeley. Hamilton complained bitterly about the I-128 short half-life, "Why can't you make me an iodine isotope with a longer half-life?" "How long a half-life do you want?" asked Seaborg. "Oh, about a week."

Seaborg and his physicist partner, Jack Livingood, prepared some tellurium targets and a week later Seaborg delivered the first and only radioisotope ever discovered to fill a physician's prescription. This sample was of a new 8-day iodine-131 (*25*).*

Hamilton, a nonpracticing physician, saw the clinical implications of the MIT-MGH collaboration. He joined forces with Mayo Soley, an internist from across the bay, and by October 1939, Hamilton, Soley, and Eichorn published the first paper on the diagnostic use of I-131 in patients (*26*). (This was not our "I-131;" it was a mixture of at least 10 isotopes of iodine.) By July 1940, autoradiograms showed the actual distribution of I-131 in normal, thyrotoxic, and nontoxic goiters, and its absence in non-functioning, malignant thyroid tissue (*27*).

Four months later the MIT cyclotron produced its first sample of I-130, a 12 hour half-life nuclide; its radio-purity seemed ideal for therapy. By January of 1941 the first patient was given a therapeutic dose of I-130 by Hertz at MIT, and a 30-patient program was started.

But radioiodine was not the first "isotope" to be used therapeutically. After much work with P-32 in animals and then tracer studies in patients, John

Lawrence gave the first therapeutic dose of a "radioisotope" to a patient with chronic lymphatic leukemia on Christmas Eve, 1937. The treatment seemed to be quite successful. One of his students, Lowell Erf, was definitely successful in treating polycythemia vera with P-32 during the next few years. In December 1939, Sr-89 was used as a convenient radioactive substitute for calcium (because calcium nuclides were not available). Excellent uptakes in metastases to bone were observed by Charles Pecher at Donner Lab. Within a year Sr-89 became the second radioisotope to be used in therapy. If diagnostic and animal physiology studies were included in a survey of radioisotope work prior to 1941, there is a hint of practically everything that would later become a part of nuclear medicine. But, on hindsight, one diagnostic study is of overriding importance.

The group at Columbia Physicians and Surgeons in New York came up against a pertinent question. Did a metastasis from thyroid carcinoma store radioiodine? Judging from some of their tissue sections, it looked possible. So they gave a patient with metastatic thyroid carcinoma a dose of radioiodine. One of their radiology residents, Robert Ball, was given a GM tube and told to find the metastases by counting the clicks. He was slowly scanning the patient's entire body (it was manual and without automatic recording, but nevertheless scanning). The work was rather boring, so he turned on the radio to ease the tedium. Suddenly the music stopped and a voice announced, "Pearl Harbor has been bombed!"

The 60-inch cyclotron at Berkeley and practically all of the personnel were soon diverted to the Manhattan District problem. Physicians in Boston, and in all the hospitals using radioiodine, were given higher priority duties. During the wartime secrecy, the MIT cyclotron, which had been dedicated to and maintained 100% medical priority, supplied millicurie amounts of radioisotopes to 36 hospitals. These 36 hospitals (plus a few that were muzzled by the atom bomb project—Berkeley, Chicago, Rochester, Boston, Oak Ridge, Columbia) represented the entire effort in medical radioisotope research for a 5-year period. Scholarly priorities cannot be ascribed because so much was kept secret.

SAM SEIDLIN SELLS CONGRESS A CANCER CURE

Shortly after the atom bombs had been dropped (August 6 and 9, 1945), Colonel K. D. Nichols of the Manhattan Project suggested that, in view of the "virtually unlimited production" of isotopes, they should be authorized for distribution to outsiders. In January 1946, Paul C. Aebersold, a physicist who had been with the Berkeley group before the war, was asked to transfer from Los Alamos to take charge of isotopes distribution from Oak Ridge. During the first months of 1946 this new isotopes branch had no methods or preparation, packaging, shipment, routes, advertising, or billing procedures. With no precedents to follow, Aebersold invented the only bureaucratic procedure that has ever worked before or since. He wrote memoranda for his superiors in Oak Ridge to send to their superiors in Washington. The next day he flew to Washington to be on hand when the memoranda were delivered. That same day he prepared directives for the superiors in Washington to send to his superiors in Oak Ridge. That same day he flew back to Oak Ridge to receive his own directions from his superiors' superiors on the now official procedure. This method has never been improved upon in the history of bureaucracy.

On June 14, 1946, six scientists and 30 newspapermen were invited to Oak Ridge to see the "isotope facilities." (Thus, a science/publicity ratio was established for the next 30 years.) An announcement was made in *Science* that radioactive isotopes were available to qualified investigators (*28*).* After months of battle in Congress over military vs. civilian control, the Atomic Energy Act of 1946 released isotopes from military control. The very next day, August 2, 1946, Pennsylvania newspapers announced the first shipment of radioisotopes to the University of Pennsylvania Hospital. But if you read the Chicago papers the real first shipment was made to the University of Chicago; and if you read the Minneapolis newspapers the real first shipment was made to the University of Minnesota; and if you read the San Francisco newspapers the real first shipment was made to the University of California. Thirty or forty orders for radioisotopes had been shipped immediately.

There was no first shipment. At a carefully staged ceremony in front of the Oak Ridge reactor, 200 mCi of carbon-14 were handed to Dr. E. V. Cowdry of Barnard Free Cancer Hospital of St. Louis. Radioisotope propaganda had been centered on the cure of cancer. The "first shipment" had been carefully selected because of the "FREE CANCER HOSPITAL" name (and, incidentally, Martin Kamen, then in St. Louis, had discovered carbon-14 back in 1941). Kamen converted the "first shipment" to a tagged acetic acid which went to Antioch College in Ohio where Dr. P. Rothemund used it to prepare a cancer-producing (not a cancer-curing) agent. The bulk of the "first shipment" was used by Dr. Simpson at Barnard Hospital for study of the production of skin cancer in mice.

Fortunately for nuclear medicine a true cancer

cure had occurred. In 1943 Samuel Seidlin, an endocrinologist in New York City, had been called in to treat a patient suffering from hyperthyroidism even though the thyroid had been removed years before for thyroid carcinoma. The hyperactive metastases were successfully destroyed with radioiodine, and this was a true cure by any definition. On December 7, 1946, the fifth anniversary of the bombing of Pearl Harbor and in the midst of congressional indecision on atomic controls, the *JAMA* published the single most important article in the history of nuclear medicine (*29*).*

Seidlin had published a preliminary article, but it was from the *JAMA* article that newspapers picked it up, and a remarkable transposition occurred into newspaperese: "CANCER CURE FOUND IN THE FIREY CANYONS OF DEATH AT OAK RIDGE." Within days, every congressman heard from his constituency. Within hours, the brand new AEC commissioners knew they now had two jobs: to stockpile bombs behind closed doors, and to pour money into cancer research out in the open. During the next 10 years, nuclear medicine was nurtured on the strength of the Seidlin article.

PAUL AEBERSOLD AND DONALEE TABERN SELL ISOTOPES

Radioisotopes suddenly became available with a built-in promoter. Paul Aebersold's isotopes division was the only safely nonsecret part of AEC. Aebersold had unlimited funds, unlimited radioisotopes and, seemingly, unlimited energy to promote the unlimited cures that had been held back from the American public for too long. The liberal establishment was in the depths of shame for having ended the war by killing people. Radioisotopes didn't kill people; they cured cancer.

Aebersold spoke at every meeting of one person or more that had one minute or more available on its program. No matter what the meeting's subject, Aebersold's topic was always the same. He sold isotopes. Aebersold had to keep an account of the progress being made with radioisotopes for the new Joint Committee on Atomic Energy in Congress. He tried to maintain a complete record of all published articles in which radioisotopes were used. (This "complete" bibliography was published by AEC in his 3-, 5-, and 8-year summaries.) By 1955 the U.S. atomic monopoly was broken, but by this time even Aebersold's office staff could not keep up with the deluge of articles.

During the first 5 years, 3,200 articles were published on the use of radioisotopes. There were 375 on the physical properties of new radionuclides and most were on some form of chemistry. But 949 papers had some relationship to medicine. Forty-three had virtually the same title—some variety of "Gee Whiz, Look at What We've Done."

The AEC did not sell drugs; they sold a radionuclide with a disclaimer on its use as a drug. A number of commercial suppliers got into the distribution business, but it was probably Abbott Laboratories who were first to sell a pharmaceutical grade of the AEC product. Then in 1948 one of their chemists, Donalee Tabern, stumbled on the first true radiopharmaceutical (in Hymer Friedell's Group at Western Reserve in Cleveland). J. P. Storaasli had measured the blood volume of 30 patients using radioiodinated human serum albumin.* Abbott trademarked a pharmaceutical grade of this as "RISA."

While the rest of us in early nuclear medicine were engulfed in details, precision, legislation, and preparing papers for publication, Aebersold toured the country extolling the virtues of radioisotopes. Tabern, however, did not give speeches. He met personally with any physician who gave the slightest hint of interest. He sold them on the value of nuclear medicine (and incidentally on the Abbott product). Then he told them which instrument to buy, taught them how to use it, and then filled out their license application to AEC. He addressed the letter, furnished the stamp, and mailed it to AEC.

In a very practical sense, nuclear medicine couldn't have advanced very far without a radiopharmaceutical industry. The industry could not have existed without AEC promotion. With 30 years of hindsight, I think Aebersold and Tabern were pioneers as much as were the Fathers of Nuclear Medicine—at least they were our Dutch Uncles.

A SOCIETY TO DISPENSE KNOWLEDGE IS FORMED

The deluge of papers, speakers, and especially publicity was not without its response from vested interests in organized medicine. A large group of radiologists highly resented cobalt-60 teletherapy, which could never take the place of 250 Kv X-ray. The annexation of thyroid therapy by an unorganized group of internists, pathologists, radiologists (and even by a physicist or two) was resented by many surgeons who felt they dominated the field. Many internists deplored the attempts at treatment of malignant effusions with Au-198 colloid by an unorganized array of radiologists, pathologists, and surgeons (and even a chemist or two). Some clinical pathologists were driven up the wall by the motley group of internists, surgeons, and radiologists (and even a technician or two) who showed disrespect for the time-tried and scientifically tested BMR. As the scintillation counter with its complex scale-of-64 electronics gained favor, physicists sneered at medics dabbling in equipment they couldn't possibly under-

Society of Nuclear Medicine

FIRST ANNUAL MEETING

BENJAMIN FRANKLIN HOTEL

May 29-30, 1954

Founders' Group

A. Kearney Atkinson, M.D.
Box 911, Great Falls, Mont.

Thomas Carlile, M.D.
1115 Terry Ave., Seattle, Wash.

Eggert T. Feldsted, M.D.
755 W. Twelfth Ave., Vancouver, Canada

William H. Hannah, B.S.
Rt. 2, Box 896, Bremerton, Wash.

Milo Harris, M.D.
252 Paulsen Bldg., Spokane, Wash.

Norman J. Holter, M.A.
Helena, Mont.

Rex L. Huff, M.D.
2418 Harvard Ave. No., Seattle, Wash.

Tyra T. Hutchens, M.D.
6623 S.W. Virginia Ave., Portland, Ore.

Robert G. Moffat, M.D.
2656 Heather St., Vancouver, Canada

Joseph P. Nealen, S.J.
Gonzaga University, Spokane, Wash.

Asa Seeds, M.D.
507 Medical Arts Bldg., Vancouver, Wash.

Charles P. Wilson, M.D.
2455 N.W. Marshall, Portland, Ore.

SATURDAY MORNING

THE SARATOGA ROOM

8:30 - 9:30 Business Session

Thomas Carlile, M.D., Seattle, Wash., *Presiding*

9:30 - 12:15 Scientific Session

A. K. Atkinson, M.D., Great Falls, Mont., *Presiding*

9:30 Estimates of Cardiac Output by In Vivo Counting of I^{131} Labeled HSA

R. L. Huff, M.D., Seattle, Wash.

10:00 I^{131} Uptake Before and After TSH in Several Small Animals

Marilyn Losli, Portland, Ore.

10:30 - 10:45 Coffee

10:45 PANEL ON THYROID TRACERS

Moderator—R. H. Williams, M.D., Seattle, Wash.

I. Methodology
E. T. Feldstad, M.D., Vancouver, Canada

II. Physical Considerations
N. J. Holter, M.A., Helena, Mont.

III. The Scintiscanner
T. T. Hutchens, M.D., Portland, Ore.

12:15 - 2:00 Society Luncheon

The Plaza Room

SATURDAY AFTERNOON

THE SARATOGA ROOM

2:00 - 5:00 Scientific Session

Milo Harris, M.D., Spokane, Wash., *Presiding*

2:00 Training of Residents in Radioisotope Techniques

D. S. Childs, Jr., M.D., Rochester, Minn.

2:30 Evaluation of the Role of Radioactive Gold in the Management of Pleural Effusion and Ascites due to Carcinomatosis

Campbell Moses, M.D., Pittsburgh, Pa.

3:00 Radioactive Phosphorus in Serous Effusions

R. G. Moffat, M.D., Vancouver, Canada

3:30 - 3:45 Recess

3:45 The Colloids: Gold, Chromic Phosphate and Yttrium

D. L. Tabern, Ph.D., North Chicago, Ill.

4:15 Chromatographic Test of Urine after Therapeutic Dosages of I^{131}: Preliminary Observations

A. F. Scott, Ph.D., Portland, Ore.

A. H. Livermore, Ph.D., Portland, Ore.

SATURDAY EVENING

6:00 - 7:00 COCKTAILS

The Saratoga Room

7:00 DINNER

The Fifth Avenue Room

Guest Speaker

Paul C. Aebersold, Ph.D.

Director, Isotopes Division
United States Atomic Energy Commission

"THE ATOMIC ENERGY PROGRAM—PAST, PRESENT and FUTURE"

Informal

SUNDAY MORNING

THE SARATOGA ROOM

9:00 - 9:30 Business Session

Thomas Carlile, M.D., Seattle, Wash., *Presiding*

9:30 - 11:45 Scientific Session

S. T. Cantril, M.D., Seattle, Wash., *Presiding*

9:30 Physical Measurements of Radioactive Cobalt Sources

H. F. Batho, Ph.D., Vancouver, Canada

10:00 The Phenomenon of Nuclear Induction: Theory and Some Applications

Warren Proctor, Ph.D., Seattle, Wash.

10:30-10:45 Coffee

10:45 Treatment of Emphysema by Inducing a Hypometabolic State: Preliminary Report

C. D. Wilson, M.D., Portland, Ore.

Huldrick Kammer, M.D., Portland, Ore.

W. L. Lehman, M.D., Portland, Ore.

11:15 Device for Routine Radioactive Analysis of Urine in Uptake Studies

J. P. Nealen, S.J., Spokane, Wash.

11:45 Closing Session

FIG. 9. Program of the first meeting of the Society of Nuclear Medicine; Benjamin Franklin Hotel, Seattle, Washington, May 29–30, 1954.

stand. An outstanding biochemist at Vanderbilt pointed out that the answer to leukemia lay in the use of semi-log graph paper and that medics counted on their fingers (he, incidentally, moved his lips when reading medical reports).

A few men in the Pacific Northwest who used "isotopes" in a small part of their regular work recognized that no one person could be competent in physics, chemistry, engineering, electronics, radiobiology, mathematics, and at least ten clinical specialties. Jeff Holter set up a "Montana Society of Nuclear Medicine" in 1953 so they could talk about their mistakes. (Holter, a physicist, was responsible for dumping the name "radioisotopes" as the first mistake to be corrected.) The Montana organization never met formally because a few friends from Seattle, Portland, and Vancouver B.C. wanted to join.

On January 19, 1954 twelve men met in the Davenport Hotel in Spokane, Washington (the compromise central point of the region). Within minutes Jeff Holter became the first officer (pre-first election) of the Society: ". . . we had a voluntary assessment of ten dollars to pay for rooms, booze, and food, and I was treasurer with an even $100.00." (Twelve men at $10 each? To this day, Jeff has not accounted for the extra $20.)

Asa Seeds was elected secretary—and on February 17, 1954, the first Newsletter of the Society of Nuclear Medicine was sent to practically everybody he could think of. I'll quote directly from the newsletter:

"The Spokane meeting was attended by Doctors R. L. Huff (Research Physician, Seattle), R. G. Moffat (Internist, Vancouver BC), E. T. Feldsted (Radiologist, Vancouver BC), C. P. Wilson (Internist, Portland), A. K. Atkinson (Radiologist, Great Falls), T. T. Hutchens (Internist, Portland), A. C. Seeds (Radiologist, Vancouver, Wash.), M. Harris (Internist, Spokane), N. J. Holter (Physicist, Helena), W. H. Hanna (Med. Physics, Bremerton, Wash.), J. P. Nealen (Physicist, Spokane), and T. Carlide (Radiologist, Seattle). These twelve individuals agreed that there was sufficient reason to organize a society, and ultimately the name "The Society of Nuclear Medicine" was adopted. It was decided that there would be no geographical designation in the name as it might have wider appeal than the Northwest. . . . Officers were elected and it was decided that the first annual meeting should be May 29th and 30th in Seattle. . . . the president, in his enthusiasm, has written a number of letters, including one to Paul Aebersold which resulted in a tentative acceptance for the speaking engagement. . . . some of you will also be interested to know that Don Tabern of Abbott Laboratories, in response to a letter from me, immediately sent a check for $10.00 and announced his intentions to come to the meeting on May 29th and 30th. [Thus, after the founding group, Tabern became the first dues-paying member of the Society.]"

The first annual meeting was opened at the Benjamin Franklin Hotel in Seattle, Washington, on Sunday morning May 29, 1954, by President Thomas Carlile. It was attended by 109 physicians, physicists, chemists and technicians. The first paper presented was by Rex Huff on "Estimates of Cardiac Output by In Vivo Counting of I-131 Labelled HSA."* Ten papers followed through Saturday and Sunday morning (Figure 9). A new instrument was described, called Ben Cassen's Scintiscanner.* Not a very important development, as most in the audience knew, but the chicken tracks it pecked out on carbon paper gave a crude impression of size, shape, and activity of the thyroid gland – and of "nodularity?" Nonsense! Nothing could ever replace the finely tuned fingers of the palpating (or was it palpitating) physician.

The first scans were crude because, as everybody in the audience realized, gamma rays could not be focused. But was this true? Bob Newell at Stanford Medical School had already discarded the optical lens concept. He cast a thick lead collimator with 19 holes focused to a point in front of it. Gamma rays from the thyroid might splay out in all directions but Newell's detector saw only those from the collimator's focus.*

Not all the gamma rays from the thyroid originated in the thyroid gland. Some were scattered from the stomach, even from the patient's hot bladder. A simple matter of electronic subtraction, said P.R. Bell in Oak Ridge: when gamma rays scatter they lose energy; Hofstadter's NaI (Tl) crystal scintillates with energy dependence.* Bell had already built a medical spectrometer that allowed a recorder to record only "primary" rays that the detector detected coming through the focused holes in the collimator.* Therefore, Cassen's sensitive scanner could achieve a high spectral resolution and the best spatial resolution ever achieved with isotopes (not good but "reasonable").

It wasn't just thyroids being scanned. George Moore in Minnesota had been using fluorescent compounds that localized in brain tumors.* One of the compounds (diiodofluorescine) could be easily labelled with radioiodine to become a brain tumor detection agent -- detection from outside the skull; few people believed it. Franz Bauer at UCLA extended the idea to spinal tumors using a more easily available agent, °IHSA; even fewer believed this. A neurosurgical resident, Eric Yuhl, noted the accumulation of °IHSA, in the liver. Abnormal spots of uptake could be distinguished in metastatic liver lesions; some noted medical physicists actively disbelieved it. Ga-72 scans of bone had already been reported from Oak Ridge (not very non-invasively but when thin slices of bone were scanned the pictures were beautiful). Thyroid, brain, spine, liver, and bone scanning, even the enthusiastic Tyra Hutchens didn't realize when he gave his talk that he was forecasting over half of the society's program material for the next quarter century. On Sunday noon at the closing session, Jeff Holter declared the meeting to be the finest ever held in the history of the Society of Nuclear Medicine.

It had taken 139 years to make such a society possible. Six generations of physicists and chemists participated in the growth of the idea.

Although the cream of London's scientific society attended that wild animal exhibition on the Strand in London in 1815, only William Prout, a practicing physician trained in scientific measurement to observe sick people, had the experience necessary to be astounded by the feces of a boa constrictor.

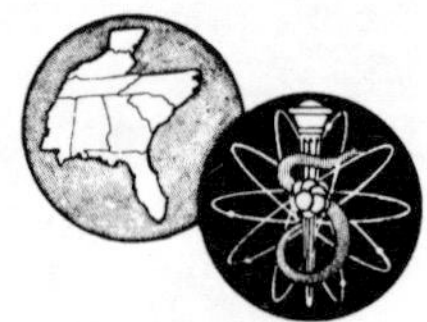

POSTSCRIPT

The logo of the Southeastern Chapter of the Society of Nuclear Medicine shows a snake entwined around a stick with some rays in the background. Most people think it symbolizes the staff of Aesculapius over a diagram of the atom. It doesn't. It is a boa constrictor in Valsalva maneuver in the rising sun.

FOOTNOTE

‡Kurie's words, but not a direct quote; I have shortened the story considerably. (From the U.S. Navy Program of the Dedication).

REFERENCES

1. I will cite only direct quotations in this summary. The stories with full references are being published during the 25th anniversary years 1978 and 1979 by Mallinckrodt, Inc., St. Louis as Vignettes in Nuclear Medicine: Vignette #91, Prout and the Whole Number Rule; Vignette #92, Evans and Radioiodine; Vignette #93, Crookes and the Radiometer; Vignette #94, Becquerel and Uranium; Vignette #95; Crookes and Uranium X; Vignette #96, Rutherford and Transmutation; Vignette #97, Hahn, Boltwood and the Natural Decay Series. A series on the periodic table and updated trilinear chart of the nuclides is scheduled for 1979.

2. Memoir of Dr. Prout FRS; *Med Times* (New Series) 1: 15–18, 1850

3. Prout W: On the relation between specific gravities of bodies . . . and the weights of their atoms. *Ann Phil* (Thomson) 6: 321, 1815

4. Crookes W: Address to Chemical Section, British Association. *Chem News* 54: 116, 1886

———: Presidential Address to Chemical Society, 1888 in Tilden WA; Obituary of Crookes. *J Chem Soc* 117: 444, 1920

5. Strutt RJ: On the Tendency of Atomic Weights to Approximate Whole Numbers. *Phil Mag* 1: 311–314, March 1901

6. Moseley HG: High-frequency spectra of the elements. I, *Phil Mag* 26: 1024, 1913; II, *Phil Mag* 27: 703, 1914

7. Fournier D'Albe EE: *Life of Sir William Crookes.* New York, Appleton, Chap 12, 1924

8. Thomson JJ: *Recollections and Reflections.* New York, Macmillan, p 373, 1937

9. Fournier D'Albe EE: *op. cit.*, p 255

10. Chalmers TW: Short history of radio-activity. *The Engineer* (London) 1951

11. Becquerel H: A series given at the Academie Des Sciences, Paris. *Compt Rend* 122: 420–501–559–689–762–1086, 1896

12. Crookes W: Uranium X. *Proc Roy Soc* 66: 409, 1900; *Chem News* 81: 253, 265, 1900

13. Rutherford E, Soddy F: Radioactivity of thorium compounds. *J Chem Soc* 81: 321, 1902

14. *Phil Mag* 81: 837, January 1902

15. Rutherford E, Soddy F: Cause and nature of radioactivity. *Phil Mag* 6 (iv): 370–396, Sept. 1902

16. Eve AS: *Rutherford.* New York, Macmillan, p 88, 1939

17. Joliot F, Curie I: Artificial production of a new kind of radio-element. *Nature* 133: 201, Feb. 10, 1934

18. Fermi E: Radioactivity induced by neutron bombardment. (Letter to the Editor) *Nature* 133: 757, May 19, 1934

19. Grosse A: Row of increasing atomic weights and the periodic law. *J Chem Educ* 14: 433, 1937

20. Sullivan WH: Trilinear Chart of Nuclear Species. New York, Wiley and Sons, 1949

21. Sullivan WH: Trilinear Chart of Nuclides. USAEC, Washington, D.C., USGPO, 1957

22. New York, Academic Press

23. Evans R: Early history of nuclear medicine at MGH. *Med Phys* 2: 105, 1969. Letter to Brucer, Oct 27, 1969

24. Hertz S, Roberts A, Evans RD: Radioactive iodine as an indicator . . . thyroid in rabbits. *Proc Soc Exp B & M* 38: 510–513, May 1938

25. Livingood JJ, Seaborg GT: Radioactive Iodine Isotopes. *Phys Rev* 53: 1015, 1938

26. Hamilton JG, Soley MH: Studies in iodine metabolism. *Am J Physiol* 127: 557–572, October 1939

27. Hamilton JG, Soley MH, Eichorn KB: Deposition of radioiodine in human thyroid tissue. *U Cal Pub Pharm* 1: 339–368, 1940

28. ———. Announcement. *Science* 103: 697, June 14, 1946

29. Seidlin SM, Marinelli LD, Oshry E: Radioactive iodine therapy. *JAMA* 132: 838, Dec. 7, 1946

30. Rutherford, ER, Geiger H: The Charge and Nature of the Alpha-particle. *Proc Roy Soc* A81: 162, 1908

31. Glasstone S: Sourcebook on Atomic Energy. Princeton, D. Van Nostrand, 3rd., p. 666, 1967

Table of Contents

*An asterisk after a paper indicates that only a portion of the whole paper has been reproduced.

The Heritage of
NUCLEAR MEDICINE

Excerpts from an Address to the Chemical Section of the British Association

By William Crookes, F.R.S., V.P.C.S.

Chemical News 54 (1397): 115-126, September 3, 1886

A glance over the Presidential Addresses delivered before this Section on former occasions will show that the occupiers of this chair have ranged over a fairly wide field. Some of my predecessors have given a general survey of the progress of chemical science during the past year; some, taking up a technological aspect of the subject, have discussed the bearings of chemistry upon our national industries; others, again, have passed in review the various institutions in this country for teaching chemistry; and in yet other cases the speaker has had the opportunity of bringing before the scientific world, for the first time, an account of some important original researches.

On this occasion I venture to ask your attention to a few thoughts on the very foundations of chemistry as a science — on the nature and the probable, or at least possible, origin of the so called elements. If the views to which I have been led may at first glance appear heretical, I must remind you that in some respects they are shared more or less, as I shall subsequently show, by not a few of the most eminent authorities, and notably by one of my predecessors in this chair, Dr. J.H. Gladstone, F.R.S., to whose brilliant address, delivered in 1883, I must beg to refer you.

Should it not sometimes strike us, chemists of the present day, that after all we are in a position unpleasantly akin to that of our forerunners, the alchemists of the Middle Ages? These necromancers of a time long past did not, indeed, draw so sharp a line as do we between bodies simple and compound; yet their life-task was devoted to the formation of new combinations, and to the attempt to transmute bodies which we commonly consider as simple and ultimate — that is, the metals. In the department of synthesis they achieved very considerable successes; in the transmutation of metals their failure is a matter of history....

The first riddle, then, which we encounter in chemistry is "What are the elements?" Of the attempts hitherto made to define or explain an element none satisfy the demands of the human intellect. The text-books tell us that an element is "a body which has not been decomposed;" that it is "a something to which we can add, but from which we can take away nothing," or "a body which increases in weight with every chemical change." Such definitions are doubly unsatisfactory: they are provisional, and may cease tomorrow to be applicable in any given case. They take their stand, not on any attribute of the things to be defined, but on the limitations of human power; they are confessions of intellectual impotence.

Just as Columbus' long philosophic meditation led him to the fixed belief of the existence of a yet untrodden world beyond that waste of Atlantic waters, so to our most keen-eyed chemists, physicists, and philosophers a variety of phenomena suggest the conviction that the elements of ordinary assumption are not the ultimate boundary in this direction of the knowledge which man may hope to attain. Well do I remember, soon after I had obtained evidence of the distinct nature of thallium, that Faraday said to me: "To discover a new element is a very fine thing, but if you could decompose an element and tell us what it is made of, that would be a discovery indeed worth making." And this was no new speculation of Faraday's, for in one of his early lectures he remarked: "At present we begin to feel impatient, and to wish for a new state of chemical elements. For a time the desire was to add to the metals, now we wish to diminish their number.... To decompose the metals, then, to reform them, to change them from one to another, and to realise the once absurd notion of transmutation are the problems now given to the chemist for solution."....

And this leads us up to a hypothesis which, if capable of full demonstration, would show us that the accepted elements are not co-equal, but have been formed by a process of expansion or evolution. I refer to the well-known hypothesis of Prout, which regards the atomic weights of the elements as multiples, by a series of whole numbers, of unity, equal the atomic weight of hydrogen. Every one is aware that the recent more accurate determinations of the atomic weights of different elements do not by any means bring them into close harmony with the values which Prout's law would require. Still, in no small number of cases the actual atomic weights approach so closely to those which the hypothesis demands, that we can scarcely regard the coincidence as accidental. Accordingly, not a few chemists of admitted eminence consider that we have here an expression of the truth, masked by some residual or collateral phenomena which we have not yet succeeded in eliminating....

Is there then, in the first place, any direct evidence of the transmutation of any supposed "element" of our existing list into another, or of its resolution into anything simpler?

To this question I am obliged to reply in the negative.

I doubt whether any chemist here present could suggest a process which would hold out a reasonable prospect of dissociating any of our accepted simpler bodies. The highest temperatures and the most powerful electric currents at our disposal have been tried, and tried in vain. At one time there seemed a possibility at least that the interesting researches of Prof. Victor Meyer might show the two higher members of the halogen group, bromine and iodine, as entering upon the path of dissociation. These hopes have not been fulfilled. It may be said, in the general opinion of the most eminent and judicious chemists, that none of the phenomena thus elicited prove that even an approach has been made to the object in view....

I have said that the original protyle* contained within itself the potentiality of all possible atomic weights. It may well be questioned whether there is an absolute uniformity in the mass of every ultimate atom of the same chemical element. Probably our atomic weights merely represent a mean value around which the actual atomic weights of the atoms vary within certain narrow limits.

Each well-defined element represents a platform of stability connected by ladders of unstable bodies. In the first accreting together of the primitive stuff the smallest atoms would form, then these would join together to form larger groups, the gulf across from one stage to another would be gradually bridged over, and the stable element appropriate to that stage

would absorb, as it were, the unstable rungs of the ladder which led up to it. I conceive, therefore, that when we say the atomic weight of, for instance, calcium is 40, we really express the fact that, while the majority of calcium atoms have an actual atomic weight of 40, there are not a few which are represented by 39 or 41, a less number by 38 or 42, and so on. We are here reminded of Newton's "old worn particles."

It is not possible, or even feasible, that these heavier and lighter atoms may have been in

---

* We require a word, analogous to protoplasm, to express the idea of the original primal matter existing before the evolution of the chemical elements. The word I have ventured to use for this purpose is compounded of προ (earlier than) and 'υλη (the stuff of which things are made). The word is scarcely a new coinage, for 600 years ago Roger Bacon wrote in his *De Arte Chymia* -- "The elements are made out of 'υλη, and every element is converted into the nature of another element."

some cases subsequently sorted out by a process resembling chemical fractionation? This sorting out may have taken place in part while atomic matter was condensing from the primal state of intense ignition, but also it may have been partly effected in geological ages by successive solutions and reprecipitations of the various earths.

This may seem an audacious speculation, but I do not think it is beyond the power of chemistry to test its feasibility. An investigation on which I have been occupied for several years has yielded results which to me appear apposite to the question, and I therefore beg permission here to allude briefly to some of the results, reserving details to a subsequest communication to the Section....

I would ask investigators not necessarily either to accept or to reject the hypothesis of chemical evolution, but to treat it as a provisional hypothesis; to keep it in view in their researches, to inquire how far it lends itself to the interpretation of the phenomena observed, and to test experimentally every line of thought which points in this direction. Of the difficulties of this investigation none can be more fully aware than myself. I sincerely hope that this my imperfect attempt may lead some minds to enter upon the study of this fundamental chemical question, and to examine closely and in detail what I, as if amidst the clouds and mists of a far distance, have striven to point out.

On the Invisible Radiations Emitted by Phosphorescent Substances

Henri Becquerel

[Translation of "Sur les radiations invisibles emises par les corps phosphorescents," *Comptes rendus de l'Academie des Sciences, Paris,* 1896, *122*: 501–503 (2 March).]

At the last session I sketched briefly the experiments I had been led to perform in order to demonstrate the invisible radiations emitted by certain phosphorescent substances, radiations which penetrate various substances which are opaque to light.

I have been able to extend these observations, and, although I propose to continue and develop the study of these phenomena, their present interest [actualite] leads me to set forth as early as today the first results I have obtained.

The experiments I shall report were made with the radiations emitted by crystalline lamellas of the double sulfate of potassium and uranium

$$[K(UO)SO_4+H_2O],$$

a substance whose phosphorescence is very lively and whose persistence of luminosity is less than 1/100 of a second. The characteristics of the luminous radiations emitted by this substance have formerly been studied by my father, and I have since had occasion to point out a few interesting peculiarities which these luminous radiations show.

It is very simple to verify that the radiations emitted by this substance when exposed to the sun or to diffuse daylight will penetrate not only sheets of black paper but even some metals, for example, an aluminum plate and a thin copper foil. In particular, I have performed the following experiment:

A Lumiere plate of silver bromide in gelatine was enclosed in an opaque plate-holder of black fabric, closed on one side by a plate of aluminum; if the plate-holder was exposed to full sunlight, even for an entire day, the plate would not be fogged; but if a lamella of the uranium salt is fastened to the outside of the aluminum plate, held down, for example, by

Translation courtesy of Dover Publications Inc.

strips of paper, and if the whole is exposed to the sun for several hours, it can be seen, after the plate has been developed in the ordinary fashion, that the silhouette of the crystalline lamella appears in black on the sensitive plate and that the silver salt has been reduced opposite the phosphorescent lamella. If the sheet of aluminum is rather thick, the intensity of the action is less than that through two sheets of black paper.

If between the lamella of the uranium salt and the aluminum sheet or the black paper we place a screen formed by a sheet of copper about 0.10 mm thick, in the shape of a cross, for example, the silhouette of this cross can be seen in the image, more transparently, but with a shading which nevertheless shows that the radiation has penetrated the sheet of copper. In another experiment, a thinner sheet of copper (0.04 mm) weakened the active radiations much less.

The phosphorescence excited no longer by the direct rays of the sun but by the solar radiations reflected on the metallic mirror of a heliostat, then refracted by a prism and lens of quartz, gave rise to the same phenomena.

I shall particularly insist on the following fact, which appears to me very important and quite outside the range of the phenomena one might expect to observe. The same crystalline lamellas, placed opposite photographic plates, under the same conditions, separated by the same screens, but shielded from excitation by incident radiation and kept in darkness, still produce the same photographic impressions. Here is the way I was led to make this observation. Among the preceding experiments, some were prepared on Wednesday the 26 and Thursday the 27 of February, and, as on those days the sun appeared only intermittently, I held back the experiments that had been prepared, and returned the plate-holders to darkness in a drawer, leaving the lamellas of the uranium salt in place. As the sun still did not appear during the following days, I developed the photographic plates on the first of March, expecting to find very weak images. To the contrary, the silhouettes appeared with great intensity. I thought at once that the action must have been going on in darkness, and I arranged the following experiment.

At the bottom of a box of opaque cardboard I placed a photographic plate; then, on the sensitive side, I placed a lamella of the uranium salt, a convex lamella, which touched the gelatine-bromide at only a few points; then nearby I arranged on the same plate another lamella of the same salt, separated from the gelatine-bromide surface by a thin slip of glass; this operation having been carried out in the dark-room, the box was closed, then shut inside another cardboard box, and then inside a drawer.

I did the same with a plate-holder closed by a sheet of aluminum, into which I put a photographic plate, and, on the outside, a lamella of the uranium salt. The whole was shut inside a cardboard box, then in a drawer. At the end of five hours I developed the plates, and the silhouettes of the crystalline lamellas appeared in black, as in the preceding experiments, and as though they had been rendered phosphorescent by light. As for the lamella laid directly on the gelatine, there was hardly any difference in action between the points of contact and the parts of the lamella which were separated by about a millimeter from the gelatine; the difference can be attributed to the differing distance of the sources of the active radiations. The action of the lamella placed on a slip of glass was very slightly weakened, but the shape of the lamella was very well reproduced. Finally, through the aluminum sheet, the action was considerably weaker but nevertheless very distinct.

It is important to notice that this phenomenon does not seem to have to be attributed to luminous radiations emitted in phosphorescence, since at the end of 1/100 of a second these radiations have become so weak that they are hardly perceptible.

A hypothesis which presents itself rather naturally to the mind would be to suppose that these radiations, whose effects possess a strong analogy with the effects produced by the radiations studied by Lenard and Roentgen might be invisible radiations emitted by phosphorescence, whose duration of persistence might be infinitely greater than that of the luminous radiations emitted by these substances. Nevertheless, the present experiments, without being contrary to this hypothesis, do not warrant our formulating it. The experiments I am prosecuting at the moment may, I hope, contribute some clarification to this new order of phenomena.

THE

LONDON, EDINBURGH, AND DUBLIN

PHILOSOPHICAL MAGAZINE

AND

JOURNAL OF SCIENCE.

[FIFTH SERIES.]

JANUARY 1900.

I. *A Radio-active Substance emitted from Thorium Compounds.* *By* E. Rutherford, *M.A., B.Sc., Macdonald Professor of Physics, McGill University, Montreal* *.

It has been shown by Schmidt † that thorium compounds give out a type of radiation similar in its photographic and electrical actions to uranium and Röntgen radiation. In addition to this ordinary radiation, I have found that thorium compounds continuously emit radio-active particles of some kind, which retain their radio-active powers for several minutes. This "emanation," as it will be termed for shortness, has the power of ionizing the gas in its neighbourhood and of passing through thin layers of metals, and, with great ease, through considerable thicknesses of paper.

In order to make clear the evidence of the existence of a radio-active emanation, an account will first be given of the anomalous behaviour of thorium compounds compared with those of uranium. Thorium oxide has been employed in
most of the experiments, as it exhibits the "emanation" 7
property to a greater degree than the other compounds; but what is true for the oxide is also true, but to a less extent, of the other thorium compounds examined, viz., the nitrate, sulphate, acetate, and oxalate.

In a previous paper ‡ the author has shown that the radiation

* Communicated by Prof J. J. Thomson, F.R.S.

† Wied. *Ann.* May 1898.

‡ Phil. Mag. Jan. 1899, p. 109.

from thorium is of a more penetrating character than the radiation from uranium. Attention was also directed to the inconstancy of thorium as a source of radiation. Owens* has investigated in more detail the radiation from thorium compounds. He has shown that the radiations from the different compounds are of the same kind, and, with the exception of thorium oxide in thick layers, approximately homogeneous in character.

The intensity of thorium radiation, when examined by means of the electrical discharge produced, is found to be very variable; and this inconstancy is due to slow currents of air produced in an open room. When the apparatus is placed in a closed vessel, to do away with air-currents, the intensity is found to be practically constant. The sensitiveness of thorium oxide to slight currents of air is very remarkable. The movement of the air caused by the opening or closing of a door at the end of the room opposite to where the apparatus is placed, is often sufficient to considerably diminish the rate of discharge. In this respect thorium compounds differ from those of uranium, which are not appreciably affected by slight currents of air. Another anomaly that thorium compounds exhibit is the ease with which the radiation apparently passes through paper. The following table is an example of the way the rate of leak between two parallel plates, one of which is covered with a *thick* layer of thorium oxide, varies with the number of layers of ordinary foolscap-paper placed over the radio-active substance.

TABLE I.

Thickness of each Layer of Paper = ·008 cm. 50 volts between plates.

8

Number of Layers of Paper.	Rate of Discharge.
0	1
1	·74
2	·74
5	·72
10	·67
20	·55

* Phil. Mag. Oct. 1899, p. 360.

In the above table the rate of leak with the thorium oxide uncovered is taken as unity. It will be observed that the first layer reduced the rate of leak to ·74, and the five succeeding layers produce very little effect.

The action, however, is quite different if we use a *thin* * layer of thorium oxide. With one layer of paper, the rate of discharge is then reduced to less than $\frac{1}{16}$ of its value. At first sight it appears as if the thorium oxide gave out two types of radiation, one of which is readily absorbed by paper, and the other to only a slight extent. If we examine the radiation given out by a thin layer of thorium oxide, by placing successive layers of thin paper upon it, we find the radiation is approximately homogeneous, as the following table shows.

TABLE II.

Thickness of Paper=·0027 cm.

Number of Layers of Thin Paper.	Rate of Discharge.
0	1
1	·37
2	·16
3	·08

The rate of leak of the bare salt is taken as unity. If the radiation is of one kind, we should expect the rate of discharge (which is proportional to the intensity of the radiation) to diminish in geometrical progression with the addition of equal thicknesses of paper. The above figures show that this is approximately the case. With a thick layer of thorium oxide, by adding successive layers of thin paper, we find the rate of 9
discharge gradually diminish, till after a few layers it reaches a constant value. The amount that is cut off by the first layer of foolscap-paper (see Table I.) is of the same kind of radiation as that which is emitted by a thin layer of oxide.

On directing a slight current of air between the test-plates, the rate of discharge due to a thick layer of thorium oxide is

* To produce a thin layer on a plate, the oxide, in the form of a fine powder, was sprinkled by means of a fine gauze, so as to cover the plate to a very small depth. By a thick layer is meant a layer of oxide over a millimetre in thickness.

greatly diminished. The amount of diminution is to a great extent independent of the electromotive force acting between the plates. Under similar conditions with uranium, the rate of leak is not appreciably affected. With a thin layer of oxide, the diminution of the rate of leak is small; but with a thick layer of oxide, the rate of leak may be reduced to less than one-third of its previous value. If two thicknesses of foolscap-paper are placed over the thorium oxide, the resulting rate of leak between the plates may be diminished to less than $\frac{1}{20}$ of its value by a slight continuous blast of air from a gasometer or bellows.

The phenomena exhibited by thorium compounds receive a complete explanation if we suppose that, in addition to the ordinary radiation, a large number of radio-active particles are given out from the mass of the active substance. This "emanation" can pass through considerable thicknesses of paper. The radio-active particles emitted by the thorium compounds gradually diffuse through the gas in its neighbourhood and become centres of ionization throughout the gas. The fact that the effect of air-currents is only observed to a slight extent with thin layers of thorium oxide is due to the preponderance, in that case, of the rate of leak due to the ordinary radiation over that due to the emanation. With a thick layer of thorium oxide, the rate of leak due to the ordinary radiation is practically that due to a thin surface-layer, as the radiation can only penetrate a short distance through the salt. On the other hand, the "emanation" is able to diffuse from a distance of several millimetres below the surface of the compound, and the rate of leak due to it becomes much greater than that due to the radiation alone.

The explanation of the action of slight currents of air is clear on the "emanation" theory. Since the radio-active particles are not affected by an electrical field, extremely minute motions of air, if continuous, remove many of the radio-active centres from between the plates. It will be
10 shown shortly that the emanation continues to ionize the gas in its neighbourhood for several minutes, so that the removal of the particles from between the plates diminishes the rate of discharge between the plates.

Duration of the Radio-activity of the Emanation.

The emanation gradually loses its radio-active power. The following method was adopted to determine the rate of decay of the intensity of the radiation of the radio-active particles emitted by thorium oxide.

A thick layer of thorium oxide was enclosed in a narrow rectangular paper vessel A (fig. 1), made up of two thicknesses of foolscap-paper. The paper cut off the regular radiation almost entirely, but allowed the emanation to pass through. The thorium thus enclosed was placed inside a

Fig. 1.

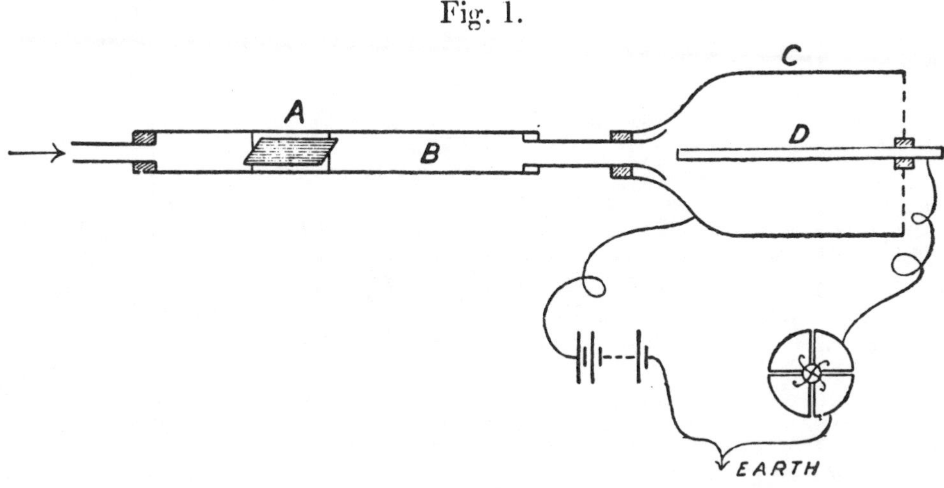

long metal tube B. One end of the tube was connected to a large insulated cylindrical vessel C, which had a number of small holes in the end for the passage of air. Inside C was fixed an insulated electrode, D, connected with one pair of quadrants of a Thomson electrometer. The cylinder, C, was connected to one terminal of a battery of 100 volts, the other terminal of which was connected to earth.

A slow current of air from an aspirator or gasometer, which had been freed from dust by its passage through a plug of cotton-wool, was passed through the apparatus. The current of air, in its passage by the thorium oxide, carried away the radio-active particles with it, and these were gradually conveyed into the large cylinder C. The electrometer-needle showed no sign of movement until the radio-active particles were carried into C. In consequence of the ionization of the 11
gas in the cylinder by the radio-active particles, a current passed between the electrodes C and D. The value of the current was the same whether C was connected with the positive or negative pole of the battery. When the current of air had been flowing for some minutes, the current between C and D reached a constant value. The flow of air was then stopped, and the rate of leak between C and D observed at regular intervals. It was found that the current between C and D persisted for over ten minutes.

The following is a series of observations.

TABLE III.

Potential-difference 100 volts.

Time in Seconds.	Current.
0	1
28	·69
62	·51
118	·23
155	·14
210	·067
272	·041
360	·018

Fig. 2.

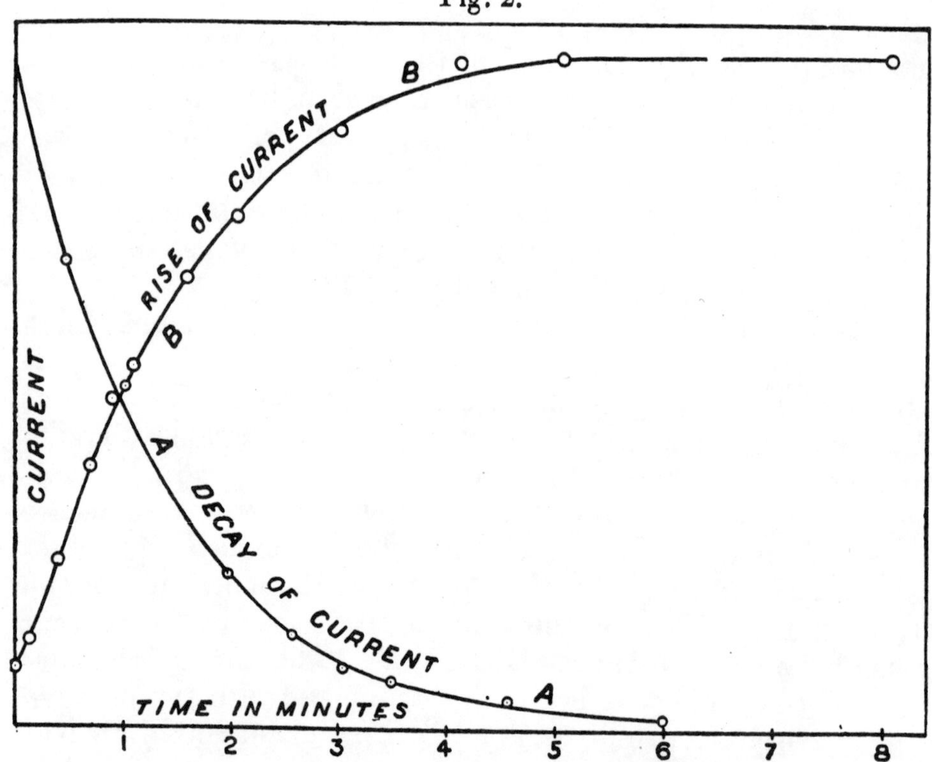

Fig. 2, curve A, shows the relation existing between the current through the gas and the time. The current, just before the flow of air is stopped, is taken as unity. It will be observed that the current through the gas diminishes in a geometrical progression with the time. It can easily be shown, by the theory of ionization, that the current through the gas is proportional to the intensity of the radiation emitted by the radio-active particles. We therefore see that the intensity of the radiation given out by the radio-active particles falls off in a geometrical progression with the time. The result shows that the intensity of the radiation has fallen to one-half its value after an interval of about *one minute*. The rate of leak due to the emanation was too small for measurement after an interval of ten minutes.

If the ionized gas had been produced from a uranium compound, the duration of the conductivity, for voltages such as were used, would only have been a fraction of a second.

The rate of decay of intensity is independent of the electromotive force acting on the gas. This shows that the radio-active particles are not destroyed by the electric field. The current through the gas at any particular instant, after stoppage of the flow of air, was found to be the same whether the electromotive force had been acting the whole time or just applied for the time of the test.

The current through the gas in the cylinder depends on the electromotive force in the same way as the current through a gas made conducting by Röntgen rays. The current at first increases nearly in proportion to the electromotive force, but soon reaches an approximate "saturation" value.

The duration of the radio-activity was also tested by another method. The paper vessel containing the thorium oxide was placed inside a long brass cylinder over 200 cms. in length. A slow current of air (with a velocity of about 2 cms. per second along the tube) was passed over the thorium oxide along the tube, and then between two insulated concentric cylinders. The rate of leak between the two concentric cylinders (potential-difference 270 volts) was observed when the air had been passing sufficiently long to produce a steady state. The rates of leak were observed for varying positions of the thorium oxide along the tube. Knowing the velocity of
the current of air along the tube, the time taken to carry the 13
radio-active particles to the testing-apparatus could be determined. In this way it was found that the rate of decay was about the same as determined by the first method, *i. e.*, the intensity fell to half its value in about one minute.

In this apparatus experiments were also tried to see whether the radio-active particles moved in an electric field. The experiments on the effect of a current of air on the rate of discharge naturally suggest that possibly one of the ions was so large that it moved extremely slowly even in strong electric fields. The results obtained showed that the particles did not move with a greater velocity than $\frac{1}{100{,}000}$ cm. per second for a potential-gradient of one volt per cm.; and it is probable that the particles do not move at all in an electric field. By blowing the emanation into an inductor, no evidence of any charge in the emanation could be detected. We may therefore conclude that the emanation is uncharged, and is not appreciably affected by an electric field.

Properties of the Emanation.

The emanation passes through a plug of cotton-wool without any loss of its radio-active powers. It is also unaffected by bubbling through hot or cold water, weak or strong sulphuric acid. In this respect it acts like an ordinary gas. An ion, on the other hand, is not able to pass through a plug of cotton-wool, or to bubble through water, without losing its charge.

The emanation is similar to uranium in its photographic and electrical actions. It can ionize the gas in its neighbourhood, and can affect a photographic plate in the dark after several days' exposure. Russell * has shown that the active agent in producing photographic action in the case of metals, paper, &c., is due to hydrogen peroxide. Hydrogen peroxide apparently has the power of passing in some way through considerable thicknesses of special substances, and in this respect the emanation resembles it. Hydrogen peroxide, however, does not ionize the gas in its neighbourhood. The action of hydrogen peroxide on the photographic plate is purely a chemical one; but it is the radiation from the emanation, and not the emanation itself, that produces ionizing and photographic actions.

The radio-active emanation passes through all metals if sufficiently thin. In order to make certain that the emanation passed through the material to be examined and did not
14 diffuse round the edges, the radio-active substance was placed in a square groove of a thick lead plate. Two layers of paper were pasted tightly over the opening to cut off the regular radiation. The material to be tested was then firmly waxed down on the lead plate.

The following numbers illustrate the effect of different metals. The rate of discharge, due to the emanation between two parallel plates 4 cms. apart, was observed.

* Proc. Roy. Soc. 1897.

Aluminium Foil, thickness = ·0008 cm.

Number of Layers.	Rate of Discharge.
0	1
1	·66
3	·42
6	·16

Cardboard, thickness ·08 cm.

Layers.	Rate of Discharge.
0	1
1	·40
2	·21

The emanation passed readily through several thicknesses of gold- and silver-leaf. A plate of mica, thickness ·006 cm., was completely impervious to the emanation.

When a thick layer of thorium oxide, covered over with several thicknesses of paper, is placed inside a closed vessel, the rate of discharge due to the emanation is small at first, but gradually increases, until after a few minutes a steady state is reached.

These results are to be expected, for the emanation can only slowly diffuse through the paper and the surrounding air. A steady state is reached when the rate of loss of intensity due to the gradual decay of the radio-activity of the emanation is recompensed by the number of new radio-active centres supplied from the thorium compound. 15

Let n = number of ions produced per second by the radio-active particles between the plates.

Let q = number of ions supplied per second by the emanation diffusing from the thorium.

The rate of variation of the number of ions at any time t is given by

$$\frac{dn}{dt} = q - \lambda n,$$

where λ is a constant.

The results given in Table III. show that the rate of diminution of the number of ions is proportional to the number present.

Solving the equation, it is seen that

$$\log_e (q-\lambda n) = -\lambda t + A,$$

where A is a constant.

When $t=0$, $n=0$;

therefore $A=\log_e q$.

Thus

$$n=\frac{q}{\lambda}(1-e^{-\lambda t}).$$

With a large potential-difference between the test-plates the current i through the gas at any time is given by

$$i=ne,$$

where e is the charge on an ion.

When a steady state is reached, $\frac{dn}{dt}=0$; and the maximum number N of ions produced per second by the radio-active particles between the plates is given by

$$N=\frac{q}{\lambda},$$

and the maximum current I is given by

$$I=Ne.$$

Therefore

$$\frac{i}{I}=1-e^{-\lambda t}.$$

The current thus increases according to the same law
16 as a current of electricity rises in a circuit of constant inductance.

This result is confirmed by an experiment on the rise of the current between two concentric cylinders. The thorium oxide enclosed in paper was placed inside the cylinder. A current of air was sent between the cylinders in order to remove the emanation as rapidly as it was formed. The current of air was then stopped and the current between the two cylinders observed, by means of an electrometer, for successive intervals after the current of air ceased. Table IV. gives the results obtained.

Table IV.

Length of cylinder = 30 cms.

Internal diameter outer cylinder = 5·5 cms.
External " inner " = ·8 cm.

100 volts between cylinders.

Time in Seconds.	Current in Scale-divisions per second.
0	2·4
7·5	3·3
2·3	6·5
4·0	10·0
5·3	12·5
6·7	13·8
9·6	17·1
12·5	19·4
18·4	22·7
24·4	25·3
30·4	25·6
48·4	25·6

The results are expressed in fig. 2, curve B, where the ordinate represents current and the abscissa time. It will be observed that the curve of rise of the current is similar in form to the rise of an electric current in a circuit of constant inductance. The current reaches half its value about one minute after the current of air has stopped,—a result which agrees with the equation given, for $e^{-\lambda t}=\frac{1}{2}$ when $t=60$ seconds (see 'able IV.). At the instant of stopping the current of air the current has a definite value, since most of the ions given off by the emanation, before it is blown out of the cylinders, reach the electrodes. 17

When the source of the emanation is removed, $q=0$, and the decay of the number of ions produced by the emanation is given by the equation

$$\frac{dn}{dt}=-\lambda n.$$

If $n=N$ when $t=0$, it is easily seen that

$$\frac{n}{N}=e^{-\lambda t},$$

or

$$\frac{i}{I} = e^{-\lambda t};$$

i. e., the current through the gas diminishes in a geometrical progression. After 20 minutes the current through the gas is only about one millionth part of its initial value.

It has been shown that $e^{-\lambda t} = \frac{1}{2}$ when $t = 60$ seconds.

Therefore $$\lambda = \frac{1}{86},$$

and $$N = \frac{q}{\lambda} = 86q;$$

or the total number of ions produced per second when a steady state is reached is 86 times the number of ions supplied per second by the emanation.

The amount of emanation from thorium oxide increases with the thickness of the layer. When 1 gramme of thorium oxide was spread over a surface of 25 cms., the amount of discharge due to the ordinary radiation had practically reached a maximum. The rate of leak due to the emanation for the same thickness was small. With 9 grammes of oxide spread over the same area, the rate of leak due to the emanation had reached about half its maximum value, which for that case corresponded to four times the rate of leak caused by the ordinary radiation. The emanation thus still preserves its radio-active properties after diffusing through several millimetres of thorium compound.

The emanation is given out whatever the gas by which the thorium is surrounded. The action is very similar whether air, oxygen, hydrogen, or carbonic acid is used.

The rate of discharge due to the emanation diminishes with lowering of the pressure of the air surrounding it. Only a few observations have been made, but the results seem to point to a uniform rate of emission of the emanation at all pressures; but since the intensity of the ionization of the gas
18 varies directly as the pressure, the rate of leak decreases with lowering of the pressure.

The amount of the emanation, so far as the experiments have gone, is also independent of the quantity of water-vapour present.

The power of emitting radio-active particles is not possessed to any appreciable extent by other radio-active substances besides thorium. All the compounds of thorium examined possess it to a marked degree, and it is especially large in the oxide. Two different specimens of the oxide have been used, one obtained from Schuchart of Germany, and the other from Eimer & Amend of New York. The oxide is prepared by the latter by igniting thorium nitrate obtained from monazite sand.

The amount of discharge caused by the emanation is increased several times by the conversion of the nitrate into the oxide; but at the same time, the rate of discharge due to the ordinary radiation emitted by the thorium is increased in about an equal ratio. The conversion of the nitrate into the oxide took place below a red heat. On heating in a muffle for some time at white heat, the amount of emanation continually diminished, till after four hours' exposure to the heat, the rate of discharge due to the emanation was only $\frac{1}{20}$ of the value immediately after its conversion into oxide.

Both thorium oxalate and sulphate act in a similar manner to the nitrate; but the emanation is still given off to a considerable extent after continued heating.

In considering the question of the origin and nature of the emanation, two possible explanations naturally suggest themselves, viz.:—

(1) That the emanation may be due to fine dust particles of the radio-active substance emitted by the thorium compounds.

(2) That the emanation may be a vapour given off from thorium compounds.

The fact that the emanation can pass through metals and large thicknesses of paper and through plugs of cotton-wool, is strong evidence against the dust hypothesis. Special experiments, however, were tried to settle the question. The experiments of Aitken and Wilson * have shown that ordinary air can be completely freed from dust particles by repeated small expansions of the air over a water-surface. The dust particles act as nuclei for the formation of small drops, and are removed from the gas by the action of gravity.

The experiment was repeated with thorium oxide present
in the vessel. The oxide was enclosed in a paper cylinder, 19
which allowed the emanation to pass through it. After repeated expansions no cloud was formed, showing that for the expansions used the particles of the emanation were too small to become centres of condensation of the water-vapour. We may therefore conclude, from this experiment, that the emanation does not consist of dust particles of thorium oxide.

It would be of interest to examine the behaviour of the emanation for greater and more sudden expansions, after the

* Trans. Roy. Soc. 1897.

manner employed by C. T. R. Wilson* in his experiments on the action of ions as centres of condensation.

The emanation may possibly be a vapour of thorium. There is reason to believe that all metals and substances give off vapour to some degree. If the radio-active power of thorium is possessed by the molecules of the substance, it would be expected that the vapour of the substance would be itself radio-active for a short time, but the radio-active power would diminish in consequence of the rapid radiation of energy. Some information on this point could probably be obtained by observation of the rate of diffusion of the emanation into gases. It is hoped that experimental data of this kind will lead to an approximate determination of the molecular weight of the emanation.

Experiments have been tried to see if the amount of the emanation from thorium oxide is sufficient to appreciably alter the pressure of the gas in an exhausted tube. The oxide was placed in a bulb connected with a Plücker spectroscopic tube. The whole was exhausted, and the pressure noted by a McLeod gauge. The bulb of thorium oxide was disconnected from the main tube by means of a stopcock. The Plücker tube was refilled and exhausted again to the same pressure. On connecting the two tubes together again, no appreciable difference in the pressure or in the appearance of the discharge from an induction-coil was observed. The spectrum of the gas was unchanged.

Experiments, which are still in progress, show that the emanation possesses a very remarkable property. I have found that the positive ion produced in a gas by the emanation possesses the power of producing radio-activity in all substances on which it falls. This power of giving forth a radiation lasts for several days. The radiation is of a more penetrating character than that given out by thorium or uranium. The emanation from thorium compounds thus has properties which the thorium itself does not possess. A more com-
20 plete account of the results obtained is reserved for a later communication.

McGill University, Montreal,
September 13th, 1899.

* Phil. Trans. Roy. Soc. vol. clxxxix. (1897).

Radiations from Radium

P. Villard

Comptes rendus de l'Academie des Sciences, Paris, 1900, 130: 1178-79.

M. and Mme. Curie having been kind enough to place at my disposal a sample of radium much more active than the one which I was using, I have undertaken with this material a series of experiments relative to the passage of the deviable rays through objects. As I have indicated previously, the principal difficulty during this study results because some of the rays not deviable by a magnet are transmitted at the same time as the others; therefore I studied, in the first place, the power of penetration of the two radiations.

The rays emitted the source traverse a suitably large slit in a bar of lead and arrive at a nearly grazing incidence on two superposed photographic plates, enveloped in doubly thick black paper, and placed in a magnetic field. The first plate thus registers the trajectories of the rays which have traversed the tube of glass containing the radium and the black paper; the subjacent plate receives only the rays which have traversed the first, at an obliquity which increases from one end of the plate to the other.

Under these conditions, the upper negative shows the trace of two distince beams: the one deviated and spread out; the other, weaker one, absolutely rectilinear and sharp on its two edges.

On the lower plate, only one of the two beams is visible: it is the non-deviable beam. The image produced by it is as intense as on the first plate and as sharp: it is even more visible because the impression is less clouded. Now, the thickness of glass traversed most distant from the source is greater than 1 cm.

Upon increasing the duration of the exposure, one succeeds in obtaining a very feeble trace of the deviable beam.

If one puts a 0.3 mm strip of lead flat on the upper plate, the trajectory of the deviable beam is abolished the full width of the strip, the non-deviable rays are only weakened. One distinguishes thus the two trajectories in the region where they are partially superposed.

Therefore the X-rays emitted by the radium have a power of penetration considerably greater than the deviable rays: this is analogous to what takes place with Crookes' tubes. A thickness of glass of 1 cm, or even a little less, practically stops the deviable rays and weakens the others very slightly. One understands from this, if the total radiations traverse successive screens, the first will produce an absorption all the more apparent from the photographic point of view, the cathodic rays appearing to be the more active; but starting from the moment when these have disappeared, the absorption by the successive screens will weaken very little the rest of the radiation.

Translation kindly provided by William G. Myers, Ph.D., Columbus, Ohio.

LONDON, EDINBURGH, AND DUBLIN

PHILOSOPHICAL MAGAZINE

AND

JOURNAL OF SCIENCE.

VOL. IV.—SIXTH SERIES.
JULY—DECEMBER 1902.

XLI. *The Cause and Nature of Radioactivity.*—Part I. *By* E. RUTHERFORD, *M.A., D.Sc., Macdonald Professor of Physics, and* F. SODDY, *B.A. (Oxon.), Demonstrator in Chemistry, McGill University, Montreal*.*

CONTENTS.

NOTE: Only sections XII and XIII are reprinted in this volume.

XII. *Summary of Results.*

The foregoing experimental results may be briefly summarized. The major part of the radioactivity of thorium—ordinarily about 54 per cent.—is due to a non-thorium type of matter, ThX, possessing distinct chemical properties, which is temporarily radioactive, its activity falling to half value in about four days. The constant radioactivity of thorium is maintained by the production of this material at a constant rate. Both the rate of production of the new material and the rate of decay of its activity appear to be independent of the physical and chemical condition of the system.

The ThX further possesses the property of exciting radioactivity on surrounding inactive matter, and about 21 per cent. of the total activity under ordinary circumstances is derived from this source. Its rate of decay and other considerations make it appear probable that it is the same as the excited radioactivity produced by the thorium emanation, which is in turn produced by ThX. There is evidence that, if from any cause the emanation is prevented from escaping in the radioactive state, the energy of its radiation goes to augment the proportion of excited radioactivity in the compound.

Thorium can be freed by suitable means from both ThX and the excited radioactivity which the latter produces, and then possesses an activity about 25 per cent. of its original value, below which it has not been reduced. This residual radiation consists entirely of rays non-deviable by the magnetic field, whereas the other two components comprise both deviable and non-deviable radiation. Most probably this residual activity is caused by a second non-thorium type of matter produced in the same change as ThX, and it should therefore prove possible to separate it by chemical methods.

XIII. *General Theoretical Considerations.*

Turning from the experimental results to their theoretical
24 interpretation, it is necessary to first consider the generally accepted view of the nature of radioactivity. It is well established that this property is the function of the atom and not of the molecule. Uranium and thorium, to take the most definite cases, possess the property in whatever molecular condition they occur, and the former also in the elementary state. So far as the radioactivity of different compounds of different density and states of division can be compared together, the intensity of the radiation appears to depend only on the quantity of active element present. It

is not at all dependent on the source from which the element is derived, or the process of purification to which it has been subjected, provided sufficient time is allowed for the equilibrium point to be reached. It is not possible to explain the phenomena by the existence of impurities associated with the radioactive elements, even if any advantage could be derived from the assumption. For these impurities must necessarily be present always to the same extent in different specimens derived from the most widely different sources, and, moreover, they must persist *in unaltered amount* after the most refined processes of purification. This is contrary to the accepted meaning of the term impurity.

All the most prominent workers in this subject are agreed in considering radioactivity an atomic phenomenon. M. and Mme. Curie, the pioneers in the chemistry of the subject, have recently put forward their views (*Comptes Rendus*, cxxxiv. 1902, p. 85). They state that this idea underlies their whole work from the beginning and created their methods of research. M. Becquerel, the original discoverer of the property for uranium, in his announcement of the recovery of the activity of the same element after the active constituent had been removed by chemical treatment, points out the significance of the fact that uranium is giving out cathode-rays. These, according to the hypothesis of Sir William Crookes and Prof. J. J. Thomson, are *material* particles of mass one thousandth of the hydrogen atom.

Since, therefore, radioactivity is at once an atomic phenomenon and accompanied by chemical changes in which new types of matter are produced, these changes must be occurring within the atom, and the radioactive elements must be undergoing spontaneous transformation. The results that have so far been obtained, which indicate that the velocity of this reaction is unaffected by the conditions, makes it clear that the changes in question are different in character from any that have been before dealt with in chemistry. It is apparent that we are dealing with phenomena outside the sphere of known atomic forces. Radioactivity may therefore be considered as a manifestation of subatomic chemical change.

The changes brought to knowledge by radioactivity, although undeniably material and chemical in nature, are of a different order of magnitude from any that have before been dealt with in chemistry. The course of the production of new matter which can be recognized by the electrometer, by means of the property of radioactivity, after the lapse of a few hours or even minutes, might conceivably require geological epochs to attain to quantities recognized by the balance. However the well-defined chemical properties of both ThX and UrX are not in accordance with the view that the actual amounts involved are of this extreme order of minuteness. On the other hand, the existence of radioactive elements at all in the earth's crust is an *à priori* argument against the magnitude of the change being anything but small.

Radioactivity as a new property of matter capable of exact quantitative determination thus possesses an interest apart from the peculiar properties and powers which the radiations themselves exhibit. Mme. Curie, who isolated from pitchblende a new substance, radium, which possessed distinct chemical properties and spectroscopic lines, used the property as a means of chemical analysis. An exact parallel is to be found in Bunsen's discovery and separation of cæsium and rubidium by means of the spectroscope.

The present results show that radioactivity can also be used to follow *chemical changes occurring in matter*. The properties of matter that fulfil the necessary conditions for the study of chemical change without disturbance to the reacting system are few in number. It seems not unreasonable to hope, in the light of the foregoing results, that radioactivity, being such a property, affords the means of obtaining information of the processes occurring within the chemical atom, in the same way as the rotation of the plane of polarization and other physical properties have been used in chemistry for the investigation of the course of molecular change.

Macdonald Physics Building,
Macdonald Chemistry and Mining Building,
McGill University, Montreal.

PROCEEDINGS

OF THE

ROYAL SOCIETY OF LONDON.

VOL. LXXI.

27

LONDON:
HARRISON AND SONS, ST. MARTIN'S LANE,
Printers in Ordinary to His Majesty.

JUNE, 1903.

"The Emanations of Radium." By Sir WILLIAM CROOKES, F.R.S.

Received March 17,—Read March 19, 1903.

A solution of almost pure radium nitrate which had been used for spectrographic work, was evaporated to dryness in a dish, and the crystalline residue examined in a dark room. It was feebly luminous.

A screen of platinocyanide of barium brought near the residue glowed with a green light, the intensity varying with the distance separating them. The phosphorescence disappeared as soon as the screen was removed from the influence of the radium.

A screen of Sidot's hexagonal blende (zinc sulphide), said to be useful for detecting polonium radiations, was almost as luminous as the platinocyanide screen in presence of radium, but there was more residual phosphorescence, lasting from a few minutes to half an hour or more according to the strength and duration of the initial excitement.

The persistence of radio-activity on glass vessels which have contained radium is remarkable. Filters, beakers, and dishes used in the laboratory for operations with radium, after having been washed in the usual way, remain radio-active; a piece of blende screen held inside the beaker or other vessel immediately glowing with the presence of radium.

The blende screen is sensitive to mechanical shocks. A tap with the tip of a penknife will produce a sudden spark of light, and a scratch with the blade will show itself as an evanescent luminous line.

A diamond crystal brought near the radium nitrate glowed with a pale bluish-green light, as it would in a "Radiant Matter" tube under the influence of cathodic bombardment. On removing the diamond from the radium it ceased to glow, but, when laid on the sensitive screen, it produced phosphorescence beneath, which lasted some minutes.

During these manipulations the diamond accidentally touched the radium nitrate in the dish, and thus a few imperceptible grains of the
28 radium salt got on to the zinc sulphide screen. The surface was immediately dotted about with brilliant specks of green light, some being a millimetre or more across, although the inducing particles were too small to be detected on the white screen when examined by daylight.

In a dark room, under a microscope with a $\frac{2}{3}$-inch objective, each luminous spot is seen to have a dull centre surrounded by a luminous halo extending for some distance around. The dark centre itself appears to shoot out light at intervals in different directions. Outside the halo, the dark surface of the screen scintillates with sparks of light. No two flashes succeed one another on the same spct, but are scattered over the surface, coming and going instantaneously, no movement of translation being seen.

The scintillations are somewhat better seen with a pocket lens magnifying about 20 diameters. They are less visible on the barium platinocyanide than on the zinc sulphide screen.

A powerful electro-magnet has no apparent effect on the scintillations, which appear quite unaffected when the current is made or broken, the screen being close to the poles and arranged axially or equatorially.

A solid piece of radium nitrate is slowly brought near the screen. The general phosphorescence of the screen as visible to the naked eye varies according to the distance of the radium from it. On now examining the surface with the pocket lens, the radium being far off and the screen faintly luminous, the scintillating spots are sparsely scattered over the surface. On bringing the radium nearer the screen the scintillations become more numerous and brighter, until when close together the flashes follow each other so quickly that the surface looks like a turbulent luminous sea. When the scintillating points are few there is no residual phosphorescence to be seen, and the sparks succeeding each other appear like stars on a black sky. When, however, the bombardment exceeds a certain intensity, the residual phosphorescent glow spreads over the screen, without, however, interfering with the scintillations.

If the end of a platinum wire which has been dipped in a solution of radium nitrate and dried is brought near the screen, the scintillations become very numerous and energetic, and cease immediately the wire is removed. If, however, the end of the wire touches the screen, a luminous spot is produced, which then becomes a centre of activity, and the screen remains alive with scintillations in the neighbourhood of the spot for many weeks afterwards.

"Polonium" basic nitrate produces a similar effect on the screen, but the scintillations are not so numerous.

Microscopic glass, very thin aluminium foil, and thin mica do not stop the general luminosity of the screen from the X-rays, but arrest the scintillations.

I could detect no variation in the scintillations when a rapid blast of air was blown between the screen and the radium salt. 29

A beam of X-rays from an active tube was passed through a hole in a lead plate on to a blende screen. A luminous spot was produced on the screen, but I could detect no scintillations, only a smooth uniform phosphorescence. A piece of radium salt brought near gave the scintillations as usual, superposed on the fainter phosphorescence caused by the X-rays, and they were not interfered with in any degree by the presence of X-rays falling on the same spot.

During these experiments the fingers soon become soiled with radium, and produce phosphorescence when brought near the screen. On turning the lens to the, apparently, uniformly lighted edge of the screen close to the finger, the scintillations are seen to be closer and more numerous; what to the naked eye appears like a uniform "milky way," under the lens is a multitude of stellar points, flashing over the whole surface. A clean finger does not show any effect, but a touch with a soiled finger is sufficient to confer on it the property. Washing the fingers stops their action.

It was of interest to see if rarefying the air would have any effect on the scintillations. A blende screen was fixed near a flat glass window in a vacuum tube, and a piece of radium salt was attached to an iron rocker, so that the movement of an outside magnet would either bring the radium opposite the screen or draw it away altogether. A microscope gave a good image of the surface of the screen, and in a dark room the scintillations were well seen. No particular difference was observed in a high vacuum; indeed, if anything, the sparks appeared a trifle brighter and sharper in air than in vacuo. A duplicate apparatus in air was put close to the one in the vacuum tube, so that the eye could pass rapidly from one to the other, and it was so adjusted that the scintillations were about equal when each was in air. The vacuum apparatus was now exhausted to a very high point, and the appearance on each screen was noticed. Here again I thought the sparks in the vacuum were not quite so bright as in air, and on breaking the capillary tube of the pump, and observing as the air entered, the same impression was left on my mind; but the differences, if any, are very minute, and are scarcely greater than might arise from errors of observation.

It is difficult to form an estimate of the number of flashes of light per second. But with the radium at about 5 cm. off the screen they are barely detectable, not being more than one or two per second. As the distance of the radium diminishes the flashes become more frequent, until at 1 or 2 cm. they are too numerous to count.

[*Added March* 18.—On bringing alternately a Sidot's blende screen and one of barium platinocyanide, face downwards, near a dish of "polonium" sub-nitrate, each became luminous, the blende screen being
30 very little brighter of the two. On testing the two screens over a crucible containing dry radium nitrate, both glowed; in this case the blende screen being much the brighter. Examined with a lens, the light of the blende screen was seen to consist of a mass of scintillations, while that of the platinocyanide screen was a uniform glow, on which the scintillations were much less apparent.

The screens were now turned face upwards so that emanations from the active bodies would have to pass through the thickness of card before reaching the sensitive surface. Placed over the "polonium" neither screen showed any light. Over the radium the platinocyanide screen showed a very luminous disc, corresponding with the opening of the crucible, but the blende disc remained quite dark.

It therefore appears that practically the whole of the luminosity on the blende screen, whether due to radium or "polonium," is occasioned by emanations which will not penetrate card. These are the emanations which cause the scintillations, and the reason why they are distinct on the blende and feeble on the platinocyanide screen, is that with the latter the sparks are seen on a luminous ground of general phosphorescence which renders the eye less able to see the scintillations.

Considering how coarse-grained the structure of matter must be to particles forming the emanations from radium, I cannot imagine that their relative penetrative powers depend on difference of size. I attribute the arrest of the scintillating particles to their electrical character, and to the ready way in which they are attracted by the coarser atoms or molecules of matter. I have shown that radium emanations cohere to almost everything with which they come into contact. Bismuth,* lead, platinum, thorium, uranium, elements of high atomic weight and density, possess this attraction in a high degree, and only lose the emanations very slowly, giving rise to what is known as "induced radio-activity." The emanations so absorbed from radium by bismuth, platinum, and probably other bodies, retain the property of producing scintillations on a blende screen, and are non-penetrating.]

It seems probable that in these phenomena we are actually witnessing the bombardment of the screen by the electrons† hurled off by radium with a velocity of the order of that of light; each scintillation rendering visible the impact of an electron on the screen. Although, at present, I have not been able to form even a rough approximation to the number of electrons hitting the screen in a given time, it is evident that this is not of an order of magnitude inconceivably great. Each electron is rendered apparent only by the enormous extent of lateral disturbance produced by its impact on the sensitive surface, just as individual drops of rain falling on a still pool are not seen as such, but by reason of the splash they make on impact, and the ripples and waves they produce in ever-widening circles.

---

* I have been quite unable to detect any lines but those of bismuth (and of known impurities) in the spectrum of the strongest and most active "polonium" salt I have been able to procure.

† Radiant matter, satellites, corpuscles, nuclei; whatever they are, they act like material masses.

THE

LONDON, EDINBURGH, AND DUBLIN

PHILOSOPHICAL MAGAZINE

AND

JOURNAL OF SCIENCE.

CONDUCTED BY

SIR OLIVER JOSEPH LODGE, D.Sc., LL.D., F.R.S.
SIR JOSEPH JOHN THOMSON, M.A., Sc.D., LL.D., F.R.S.
JOHN JOLY, M.A., D.Sc., F.R.S., F.G.S.
GEORGE CAREY FOSTER, B.A., LL.D., F.R.S.

AND

WILLIAM FRANCIS, F.L.S.

"Nec aranearum sane textus ideo melior quia ex se fila gignunt, nec noster vilior quia ex alienis libamus ut apes." JUST. LIPS. *Polit.* lib. i. cap. 1. Not.

VOL. XXI.—SIXTH SERIES.
JANUARY—JUNE 1911.

LONDON:

TAYLOR AND FRANCIS, RED LION COURT, FLEET STREET.

SOLD BY SIMPKIN, MARSHALL, HAMILTON, KENT, AND CO., LD.
SMITH AND SON, GLASGOW;—HODGES, FIGGIS, AND CO., DUBLIN;
VEUVE J. BOYVEAU, PARIS;—AND ASHER AND CO., BERLIN.

LXXIX. *The Scattering of α and β Particles by Matter and the Structure of the Atom.* *By* Professor E. RUTHERFORD, *F.R.S., University of Manchester* *.

§ 1. IT is well known that the α and β particles suffer deflexions from their rectilinear paths by encounters with atoms of matter. This scattering is far more marked for the β than for the α particle on account of the much smaller momentum and energy of the former particle. There seems to be no doubt that such swiftly moving particles pass through the atoms in their path, and that the deflexions observed are due to the strong electric field traversed within the atomic system. It has generally been supposed that the scattering of a pencil of α or β rays in passing through a thin plate of matter is the result of a multitude of small scatterings by the atoms of matter traversed. The observations, however, of Geiger and Marsden † on the scattering of α rays indicate that some of the α particles must suffer a deflexion of more than a right angle at a single encounter. They found, for example, that a small fraction of the incident α particles, about 1 in 20,000, were turned through an average angle of 90° in passing through a layer of gold-foil about ·00004 cm. thick, which was equivalent in stopping-power of the α particle to 1·6 millimetres of air. Geiger ‡ showed later that the most probable angle of deflexion for a pencil of α particles traversing a gold-foil of this thickness was about 0°·87. A simple calculation based on the theory of probability shows that the chance of an α particle being deflected through 90° is vanishingly small. In addition, it will be seen later that the distribution of the α particles for various angles of large deflexion does not follow the probability law to be expected if such large deflexions are made up of a large number of small deviations. It seems reasonable to suppose that the deflexion through a large angle is due to a single atomic encounter, for the chance of a second encounter of a kind to produce a large deflexion must in most cases be exceedingly small. A simple calculation shows that the atom must be a seat of an intense electric field in order to produce such a large deflexion at a single encounter.

Recently Sir J. J. Thomson § has put forward a theory to

* Communicated by the Author. A brief account of this paper was communicated to the Manchester Literary and Philosophical Society in February, 1911.

† Proc. Roy. Soc. lxxxii. p. 495 (1909).

‡ Proc. Roy. Soc. lxxxiii. p. 492 (1910).

§ Camb. Lit. & Phil. Soc. xv. pt. 5 (1910).

explain the scattering of electrified particles in passing through small thicknesses of matter. The atom is supposed to consist of a number N of negatively charged corpuscles, accompanied by an equal quantity of positive electricity uniformly distributed throughout a sphere. The deflexion of a negatively electrified particle in passing through the atom is ascribed to two causes—(1) the repulsion of the corpuscles distributed through the atom, and (2) the attraction of the positive electricity in the atom. The deflexion of the particle in passing through the atom is supposed to be small, while the average deflexion after a large number m of encounters was taken as $\sqrt{m} \,.\, \theta$, where θ is the average deflexion due to a single atom. It was shown that the number N of the electrons within the atom could be deduced from observations of the scattering of electrified particles. The accuracy of this theory of compound scattering was examined experimentally by Crowther * in a later paper. His results apparently confirmed the main conclusions of the theory, and he deduced, on the assumption that the positive electricity was continuous, that the number of electrons in an atom was about three times its atomic weight.

The theory of Sir J. J. Thomson is based on the assumption that the scattering due to a single atomic encounter is small, and the particular structure assumed for the atom does not admit of a very large deflexion of an α particle in traversing a single atom, unless it be supposed that the diameter of the sphere of positive electricity is minute compared with the diameter of the sphere of influence of the atom.

Since the α and β particles traverse the atom, it should be possible from a close study of the nature of the deflexion to form some idea of the constitution of the atom to produce the effects observed. In fact, the scattering of high-speed charged particles by the atoms of matter is one of the most promising methods of attack of this problem. The development of the scintillation method of counting single α particles affords unusual advantages of investigation, and the researches 35
of H. Geiger by this method have already added much to our knowledge of the scattering of α rays by matter.

§ 2. We shall first examine theoretically the single encounters † with an atom of simple structure, which is able to

* Crowther, Proc. Roy. Soc. lxxxiv. p. 226 (1910).

† The deviation of a particle throughout a considerable angle from an encounter with a single atom will in this paper be called "single" scattering. The deviation of a particle resulting from a multitude of small deviations will be termed "compound" scattering.

produce large deflexions of an α particle, and then compare the deductions from the theory with the experimental data available.

Consider an atom which contains a charge $\pm Ne$ at its centre surrounded by a sphere of electrification containing a charge $\mp Ne$ supposed uniformly distributed throughout a sphere of radius R. e is the fundamental unit of charge, which in this paper is taken as $4{\cdot}65 \times 10^{-10}$ E.S. unit. We shall suppose that for distances less than 10^{-12} cm. the central charge and also the charge on the α particle may be supposed to be concentrated at a point. It will be shown that the main deductions from the theory are independent of whether the central charge is supposed to be positive or negative. For convenience, the sign will be assumed to be positive. The question of the stability of the atom proposed need not be considered at this stage, for this will obviously depend upon the minute structure of the atom, and on the motion of the constituent charged parts.

In order to form some idea of the forces required to deflect an α particle through a large angle, consider an atom containing a positive charge Ne at its centre, and surrounded by a distribution of negative electricity Ne uniformly distributed within a sphere of radius R. The electric force X and the potential V at a distance r from the centre of an atom for a point inside the atom, are given by

$$X = Ne\left(\frac{1}{r^2} - \frac{r}{R^3}\right)$$

$$V = Ne\left(\frac{1}{r} - \frac{3}{2R} + \frac{r^2}{2R^3}\right).$$

Suppose an α particle of mass m and velocity u and charge E shot directly towards the centre of the atom. It will be brought to rest at a distance b from the centre given by

36

$$\tfrac{1}{2}mu^2 = NeE\left(\frac{1}{b} - \frac{3}{2R} + \frac{b^2}{2R^3}\right).$$

It will be seen that b is an important quantity in later calculations. Assuming that the central charge is $100\,e$, it can be calculated that the value of b for an α particle of velocity $2{\cdot}09 \times 10^9$ cms. per second is about $3{\cdot}4 \times 10^{-12}$ cm. In this calculation b is supposed to be very small compared with R. Since R is supposed to be of the order of the radius of the atom, viz. 10^{-8} cm., it is obvious that the α particle before being turned back penetrates so close to the central charge, that the field due to the uniform distribution of negative electricity may be neglected. In general, a simple calculation shows that for all deflexions greater than a degree, we may without sensible error suppose the deflexion due to the field of the central charge alone. Possible single deviations due to the negative electricity, if distributed in the form of corpuscles, are not taken into account at this stage of the theory. It will be shown later that its effect is in general small compared with that due to the central field.

Consider the passage of a positive electrified particle close to the centre of an atom. Supposing that the velocity of the particle is not appreciably changed by its passage through the atom, the path of the particle under the influence of a repulsive force varying inversely as the square of the distance will be an hyperbola with the centre of the atom S as the external focus. Suppose the particle to enter the atom in the direction PO (fig. 1), and that the direction of motion

Fig. 1.

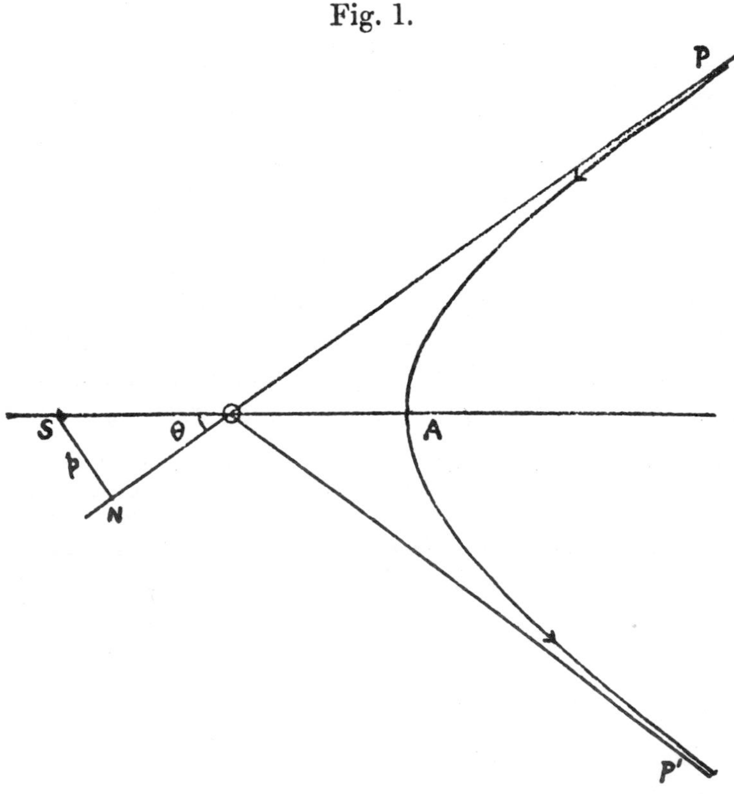

on escaping the atom is OP′. OP and OP′ make equal angles with the line SA, where A is the apse of the hyperbola. p=SN=perpendicular distance from centre on direction of initial motion of particle.

Let angle POA $=\theta$.

Let V = velocity of particle on entering the atom, v its velocity at A, then from consideration of angular momentum

$$pV = SA \, . \, v.$$

From conservation of energy

$$\tfrac{1}{2}mV^2 = \tfrac{1}{2}mv^2 + \frac{NeE}{SA},$$

$$v^2 = V^2\left(1 - \frac{b}{SA}\right).$$

Since the eccentricity is sec θ,

$$SA = SO + OA = p \operatorname{cosec} \theta (1 + \cos \theta)$$

$$= p \cot \theta/2,$$

$$p^2 = SA(SA - b) = p \cot \theta/2 (p \cot \theta/2 - b),$$

$$\therefore \quad b = 2p \cot \theta.$$

The angle of deviation ϕ of the particle is $\pi - 2\theta$ and

$$\cot \phi/2 = \frac{2p}{b} \text{*} \quad \ldots \ldots \quad (1)$$

This gives the angle of deviation of the particle in terms of b, and the perpendicular distance of the direction of projection from the centre of the atom.

For illustration, the angle of deviation ϕ for different values of p/b are shown in the following table :—

p/b	10	5	2	1	·5	·25	·125
ϕ	5°·7	11°·4	28°	53°	90°	127°	152°

§ 7. *General Considerations.*

In comparing the theory outlined in this paper with the experimental results, it has been supposed that the atom consists of a central charge supposed concentrated at a point, and that the large single deflexions of the α and β particles are mainly due to their passage through the strong central field. The effect of the equal and opposite compensating charge supposed distributed uniformly throughout a sphere has been neglected. Some of the evidence in support of these assumptions will now be briefly considered. For concreteness, consider the passage of a high speed α particle through an atom having a positive central charge Ne, and surrounded by a compensating charge of N electrons. Remembering that the mass, momentum, and kinetic energy of the α particle are very large compared with the corresponding values for an electron in rapid motion, it does not seem possible from dynamic considerations that an α particle can be deflected through a large angle by a close approach
to an electron, even if the latter be in rapid motion and 39
constrained by strong electrical forces. It seems reasonable to suppose that the chance of single deflexions through a large angle due to this cause, if not zero, must be exceedingly small compared with that due to the central charge.

It is of interest to examine how far the experimental evidence throws light on the question of the extent of the

* *Annal. d. Phys.* iv. 23. p. 671 (1907).

distribution of the central charge. Suppose, for example, the central charge to be composed of N unit charges distributed over such a volume that the large single deflexions are mainly due to the constituent charges and not to the external field produced by the distribution. It has been shown (§ 3) that the fraction of the α particles scattered through a large angle is proportional to $(Ne\mathrm{E})^2$, where Ne is the central charge concentrated at a point and E the charge on the deflected particle. If, however, this charge is distributed in single units, the fraction of the α particles scattered through a given angle is proportional to Ne^2 instead of N^2e^2. In this calculation, the influence of mass of the constituent particle has been neglected, and account has only been taken of its electric field. Since it has been shown that the value of the central point charge for gold must be about 100, the value of the distributed charge required to produce the same proportion of single deflexions through a large angle should be at least 10,000. Under these conditions the mass of the constituent particle would be small compared with that of the α particle, and the difficulty arises of the production of large single deflexions at all. In addition, with such a large distributed charge, the effect of compound scattering is relatively more important than that of single scattering. For example, the probable small angle of deflexion of a pencil of α particles passing through a thin gold foil would be much greater than that experimentally observed by Geiger (§ *b*–*c*). The large and small angle scattering could not then be explained by the assumption of a central charge of the same value. Considering the evidence as a whole, it seems simplest to suppose that the atom contains a central charge distributed through a very small volume, and that the large single deflexions are due to the central charge as a whole, and not to its constituents. At the same time, the experimental evidence is not precise enough to negative the possibility that a small fraction of the positive charge may be carried by satellites extending some distance
40 from the centre. Evidence on this point could be obtained by examining whether the same central charge is required to explain the large single deflexions of α and β particles; for the α particle must approach much closer to the centre of the atom than the β particle of average speed to suffer the same large deflexion.

The general data available indicate that the value of this central charge for different atoms is approximately proportional to their atomic weights, at any rate for atoms heavier than aluminium. It will be of great interest to examine experimentally whether such a simple relation holds also for the lighter atoms. In cases where the mass of the deflecting atom (for example, hydrogen, helium, lithium) is not very different from that of the α particle, the general theory of single scattering will require modification, for it is necessary to take into account the movements of the atom itself (see § 4).

It is of interest to note that Nagaoka * has mathematically considered the properties of a "Saturnian" atom which he supposed to consist of a central attracting mass surrounded by rings of rotating electrons. He showed that such a system was stable if the attractive force was large. From the point of view considered in this paper, the chance of large deflexion would practically be unaltered, whether the atom is considered to be a disk or a sphere. It may be remarked that the approximate value found for the central charge of the atom of gold (100 e) is about that to be expected if the atom of gold consisted of 49 atoms of helium, each carrying a charge 2 e. This may be only a coincidence, but it is certainly suggestive in view of the expulsion of helium atoms carrying two unit charges from radioactive matter.

The deductions from the theory so far considered are independent of the sign of the central charge, and it has not so far been found possible to obtain definite evidence to determine whether it be positive or negative. It may be possible to settle the question of sign by consideration of the difference of the laws of absorption of the β particle to be expected on the two hypotheses, for the effect of radiation in reducing the velocity of the β particle should be far more marked with a positive than with a negative centre. If the central charge be positive, it is easily seen that a positively charged mass if released from the centre of a heavy atom, would acquire a great velocity in moving through the electric field. It may be possible in this way to account for the high velocity of expulsion of α particles without supposing that
they are initially in rapid motion within the atom. 41

Further consideration of the application of this theory to these and other questions will be reserved for a later paper, when the main deductions of the theory have been tested experimentally. Experiments in this direction are already in progress by Geiger and Marsden.

University of Manchester,
April 1911.

* Nagaoka, Phil. Mag. vii. p. 445 (1904).

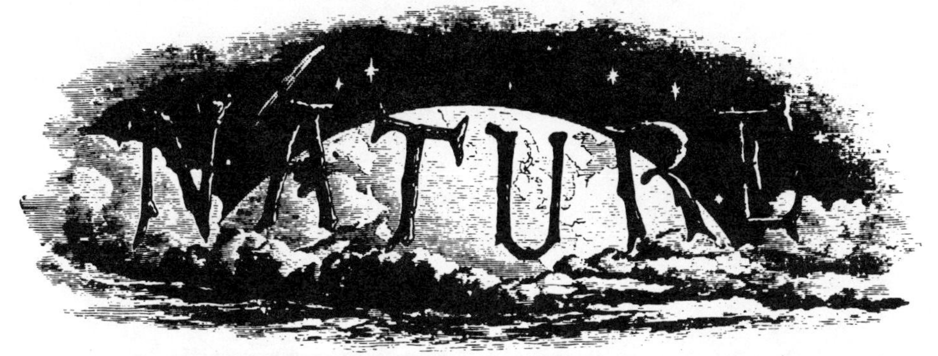

A WEEKLY ILLUSTRATED JOURNAL OF SCIENCE.

" To the solid ground
Of Nature trusts the mind which builds for aye."—WORDSWORTH.

THURSDAY, SEPTEMBER 4, 1913.

Intra-atomic Charge.

THAT the intra-atomic charge of an element is determined by its place in the periodic table rather than by its atomic weight, as concluded by A. van der Broek (NATURE, November 27, p. 372), is strongly supported by the recent generalisation as to the radio-elements and the periodic law. The successive expulsion of one α and two β particles in three radio-active changes in any order brings the intra-atomic charge of the element back to its initial value, and the element back to its original place in the table, though its atomic mass is reduced by four units. We have recently obtained something like a direct proof of van der Broek's view that the intra-atomic charge of the nucleus of an atom is not a purely positive charge, as on Rutherford's tentative theory, but is the difference between a positive and a smaller negative charge.

Fajans, in his paper on the periodic law generalisation (*Physikal. Zeitsch.*, 1913, vol. xiv., p. 131), directed attention to the fact that the changes of chemical nature consequent upon the expulsion of α and β particles are precisely of the same kind as in ordinary electrochemical changes of valency. He drew from this the conclusion that radio-active changes must occur in the same region of atomic structure as ordinary chemical changes, rather than with a distinct inner region of structure, or "nucleus," as hitherto supposed. In my paper on the same generalisation, published immediately after that of Fajans (*Chem. News*, February 28), I laid stress on the absolute identity of chemical properties of different elements occupying the same place in the periodic table.

A simple deduction from this view supplied me with a means of testing the correctness of Fajans's conclusion that radio-changes and chemical changes are concerned with the same region of atomic structure. On my view his conclusion would involve nothing else than that, for example, uranium in its tetravalent uranous compounds must be chemically identical with and non-separable from thorium compounds. For uranium X, formed from uranium I by expulsion of an α particle, is chemically identical with thorium, as also is ionium formed in the same way from uranium II. Uranium X loses two β particles and passes back into uranium II, chemically identical with uranium. Uranous salts also lose two electrons and pass into the more common hexavalent uranyl compounds. If these electrons come from the same region of the atom uranous salts should be chemically non-separable from thorium salts. But they are not.

There is a strong resemblance in chemical character between uranous and thorium salts, and I asked Mr. Fleck to examine whether they could be separated by chemical methods when mixed, the uranium being kept unchanged throughout in the uranous or tetravalent condition. Mr. Fleck will publish the experiments separately, and I am indebted to him for the result that the two classes of compounds can readily be separated by fractionation methods.

This, I think, amounts to a proof that the electrons expelled as β rays come from a nucleus not capable of supplying electrons to or withdrawing them from the ring, though this ring is capable of gaining or losing electrons from the exterior during ordinary electrochemical changes of valency.

I regard van der Broek's view, that the number representing the net positive charge of the nucleus is the number of the place which the element occupies in the periodic table when all the possible places from hydrogen to uranium are arranged in sequence, as practically proved so far as the relative value of the charge for the members of the end of the sequence, from thallium to uranium, is concerned. We are left uncertain as to the absolute value of the charge, because of the doubt regarding the exact number of rare-earth elements that exist. If we assume that all of these are known, the value for the positive charge of the nucleus of the uranium atom is about 90. Whereas if we make the more doubtful assumption that the periodic table runs regularly, as regards numbers of places, through the rare-earth group, and that between barium and radium, for example, two complete long periods exist, the number is 96. In either case it is appreciably less than 120, the number were the charge equal to one-half the atomic weight, as it would be if the nucleus were made out of α particles only. Six nuclear electrons are known to exist in the uranium atom, which expels in its changes six β rays. Were the nucleus made up of α particles there must be thirty or twenty-four respectively nuclear electrons, compared with ninety-six or 102 respectively in the ring. If, as has been suggested, hydrogen is a second component of atomic structure, there must be more than this. But there can be no doubt that there must be some, and that the central charge of the atom on Rutherford's theory cannot be a pure positive charge, but must contain electrons, as van der Broek concludes.

So far as I personally am concerned, this has resulted in a great clarification of my ideas, and it may be helpful to others, though no doubt there is little originality in it. The same algebraic sum of the positive and negative charges in the nucleus, when the arithmetical sum is different, gives what I call "isotopes" or "isotopic elements," because they occupy the same place in the periodic table. They are chemically identical, and save only as regards the relatively few physical properties which depend upon atomic mass directly, physically identical also. Unit changes of this nuclear charge, so reckoned algebraically, give the successive places in the periodic table. For any one "place," or any one nuclear charge, more than one number of electrons in the outer-ring system may exist, and in such a case the element exhibits variable valency. But such changes of number, or of valency, concern only the ring and its external environment. There is no in- and out-going of electrons between ring and nucleus.

FREDERICK SODDY.

Physical Chemistry Laboratory,
University of Glasgow.

LIII. THE ABSORPTION AND TRANSLOCATION OF LEAD BY PLANTS.

A CONTRIBUTION TO THE APPLICATION OF THE METHOD OF RADIOACTIVE INDICATORS IN THE INVESTIGATION OF THE CHANGE OF SUBSTANCE IN PLANTS.

By GEORGE HEVESY.

From the Institute of Plant Physiology of the Agricultural High School, and Institute of Theoretical Physics of the University, Copenhagen.

(*Received May 4th, 1923.*)

The investigation of the absorption of lead by plants can be carried out quite simply by dipping them into a solution which contains a radioactive isotope of lead, and determining the radioactivity of the ash from various parts of the plant. In addition to its simplicity and the extraordinary rapidity with which the work can be carried out this method possesses the following advantages:—(*a*) By mixing suitable amounts of ordinary lead with the radioactive lead isotope, one can vary the lead concentration of the solution, as it were, between very wide limits. The assimilation of lead from a $N/1$ solution can be just as readily investigated as that from a solution many million times more dilute. (*b*) One can follow the change in localisation of the lead taken up by the plant, and thence draw conclusions as to the nature of its combination.

The experiments described in this paper were so carried out, that the plants, which had been cultivated in a culture solution, were washed with distilled water, and then the roots were immersed from 1 to 48 hours in a solution containing a mixture of lead nitrate and thorium *B* nitrate. In most cases *Vicia Faba* (horse-bean) was used. After this period of immersion the
individual parts of the plant were first well rinsed with distilled water, and 45
then ignited, and the intensity of the radioactivity of the ash was determined by means of an electroscope. This latter magnitude gives directly the lead content of the ash and thus also that of the corresponding part of the plant, when we know the radioactivity and the lead content of the solution in which the plant has been immersed.

Thorium *B* is a transformation product of thorium emanation, and is obtained in a very simple manner. A piece of platinum foil is charged negatively to a potential of 110 volts, say, and suspended in a vessel containing the preparation (radio-thorium, thorium X, etc.) from which the thorium emanation is generated. Under these circumstances the thorium B collects on the platinum surface, and can be removed with the aid of a few drops of dilute nitric acid. The normality as regards lead of a solution (thorium B is an isotope of lead, *i.e.* a substance showing completely the chemical properties of lead) prepared in this way is about 10^{-12}, and if we wish to increase it we only need add to the solution a known amount of lead nitrate. For example, if we assume that we have prepared in this manner a 10^{-6} N solution of lead nitrate, and that after evaporating it to dryness it shows a radioactivity of 10,000 relative units, then each relative radioactive unit would correspond to an amount of $2 \cdot 10^{-5}$ mg. of lead. We must of course take account of the fact that the material of the ash of the parts of the plants absorb part of the rays from the contained thorium B, but we can easily eliminate this disturbance by mixing the preparation used for comparison with the same quantity of ash as is contained in the sample the radioactivity of which we desire to know.

The following example shows the procedure during an experiment: *Vicia Faba* that had undergone cultivation in a nutrient solution for a fortnight was introduced, after careful washing, into 500 cc. of a 10^{-5} N radioactive solution of lead nitrate, which also contained 1/200 mol. of sodium nitrate. The temperature was 17°. The usual precautions such as screening the roots from light, etc., were also attended to. After 22 hours the plant was removed from the solution, and after careful washing with distilled water, the various parts—root, fruit, stem and leaves—were dried separately, ignited after the addition of a drop of concentrated sulphuric acid, and measured electroscopically[1]. The result of the experiment is shown in the following table.

Experiment (*a*):

Part of plant	Weight of ash in mg.	% of the total lead in the solution contained in the ash	Mg. of lead in the ash	Lead content of the ash in %
Roots	45	13·1	0·11	0·25
Fruit	5	0·10	0·0008	0·016
Stem	46	0·05	0·0004	0·001
Leaves	36	0·013	0·0001	0·0003

46 The purpose of the following experiments was to investigate the manner in which the assimilation of lead in the case of *Vicia Faba* varies with the lead concentration of the solution. In all of these experiments the volume of the lead solution was 200 cc. and the duration of the experiment was 24 hours.

The following collection of results shows that the individual experiments can be repeated, the agreement being quite satisfactory. Per cent. of the

[1] Before the measurement one must wait about six hours in order to be certain that radioactive equilibrium has been established between thorium B and thorium C. The reasons for this are outside the scope of this paper.

lead content taken up by the root from a 10^{-6} N solution: 61·2, 62·3, 57·4, 59·6, 55·4, 57·8, 47·3, 62·2, 61·7, 62·6, 60·0, 51·2, 68·7, 57·6.

Experiment (*b*). With 10^{-6} N lead solution:

Part of plant[1]	Weight of ash in mg.	% of the total lead in the solution contained in the ash	Mg. of lead in the ash	Lead content of the ash in %
Root	41	60·0	0·02	0·052
Stem	12·6	0·04	0·000013	0·0001
Leaves	5·5	0·004	0·000001	0·00002
Experiment (*c*). With 10^{-5} N lead solution:				
Root	43	31·7	0·11	0·26
Stem	18	0·015	0·0004	0·002
Leaves	9·8	0·0012	0·00003	0·0003
Experiment (*d*). With 10^{-3} N lead solution:				
Root	39	11·9	3·9	10
Stem	18	0·02	0·007	0·04
Leaves	18	0·002	0·0007	0·004
Experiment (*e*). With 10^{-1} N lead solution:				
Roots	26	0·30	9·9	38
Fruit	18	0·11	3·6	20
Stem	11	0·065	2·2	20
Leaves	10	0·035	1·2	12

[1] The fruit was removed when the plant was introduced into the culture solution, since it constitutes a particularly good nutritive medium for troublesome moulds.

From the above experimental data it is seen that, whereas in the case of a 10^{-6} N solution more than half of the lead is taken up by the root, the percentage loss when a 10^{-1} N solution is used only amounts to 0·3, although the quantities of lead taken up by the root in the latter case are very much greater than in the former case. It is of interest to note that the *percentage* of lead which passes over into the stem and leaves from the concentrated solution of lead is not smaller than that from dilute solutions. This can be interpreted as meaning that with very dilute solutions the root itself is able to bind almost the whole quantity of lead, and thus renders extremely difficult the ascent of lead into the stem and leaves. On the other hand, when a concentrated lead solution is used, an ample sufficiency of unbound lead is available, and this can be carried upwards by the transpiration current. Except in the case of concentrated solutions, the root thus protects, as it were, the remaining parts of the plant, and this marked ability for "binding" lead is probably connected with an explanation of the relatively small toxicity of
lead for plants, discussed on p. 444[1] [cf. Strasburger, 1891]. 47

On the mode of combination of lead in the root.

The question as to whether the assimilated lead enters into an organic molecule, or whether it is retained by the plant in the form of a saline com-

[1] Trees placed in solutions of copper sulphate or picric acid, etc., do not die until the poisonous substance has reached the highest points of the crown.

pound can easily be decided. In the first case, lead atoms which had once been taken up by the root would not be able to interchange places with other lead atoms, whereas in the second case an active kinetic interchange between the lead atoms bound in the plant and those present in the solution would necessarily take place.

In order to make the argument clearer, we shall designate the atoms of lead in molecules such as those of lead tetraphenyl as "red" ones, and those which occur in such a form as lead nitrate as "blue" ones. If we dissolve both compounds in the same solvent and then separate them by crystallisation, we should find only *red* atoms in the lead tetraphenyl and only *blue* ones in the lead nitrate, since the lead atoms in the lead tetraphenyl are available in an undissociable form. If, on the other hand, we dissolve equi-molecular amounts of lead chloride (with *red* lead) and lead nitrate (with *blue* lead), *i.e.* two salts in the same solvent, then after separation the two compounds would be composed half of *red* and half of *blue* lead atoms [Hevesy and Zechmeister, 1920]. The distinction between *red* and *blue* corresponds here to radioactive and to inactive lead.

If the root has taken up active lead and we place it in a solution of inactive lead, then, if the active lead lies stably embedded in organic molecules, no active lead will be able to pass over into the solution, or in other words we shall not be able to displace the active lead with the aid of inactive lead. Now experiment shows that, with the help of a solution which is relatively rich in lead (10^{-2} N), we can remove almost quantitatively the lead taken up by the root, whence we must conclude that *the lead in the plant root exists in the form of a dissociable saline compound*, perhaps attached to the cell walls.

For example, if we introduce a *Vicia Faba* (after careful rinsing) which has stood 24 hours in 200 cc. of an active 10^{-6} N lead nitrate solution into a much more concentrated 10^{-2} N inactive lead nitrate solution of the same volume, we find that 95 % of the active lead taken up by the root passes over into the 10^{-2} N solution; *i.e.* the active Pb-atoms are almost completely displaced from their places in the root by inactive atoms, which, of course, preponderate strongly (about 20,000 times), from the statistical viewpoint.

Now a 10^{-2} N lead nitrate solution is partially split up hydrolytically, and one might be inclined to ascribe the inverse dissolving action of lead nitrate to its acid content. However, with the aid of a 10^{-3} N HNO_3 solution it was
48 possible to remove only 29 % of the lead content of the root, and by the use of distilled water as solvent only 18 % could be removed. The investigation of the assimilation of lead from solutions of different lead content showed that from 10^{-4} N HNO_3 64 %, and from 10^{-3} N HNO_3 practically the same amount, viz. 62 % is taken up by the root, when the normality of the lead ions in the solution is 10^{-6} N. From a 10^{-2} N HNO_3 solution, a concentration sufficient, in general, to kill the plant, only 26 % is assimilated by the root.

THE DISPLACEMENT OF THE LEAD TAKEN UP BY THE ROOT BY OTHER IONS.

Since it has been established that we can displace the lead taken up by the root by other lead atoms, it seemed to be of interest to investigate the ability of other ions to displace the assimilated lead. 10^{-2} *N* solutions were used throughout these experiments. The plant containing lead was placed for 24 hours in the solution under consideration and then both the amount of lead remaining in the plant and the amount displaced into the solution were determined. The results of these experiments are shown in the following table:

Solution used	% of the lead initially present in the root which remained after treatment
Lead nitrate (inactive)	5
Cupric nitrate	3
Cadmium nitrate	34
Zinc nitrate	38
Chromium nitrate	43
Barium nitrate	74
Sodium nitrate	76

When the reverse solution took place with the help of a 10^{-3} *N* $Pb(NO_3)_2$ solution, 14 % of the originally assimilated lead were still present in the root after 24 hours' treatment.

Only copper is able to displace lead in a similar degree to lead itself; all the other cations investigated show an appreciably smaller displacing power.

The extent of the re-solution of the lead taken up by the stem and leaves was not determined. Experiments which are being undertaken on the assimilation of lead by *algae* will, amongst other things, also serve to shed light on this point.

As is well known, different ions are assimilated to quite different degrees by plants, according to what other ions are present in the culture solution. The toxicity of individual types of ions is also arrested by others. One of the best known cases of this "antagonism" is probably that between $CaCl_2$ and NaCl. In this case the phenomenon of the suspension of the toxicity of NaCl by $CaCl_2$ is attributed to the ability of the $CaCl_2$ to alter the plasma-membrane in such a way that it is less permeable to NaCl [Osterhout, 1912]. Since it has been possible to show that in the case of lead a kinetic displacement of the assimilated ions by other ions occurs, we shall certainly have to reckon with
the possibility that the antagonism is in individual cases occasioned by such 49
kinetic effects.

LEAD ASSIMILATION AND TRANSPIRATION CURRENT.

From the fact that more than 50 % of the lead is taken up in 24 hours by the root in very dilute solutions of lead, *i.e.* a quantity of lead which was present in more than 100 cc. of liquid, we can conclude that it is *not the transpiration current* which transmits the assimilated lead, since the daily loss of water of *Vicia Faba* under present conditions is less than 1 cc. This independence is also shown in the following experiment. In one case the percentage assimilation of lead by the root was determined in the usual way, and in another after the root had been first separated from the stem under water. The volume of water was 500 cc., the lead concentration was 10^{-6} *N*, and $p_H = 4$. Duration of experiment = 1 hour.

Root as usual	6·8 and 7·5 %.
Root cut off	6·5 and 7·1 %.

It is seen that the amount of lead taken up was in both cases the same. Moreover, the lack of dependence of the assimilation of salt on the absorption of water by the plant has repeatedly been established [cf. Arrhenius, 1922].

The toxicity of lead.

In connection with the experiments described in the previous section it is of interest to note that, as has been shown by Bonnet [1922], the introduction of plants into 10^{-1} *N* $Pb(NO_3)_2$ solution unfavourably influences the transpiration current. In contrast to more dilute solutions, such an appreciable concentration of lead shows distinct toxic effects on the plant[1]. *Vicia Faba* which had stood 24 hours in a 10^{-1} *N* $Pb(NO_3)_2$ solution already showed a slight deviation from the geotropic direction, and the leaves situated closest to the root showed signs of withering.

The toxic action of lead on different plants, such as wheat, radishes, lentils, cabbage, etc., has been investigated quite recently by Bonnet [1922]. Just as in the present case, he introduced the plants into 200 cc. of water after their roots had attained a length of several centimetres. The water contained in solution a definite amount of lead acetate or lead nitrate, and he obtained the following results:

(1) After the plants had stood in 10^{-1} *N* solutions of lead salts, lead could readily be detected qualitatively in the root.

(2) Only traces of lead were found in the stem and in the leaves.

(3) 10^{-1} *N* solutions of lead killed, *e.g.* the wheat plant after 20 days, balsam after two days.

(4) Mg, Ca and K showed no antagonistic action to lead.

50 (5) The greater the dilution, the less lead was taken up by the plant.

Our present results confirm those of Bonnet. As regards the first result, we were able, thanks to the sensitiveness of the radioactive method, to detect with ease and quantitatively to determine the presence of lead even in the stem and in the leaves. It is interesting to note that Mg, Ca and K, which do not have an antitoxic action, have only a slight capacity of displacing lead, according to the experiments of the present author. In reference to

[1] Cf. also Lavison [1911] and older experiments of Phillips [1883], Knop [1885], Nolle, Bässler and Will [1884].

point (5), the radioactive methods enable us to carry out a quantitative investigation of the dependence of the assimilation of lead on the concentration of the solution within wide limits, in which all other methods fail. In this manner, it is found that only 1/500 part of the amount of lead is taken up from a 10^{-6} N solution as compared with a 10^{-1} N solution. Those experiments of Bonnet should be mentioned, from which we can see the influence of the assimilation of lead on the growth of plants. He finds the following values:

Plant: The bean.

	Length of root in mm.		
	Initially	After 1 week	After 1 month
In water	25	100	1000
In 10^{-3} N $Pb(NO_3)_2$	31	31	32

SUMMARY.

(1) The assimilation of lead from lead nitrate solutions by *Vicia Faba* has been investigated. A radioactive isotope of lead was mixed with the lead nitrate, and the amount of lead taken up was determined after ignition from the radioactive intensity of the ash of the various parts. This method makes possible the determination of exceedingly small amounts of assimilated lead.

(2) Whereas 0·3 % of the lead is taken up by the root from 200 cc. of a 10^{-1} N lead nitrate solution in the course of 24 hours, 60 % of the lead content of a 10^{-6} N solution is taken up in the same time. The leaves show a lead content of only a few hundredths or thousandths of 1 % of the amount of lead present in the solution.

(3) The assimilated (radioactive) lead can be displaced by introduction of the plant containing lead into another lead solution, whereby inactive lead atoms now take the place of the radioactive ones. From this it follows that the lead is not combined with carbon within the plant, but that it exists in the form of a dissociable salt which is soluble with difficulty.

(4) Even after 24 hours, a 10^{-1} N solution of a lead salt produces toxic effects on the plant, whilst more dilute solutions do not. Lead belongs to the least poisonous of the heavy metals.

I am indebted primarily to Professor Fr. Weis for so kindly placing at my disposal the facilities of his Institute, furthermore to Dr B. Krause for his help, and to my friend Professor L. Zechmeister for numerous suggestions. 51

REFERENCES.

Arrhenius (1922). *J. Gen. Phys.* **5**, 87.
Bonnet (1922). *Compt. Rend. Acad. Sci.* **174**, 488.
Hevesy and Zechmeister (1920). *Ber. deutsch. chem. Ges.* **53**, 410.
Knop (1885). *Ber. sächs. Ges.* 51.
Lavison (1911). *Ann. Sci. Nat. Bot.* **14**.
Nolle, Bässler and Will (1884). *Landw. Versuchsamt*, **30**, 382.
Osterhout (1912). *Science*, **35**, 112.
Phillips (1883). *Bot. Centralb.* **13**, 364.
Strasburger (1891). *Histologische Beiträge*, **3**, 607.

STUDIES ON THE VELOCITY OF BLOOD FLOW

I. The Method Utilized[1]

By HERRMANN L. BLUMGART and OTTO C. YENS

(From the Thorndike Memorial Laboratory, Boston City Hospital and the Department of Medicine, Harvard Medical School)

(Received for publication October 4, 1926)

An adequate flow of blood to the tissues implies two things. In the first place an adequate amount of blood must be expelled from the heart per unit of time. In the second place this blood must be transported to the site of utilization at an adequate speed. The former aspect of the circulation, the minute volume output, has received considerable study. The second aspect, the velocity of blood flow, has not. Nevertheless, discussions of the probable velocity and its significance in maintaining the physiological integrity of the body have frequently been reported.

HISTORICAL RÉSUMÉ OF METHODS EMPLOYED IN STUDYING THE VELOCITY OF BLOOD FLOW

With the discovery by Harvey in 1628 (1) of the movement of blood in a circuit, the problem of the velocity at which the blood flows first presented itself. Not until 1733, however, when Stephen Hales (2) published his penetrating inquiries was the question of the velocity of blood flow discussed in quantitative terms. His grasp of the essentials of the problem was extraordinary. From his estimation of the capacity of the left ventricle, the diameter of the base of the aorta, and the pulse rate he computed the velocity of blood flow in the aorta of the horse.

The problem of the velocity of blood flow received its next impetus in 1827, when Eduard Hering (3) measured the velocity of blood flow by injecting a solution of potassium ferrocyanide at one point and

[1] This study was aided by a grant from the Proctor Fund of the Harvard Medical School for the Study of Chronic Disease.

determining its time of arrival in the blood at another point in the vascular circuit by testing the samples of withdrawn blood for prussian blue. He measured in this way the circulation time from the right to the left external jugular vein.

In 1850, Volkman (4) constructed the haemodromometer, a pendulum device which gauged the velocity of blood flow by recording the movement of a pendulum placed in the lumen of a blood vessel. The inertia of the instrument was sufficient to distort the results. But aside from this defect the obstruction imposed by the instrument to the onward flow of blood must have altered the velocity.

The haemotachometer designed by Vierordt (5) was a distinct improvement. His method resembled Hering's, but whereas Hering's observations were confined solely to horses, Vierordt extended his to rabbits, hedgehogs, squirrels, cats, dogs, ducks, cocks and geese. Actually, he observed the time necessary for the fastest particle of blood to traverse various paths. From these data he attempted to estimate the mean velocity (page 119). Vierordt improved Hering's method by affixing a number of cups to a disc (page 56), which was rotated at a uniform and known rate. In each of the cups he collected samples of blood drawn at intervals of one second.

In the latter part of the nineteenth century, there were repeated attempts to estimate the velocity of the blood in the arteries and veins by means of Cybulski's photohaemotachometer and O. Frank's differential manometer. The insertion of such devices into the blood stream demanded much manipulation and introduced so many extraneous physical factors that the results were difficult of accurate interpretation, and therefore failed to clarify the problem.

More fruitful was the approach of G. N. Stewart (6) who studied the circulation time by injecting a hypertonic solution of sodium chloride into one jugular vein, and by ascertaining its time of arrival
54 in another vessel. The time of arrival was signalled by a change in the electrical conductivity of the blood in the vessel, which was placed between two non-polarizable electrodes. He also utilized methylene blue injections observing by transillumination the time at which the dye appeared in the common carotid artery. He studied the circulation times of many pathways in various animals and also studied the circulation times of individual organs.

In 1922, E. Koch (7) presented his measurements of the circulation time in man in both normal and pathological states. His method consisted of the injection of 1.0 cc. of a 1.6 per cent solution of fluorescein into the cubital vein of one arm and then obtaining samples of blood at five second intervals from the cubital vein of the other arm. The dye, therefore, traversed the veins to the right ventricle, the lung circulation to the left ventricle, the aorta, the arteries of the arm, the peripheral capillaries of the arm, and then finally, the vein from which the blood was collected. His results will be discussed later. It should be noted, however, that withdrawal of blood is feasible only from the cubital vein. In order to determine the time of arrival of such a dyestuff, it is necessary that a constant stream of blood flow from the arm through the needle to the collecting tubes. The formation of clots, the inaccessibility of veins, alteration of flow by the introduction of the needle into the vein, all necessarily interfere with the trustworthiness of such a method.

Because of the inaccuracies and limitations of previous methods, we felt the necessity of developing a more satisfactory approach to this fundamental problem.

Theoretically the most desirable measurement of the velocity of blood flow consists in establishing the separate velocities of each minute portion of the blood along the many separate paths. When one considers that the innumerable vessels in the body are constantly changing in size and elasticity and that the blood is a suspension of corpuscles in a fluid medium, the impossibility of fulfilling the ideal requirements becomes obvious. The problem is further complicated; any mean velocity measurements which depend on the insertion of a mechanical device into the blood stream defeats its ends and can therefore, not be considered for clinical application. The most feasible method appears to be the injection of some substance at one point in the body, and the measurement of the time of its arrival at another 55
point. Consideration of the problem shows that the substance to be used must fulfill the following requirements.

1. The substance must not be toxic in the amounts utilized. Toxicity is of course a relative quality, for any substance, if given in sufficiently large amounts, may bring about grave consequences.

2. The substance should not be present previously in the body.

Estimation of additional amounts of substances already within the body is always subject to error. Weber's law, moreover, is applicable. According to this law, the increase of stimulus necessary to produce an appreciable increase in sensation must always bear the same ratio to the whole stimulus. If, accordingly, a substance were already present, greater amounts of that substance must be injected to produce appreciable changes at the point of detection.

3. The substance must not in any way disturb the very phenomena under investigation. Toxicity would introduce such an error. The introduction of hypertonic salt solution would also cause an error for it would alter the blood volume, vary the speed of blood flow, and thereby modify the very phenomenon under investigation.

4. It is desirable that the substance disappear from the body with sufficient rapidity to allow of repeated measurements.

5. The substance must be readily detectable in minute amounts. Were this impossible, varying dilutions of the substance would be all the more likely to produce correspondingly variable results.

Initial attempts were made in animals to test the usefulness of various substances. We injected intravenously salts such as those of lithium and strontium, and examined spectroscopically drops of blood from various parts of the body. The results were unsatisfactory.

The use of the active deposit of radium (or radium C) had yielded a method which fulfills the foregoing criteria and has proved entirely satisfactory.[2]

The method consists of the injection of the active deposit of radium at one point in the body, and the detection of its time of arrival at another point. The active deposit is particularly suited to the purpose because of the following properties. In the first place, it is non-toxic in the amounts necessary for the purpose. Quick and Duffy (8) at the Memorial Hospital in New York in studying the possible thera-
56 peutic effects of radium C in patients with advanced generalized carcinomatosis gave repeatedly intravenous injections of 50, and 75 millicuries without any consequent ill effects. They studied the urine for signs of renal irritation, and the blood for evidence of nitrogen retention, without noting any untoward effects. No significant

[2] In a forthcoming paper, we intend to describe the method of preparation of radium C.

changes were noted in the red blood cell count or hemoglobin. Our own experiments on animals and, as will appear below, our subsequent study of the effect of radium C in ourselves and in patients has uniformly showed an absence of any objective or subjective ill effects. In a few patients with generalized carcinomatosis large amounts of radium C were administered; the amount necessary, however, for a measurement is only one to four millicuries.

Active deposit fulfills the other requirements previously mentioned. It is not present normally in the body. The injection of radium C into animals and later into human beings has shown a uniform absence

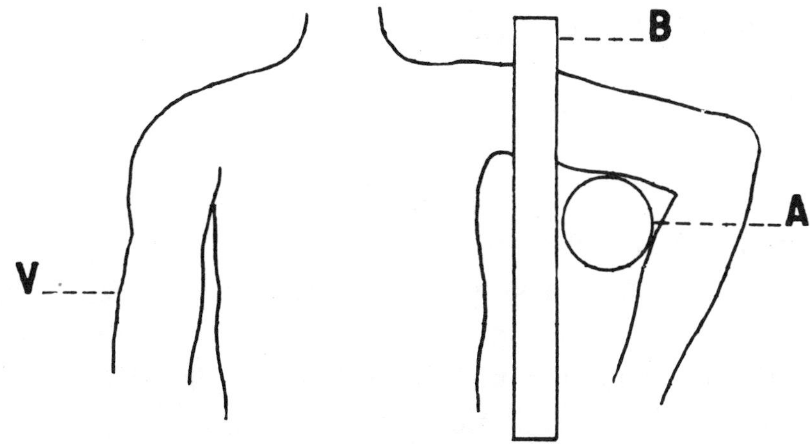

Fig. 1. Diagram of Relation of the Lead Shield and the Detecting Device to the Patient

A, detecting device; *B*, lead shield through which the left arm passes; *V*, right arm.

of any discernible alterations in the blood pressure or the ventricular rate or the ventricular rhythm. The properties of the active deposit of radium are such, moreover, that observations can be repeated after approximately three hours, inasmuch as the active deposit decomposes
to within 3 per cent of its initial value at the end of that time. 57
As to its detectability in small amounts, the active deposit leaves nothing to be desired since the presence of a single atom can be detected.

The active deposit lends itself particularly to the purpose of measuring the velocity of blood flow because of its radiation; for, being a member of the radium family, it gives out penetrating radiation in the form of beta particles or electrons, and gamma rays which are comparable to hard x-rays. These radiations penetrate ordinary materials such as tissues and air, but can be stopped by lead. If the active deposit of radium is injected into the vein of one arm (fig. 1), it gives off radiation as it is carried up the arm to the right side of the heart and thence through the lungs to the left side of the heart. The lead shield *B*, prevents the radiation from reaching the detecting device *A*. As soon as the radium active deposit reaches the arterial vessels of the arm beyond the lead block, the radiations are no longer separated from the detector *A*, by lead. Instead, they penetrate the tissues, traverse the air, and enter the detecting device, where they appear as definite white streaks.

DESCRIPTION OF THE APPARATUS

1. The detecting device

To secure a suitable detecting device proved to be a formidable undertaking. The usefulness of instruments for detecting minute amounts of radioactive substances depends on their ability to detect the characteristic beta and gamma radiations which are emitted from within the atom. These radiations cause ionization of any gas they traverse. Conversely, under suitable conditions, the onset of ionization in a gas can therefore be assumed to indicate the presence of the radiation of a member of a radioactive series.

The use of an electroscope as a detector was attended with great difficulties. Perfectly satisfactory shielding of the electroscope from the radiations of the active deposit as it coursed through the body was impracticable. Morever, the precise instant at which the radium active deposit arrived was extraordinarly difficult to ascertain by this device.

58 Kovarik's modification of the Geiger counting chamber was likewise tested (9). The necessity of a source of constant high potential, the instability of the steel needle electrode; and the relatively high number of spontaneous discharges discouraged the choice of this mode of detection.

We also attempted to use parallel plate ionization chambers. We found, however, that the large electrical capacity of the plates reduced the sensitivity of the ionization chambers, even when we used low pressures and introduced various vapors to obtain the greatest possible amount of ionization by collision.

The use of a cloud chamber of the C. T. R. Wilson type (10) approached more closely our requirements. In principle this apparatus consists of an air-tight chamber saturated with water vapor. At the bottom of the chamber is a piston which falls periodically, and in so doing produces an adiabatic expansion of the enclosed volume of air and water vapor. The vapor is cooled to such an extent by this expansion that it becomes critically supersaturated. In this state, the vapor condenses in the form of minute droplets upon any small particles such as dust, which are suspended in the gas. If no dust particles are present, the water vapor condenses in minute droplets upon any electrically charged bodies such as ionized molecules. If, for instance, a gamma ray or beta particle should traverse the chamber and create an ionized path, while the chamber is in the condition of critical supersaturation, the water vapor would condense as minute droplets along the ionized path. With proper illumination, this ionized path appears as a white streak. Unfortunately, a constant state of supersaturation can not be maintained, but by the use of a reciprocating piston device of the Shimizu type (11), the chamber can be rendered periodically susceptible to the formation of droplets along any ionized path. The critical degree of supersaturation, therefore, is attained on each descent of the piston.

The detecting device which we finally adapted from that of C. T. R. Wilson may be represented diagramatically (fig. 2). Letter *F* is a brass cylinder into which a duralumin piston, *D*, is accurately fitted. This piston is connected below to a shaft, *R*, which is moved up and down by a cam, *P*. Every revolution of the cam *P* causes the piston, *D*, to drop suddenly from a high to a low position. The top and the bottom positions and therefore the extent of the fall are all adjustable 59
by the bearing *S*. This device is of considerable importance, for the degree of vapor supersaturation required is a critical one. It is dependent on variable conditions such as room temperature and the amount of water vapor initially present in the chamber. Once the adjustments are made, however, by means of varying *S*, no further manipulations are necessary during the time of an experiment.

Upon the top of a cylinder is screwed the chamber consisting of a threaded brass collar, *B*, celluloid ring, *C*, and glass top plate *A*. The celluloid ring consists of a strip of celluloid 0.005 inch in thickness, the ends of which are stuck together with amyl acetate. By means of rosin it is rigidly set into a groove in the brass collar below, and into a corresponding groove in the glass plate above. The rosin must

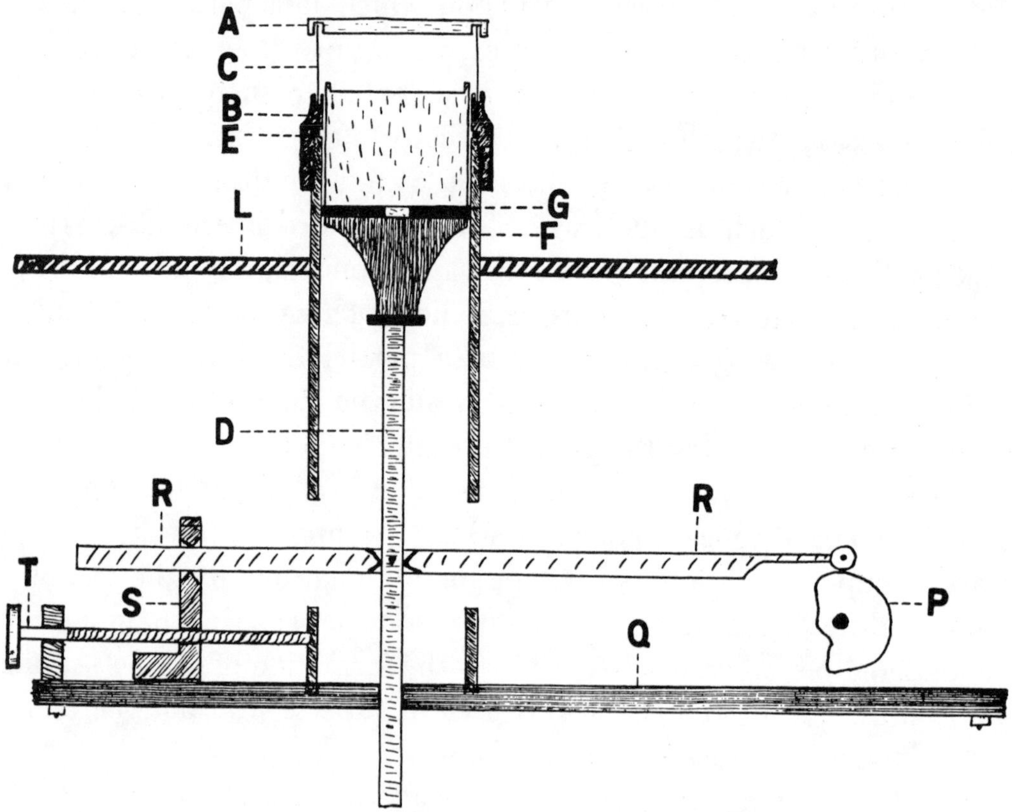

FIG. 2. DIAGRAM OF DETECTING DEVICE

A, glass top plate; *B*, threaded brass collar; *C*, celluloid ring; *D*, duralumin piston; *E*, rubber washer; *F*, brass cylinder; *G*, leather washer; *P*, cam; *Q*, steel bottom plate; *R*, duralumin shaft; *S*, support and bearing for shaft; *T*, adjusting screw; *L*, shelf for arm rest.

60 be heated to a temperature of 110° to 130°C. and it must be free of air bubbles.

The top of the piston and the bottom of the cover glass are coated with gelatin. The gelatin covering the piston is blackened with India ink. The gelatin covering the top glass plate contains a small amount of copper sulphate and can therefore, be used to establish an electrically negative charge. The charge passes into the chamber by means of a tongue of lead foil, leading to a thin ring imbedded in the copper sulphate gelatin. The charge established on the top plate consists of about minus fifty volts. It serves to dispel the tracks formed at each descent of the piston. In this way the chamber is cleared for the new tracks of the next expansion. The piston is at ground potential. The charge on the top plate is applied during only a portion of the upstroke. During the rest of the time the top plate is grounded. The regulation of the charge on the top plate is accomplished by means of an adjustable commutator operated from another cam, not shown in the diagram but concentric with the cam, *P*.

The cycle of events is therefore as follows. During the downstroke of the piston the gas in the chamber is suddenly expanded and becomes supersaturated for an instant. If, during this instant, any primary or secondary beta particles are travelling through the chamber, the water vapor condenses along that path and when properly illuminated appears as thin, white streaks. The streaks or tracks settle slowly under gravity, but before they have moved far the piston returns to its former high position and the gas is again at its initial volume. Part of the drops immediately evaporate. The others are swept to the top of the piston below by the repelling force of the negative electric charge on the top plate. The chamber is again clear and ready for another expansion.

The instrument may be operated at any rate up to three or five expansions per second, but about one per second has proven most satisfactory. The moving parts are placed below the cylinder head so that the patient's arm may be conveniently laid upon the iron plate, *L*, and brought against the thin celluloid rim *C*.

In the actual observations we have placed the detecting device within the bend of the elbow, so that the ionization chamber is exposed to the radiation from the brachial artery and its branches. The arm 61
of the patient passes through a lead block 8 cm. in thickness, which serves to prevent radiations from the rest of the body from reaching the detector.

PROCEDURE OF THE MEASUREMENTS

Sodium chloride is exposed to radium emanation for an appropriate length of time, during which radium C is deposited upon the salt.

The method utilized is that described by Theis and Bagg (12). The sodium chloride is then dissolved in sterile distilled water and its radioactivity measured by means of a gamma ray electroscope. The volume of the solution, which is contained in the syringe is usually about 0.5 cc.

The measurement of the velocity of blood flow is made under basal metabolic conditions, no food being taken by the patient after supper on the preceding evening. The patient lies down in bed and rests for at least twenty minutes. The left arm is passed through the lead block and arranged around the cylinder of the cloud chamber. The active deposit is not injected for at least twenty minutes after it has been removed from exposure to the emanation to allow the alpha ray activity to decay to four per cent of its initial activity (13). The cubital vein of the right arm is entered with a sharp needle to which is attached a three-way stopcock. A small amount of blood is withdrawn in order to be certain that the needle lies free within the vein. The stopcock is then turned so that the needle communicates with a manometer filled with a solution of sodium citrate. The level of the top of the sodium citrate in the manometer is then compared with the level of the right auricle. The details of the measurement of venous pressure are practically those published originally by Moritz and Tabora (14).

The syringe into which the blood was drawn is replaced by one containing the radium active deposit. The stopcock is then turned and the 0.5 cc. solution containing a minute volume of active deposit is quickly injected into the vein. The injection time is always less than one second. As the active deposit courses through the body an occasional track is visible within the cloud chamber. With the arrival of active deposit within the arterial vessels of the arm, beta particles and gamma rays pass through the tissues of the arm, traverse the thin
62 celluloid rim, enter the cloud chamber, and there become visible. Instead of an occasional track, at least two or more tracks are visible at succesive expansions. The time of arrival of the active deposit in the arterial vessels of the left arm is registered by means of a stop watch. The difference between the time of injection and the time of arrival gives the velocity of blood flow between the two points. The amount of active deposit utilized for a determination has been from

1 to 6 millicuries. On theoretical grounds it is difficult to conceive of such amounts causing any toxic effects. In practice we have verified the theoretical expectation.

RESULTS

The primary purpose of the preliminary measurements was rather to test the method than to gain additional knowledge of the circulation. The velocity of blood flow (measurement numbers 1, 2, 3, 4, 5, 6)

TABLE 1

Number	Date	Diagnosis	Millicuries injected	Circulation time
2	February 28, 1925	Carcinoma of esophagus	52	18
5	March 2, 1925	Metastatic carcinoma of liver	17	20
10	March 2, 1925	Chronic myocarditis	18	32
3	March 3, 1925	Carcinoma of stomach	33	18
9	March 3, 1925	Jaundice, bradycardia	5	30
8	August 22, 1925	Emphysema	35	28
7	August 22, 1925	Emphysema	5	25
13	August 28, 1925	Auricular fibrillation	38	55
12	September 1, 1925	Auricular fibrillation	4	53
1	August 28, 1925	Chronic arthritis	2	15
4	August 29, 1925	Normal	2	18
6	September 1, 1925	Normal	1	21
14	August 29, 1925	Cardiac decompensation	4	65
15	September 1, 1925	Chronic myocarditis Cardiac decompensation	2	71
11	September 1, 1925	Auricular fibrillation Cardiac decompensation	7	50

(table 1) was studied in patients in whom the cardio-respiratory system
was normal. The time required for the substance to flow from one
arm to the other arm was found to be from fifteen to twenty-one
seconds. These results are in contrast with the velocities recorded in 63
three patients who showed signs or symptoms of cardiac decompensa-
tion. In these patients (numbers 12, 14 and 11), the times noted 53,
65 and 50 seconds clearly belong to a different order.

Observations were repeated in the same individuals to test the reliability of the method. Measurements 7 and 8, 4 and 6, 12 and 13 all show agreement within three seconds. Of particular interest are numbers 7 and 8, for the amount of deposit utilized in the first is sevenfold that injected for the second measurement.

In all these patients the urine was carefully examined immediately before and immediately after injection, and uniformly failed to show any signs of renal irritation. No anemia followed the injection of radium C in the amounts used.

CONCLUSIONS

A new method is presented for the measurement of the velocity of blood flow in man. The active deposit of radium is injected into the antecubital vein of one arm and its time of arrival in the other arm is detected by means of a modified C. T. R. Wilson cloud chamber device. The advantages of the method are as follows:

1. The volume of fluid injected is very small.
2. The substance injected is non-toxic in the amounts utilized.
3. The presence of extraordinarily minute amounts of the substance can be detected with certainty.
4. The radiations by traversing the tissues of the arm automatically indicate the time of arrival of the active deposit.
5. No withdrawal of blood is necessary.
6. The method is objective requiring no coöperation on the part of the patient.
7. The method gives a quantitative estimate of a fundamental aspect of the circulation.

We wish to express our appreciation to Dr. Francis W. Peabody for his constant advice and encouragement.

BIBLIOGRAPHY

1. Harvey, William, Exercitatio Anatomica De Motu Cordis et Sanguinis in
64 Animalibus. In A. Spizelius' opera quae extant omnia. Amsterdam, 1645.
2. Hales, Stephen, Statical Essays, Vol. ii. London, 1733.
3. Hering, Eduard, Ztschr. f. Physiol., 1827, iii, 85. Quoted by Tigerstedt, R. Die Physiologie der Kreislaufes, 1923, iv, 57.
4. Volkmann, Alfred W., Die Hämodynamik nach Versuchen. 185. Leipzig, 1850.
5. Vierordt, Karl, Die Erscheinungen und Gesetze der Stromgeschwindigkeiten des Blutes. Berlin, 1862.

6. Stewart, G. N., J. Physiol., 1893, xv, 31. Researches on the Circulation Time in Organs and on the Influences which Affect It.
7. Koch, E., Deutsches, Arch. f. klin. Med., 1922, cxl, 39. Die Stromgeschwindigkeit des Blutes.
8. Duffy, H., Personal Communication.
9. Kovarik, A. F., Physical Rev., 1919, xiii, 272. On the Automatic Registration of α-Particles, β-Particles and γ-Ray and X-Ray Pulses.
10. Wilson, C. T. R., Proc. Roy. Soc., Series A, 1911, lxxxv, 285. On a Method of Making Visible the Paths of Ionizing Particles through a Gas.
11. Shimizu, Takeo, Proc. Roy. Soc., Series B, 1921, xcix, 425. A Reciprocating Expansion Apparatus for Detecting Ionizing Rays.
12. Theis, R. C., and Bagg, H. J., Jour. Biol. Chem., 1920, xli, 525. The Effect of Intravenous Injections of Active Deposit of Radium on Metabolism in the Dog.
13. Rutherford, E. F., Radioactive Substances and Their Radiations. London, 1913, page 491.
14. Moritz, F., and Tabora, D. v., Deut. Arch. f. klin. Med., 1910, xcviii, 475. Ueber eine Methode, beim Menschen den Druck in Oberflächlichen Venen exakt zu bestimmen.

The Electron Counting Tube

Hans Geiger and Walther Muller

Physik Zeitschr 29: 839-841, 1928

1. Mode of Operation and Preparation of a Counting Tube

Along the axis of a metal tube, a thin wire is stretched; its surface is covered with a uniform layer of a poorly conducting material. Because of the insulating effect of this layer, the electric tension between wire and tube can be increased beyond the sparking potential. A small number of ions formed anywhere within the tube actuates the instantaneous flow of a considerable amount of electricity towards the wire caused by the intense ion avalanche. In the case of a bare wire, such an electric pulse would cause a continuous discharge; the surface of the treated wire, however, is charged only for a short time followed by a breakdown of the electric field and a rupture of the electric current. Since the electric pulse can be easily registered with a string electrometer, the possibility arises to use this device, which we will call a counting tube, for the detection of corpuscular radiation. In contrast to the spark counter with a sensitive area limited to a diameter of a few millimeters, the electron counting tube has the advantage that radiation within areas of 100 cm^2 and larger can be counted. Therefore, for the detection of an extremely weak radiation from a radioactive material or an X-ray tube, the sensitivity of the counting tube exceeds that of all previously known systems. Furthermore, the counting tube can be produced without difficulties in greatly different dimensions and it will operate with surprising reliability and consistency over long periods of time.

The production of the wire can be accomplished by various methods. For a first trial we like to suggest the following procedure that assures success: a 0.2 mm thick steel wire is submerged in nitric acid until it is covered with a uniform, clearly visible black coating. The wire is then centered with hard rubber stoppers along the axis of a brass tube which is evacuated and filled with dry air to a pressure of about 5 cm Hg. Under those conditions, the required potential is about 1200 volts and it is advisable to connect the tube to the negative pole of the voltage supply. The wire is coupled to a string electrometer and is simultaneously grounded through a resistor of 100–1,000 Megohm. Instead of the acid treated wire, annealed or varnished wires can also be used.

A good counting tube exposed to a radium source produces a deflection number independent of the electric potential over a range of about 50 Volt. How many deflections are to be expected can be calculated from specifications given in Section 2. The deflections are very large and uniform even with an electrometer of reduced sensitivity. Any kind of movements of the strings that could be mistaken for deflections do not occur even during series of observations if the construction is carefully executed.

2. Sensitivity of Counting Tube

Depending on the specific application of the counting tube, its dimension will be chosen differently. In Table 1, the length, diameter and wall thickness are given in columns 2 to 4 for three counting tubes that have been used for experiments to be described. The sensitivity given in column 5 is defined by the number of deflections per minute produced by the gamma radiation of 1 mg radium at 1 m distance. Notice that on the average 20–30 de-

Translation kindly provided by Gerald J. Hine, Ph.D., Boulder, Colorado.

flections are observed per cm^2 surface of the counting tube. Unfortunately it is not possible to calculate with sufficient accuracy the expected number of deflections to investigate the quantitative properties of the counting tube. Nevertheless, there appears to be no doubt that the number of observed deflections corresponds closely to the number of secondary electrons passing the counting tube; this is quite surprising considering that the radiation can produce only very few ion pairs within the gas because of the low pressure and the short path within the tube. However, it may be possible that at the low pressure the pulses are caused less by gas ionization than by tertiary radiation induced within the walls of the tube. We hope to clarify this question soon by varying the gas pressure and the wall material.

For the practical application of a counting tube, the magnitude of the so-called natural effects (background radiation) given in column 6 of Table 1 is of decisive importance besides the sensitivity in column 5. All counting tubes built by us produced up to 4 spontaneously grounded through a resistor of 100–1,000 megohm. Instead of the acid treated protective precautions. A complete iron shield of 20-cm thickness reduced the number of spontaneous deflections to one third and in some cases to considerably less, proving that

TABLE 1. SENSITIVITY AND BACKGROUND FOR DIFFERENT COUNTING TUBES

					Number of background deflexions	
No.	Length cm	Inside Diameter cm	Wall Thickness mm	Sensitivity	Counting Tube Shielded	Counting Tube With 20-cm Fe Shield
1	4.2	1	0.07	300	12	3.8
2	5	1	0.15	450	23	3.8
3	17	3	1	5500	150	40

the background radiation consists to a considerable degree of radiation from the surrounding brick walls, the earth below and the cosmic radiation. Increasing the thickness of the iron shield resulted in a further reduction of the background radiation. It remains to be seen what fractions of the radiation still observed with the thickest iron shielding comes from not absorbed cosmic radiation, activity in the tube wall or the iron shield or other unknown sources.

3. Examples for Applications of the Counting Tube

We will describe some simple experiments to illustrate the application of the counting tube's sensitivity for different types of radiation.

Potassium radiation. The intensity of the potassium β-radiation is so minute that its effect on an ordinary leaf electrometer remains smaller than that of the background radiation even for a large potassium surface. Using the generally known apparatus of Hoffman which greatly exceeds the sensitivity of all other electrometric methods of current detection, the measurements of Biltz and Ziegert of the activity from a bare potassium chloride surface of 12.5 cm^2 yielded four times the background radiation. This favorable ratio of potassium activity to background radiation could be achieved only with special precautions to eliminate the α-component of the background radiation.

Using counting tube number 2, the number of deflections was increased from 3.8 to 36.2 by surrounding it completely (15.7 cm^2) with potassium chloride. This shows that the activity of potassium relative to the natural background radiation is in our case even greater than with the apparatus of Hoffmann. These favorable results with the counting tube are based on the fact that it registers α-and β-radiation independent of their ionization, while in an ionization chamber an α-particle contributes about a thousand times more to the current that a β-particle. The ratio could be further improved by using a tube with a thinner wall and increasing the shielding conditions.

Cosmic radiation of Hess. Counting tube number 3 was installed on the ground floor of the institute and it was protected against radiation from below and all sides by 20 cm iron: therefore at the beginning of the experiment radiation could enter unobstructed only from above. By adding layers of iron of about 60×90 cm^2 surface, this radiation was then attenuated gradually. Figure 1 shows the reduction of the deflection rate with increasing absorber thickness; this is then followed by a slow decrease as soon as the radiation of Hess is the main component. A more detailed discussion of the curve should be postponed until the background radiation remaining with the greatest shielding can be explained.

The accuracy of such measurements depends solely on the number of particles being counted. In the present case, about 2,000 particles were counted for every point on the

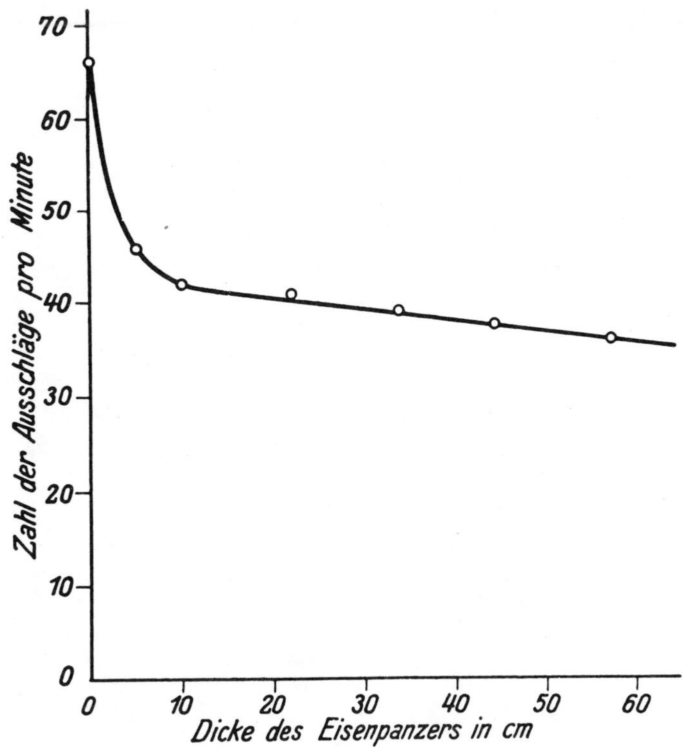

Absorption of cosmic radiation measured with the electron counting tube (number of deflections per minute vs thickness of iron shielding in cm).

curve. Therefore the measurement of the whole curve required a counting time of 6–7 hours. This time could be reduced significantly by using photographic or automatic methods for registering the counts since the deflections per minute could be greatly increased by the choice of a correspondingly larger counting tube. Especially for the cosmic ray problem the speed with which the measurements can be made is of particular importance.

We have checked the stability of counting tube number 3 during 14 days by measurements of the deflection rate with the thickest iron shield. The observed deflection rate remained constant within the expected statistical fluctuations.

X-radiation. We have limited ourselves in this area to a few simple demonstrations. The radiation from a small model X-ray tube driven by a commercial children's toy electrifying machine produced a major effect with counting tube number 1 at several meters distance. Driving the X-ray tube by a small induction coil the radiation was still easy to detect at a distance of 20 m. It should be noticed that the counting tube presented only a surface of 4 cm^2 for the radiation and that the solid angle therefore was extremely small. We believe that the counting tube combining a small solid angle with a high sensitivity will be particularly suited for many X- and φ-radiation problems.

Letters to the Editor

[The Editor does not hold himself responsible for opinions expressed by his correspondents. Neither can he undertake to return, nor to correspond with the writers of, rejected manuscripts intended for this or any other part of NATURE. *No notice is taken of anonymous communications.]*

Possible Existence of a Neutron

IT has been shown by Bothe and others that beryllium when bombarded by α-particles of polonium emits a radiation of great penetrating power, which has an absorption coefficient in lead of about 0·3 (cm.)$^{-1}$. Recently Mme. Curie-Joliot and M. Joliot found, when measuring the ionisation produced by this beryllium radiation in a vessel with a thin window, that the ionisation increased when matter containing hydrogen was placed in front of the window. The effect appeared to be due to the ejection of protons with velocities up to a maximum of nearly 3×10^9 cm. per sec. They suggested that the transference of energy to the proton was by a process similar to the Compton effect, and estimated that the beryllium radiation had a quantum energy of 50×10^6 electron volts.

I have made some experiments using the valve counter to examine the properties of this radiation excited in beryllium. The valve counter consists of a small ionisation chamber connected to an amplifier, and the sudden production of ions by the entry of a particle, such as a proton or α-particle, is recorded by the deflexion of an oscillograph. These experiments have shown that the radiation ejects particles from hydrogen, helium, lithium, beryllium, carbon, air, and argon. The particles ejected from hydrogen behave, as regards range and ionising power, like protons with speeds up to about $3{\cdot}2 \times 10^9$ cm. per sec. The particles from the other elements have a large ionising power, and appear to be in each case recoil atoms of the elements.

If we ascribe the ejection of the proton to a Compton recoil from a quantum of 52×10^6 electron volts, then the nitrogen recoil atom arising by a similar process should have an energy not greater than about 400,000 volts, should produce not more than about 10,000 ions, and have a range in air at N.T.P. of about 1·3 mm. Actually, some of the recoil atoms in nitrogen produce at least 30,000 ions. In collaboration with Dr. Feather, I have observed the recoil atoms in an expansion chamber, and their range, estimated visually, was sometimes as much as 3 mm. at N.T.P.

These results, and others I have obtained in the course of the work, are very difficult to explain on the assumption that the radiation from beryllium is a quantum radiation, if energy and momentum are to be conserved in the collisions. The difficulties disappear, however, if it be assumed that the radiation consists of particles of mass 1 and charge 0, or neutrons. The capture of the α-particle by the Be^9 nucleus may be supposed to result in the formation of a C^{12} nucleus and the emission of the neutron. From the energy relations of this process the velocity of the neutron emitted in the forward direction may well be about 3×10^9 cm. per sec. The collisions of this neutron with the atoms through which it passes give rise to the recoil atoms, and the observed energies of the recoil atoms are in fair agreement with this view. Moreover, I have observed that the protons ejected from hydrogen by the radiation emitted in the opposite direction to that of the exciting α-particle appear to have a much smaller range than those ejected by the forward radiation. This again receives a simple explanation on the neutron hypothesis.

If it be supposed that the radiation consists of quanta, then the capture of the α-particle by the Be^9 nucleus will form a C^{13} nucleus. The mass defect of C^{13} is known with sufficient accuracy to show that the energy of the quantum emitted in this process cannot be greater than about 14×10^6 volts. It is difficult to make such a quantum responsible for the effects observed.

It is to be expected that many of the effects of a neutron in passing through matter should resemble those of a quantum of high energy, and it is not easy to reach the final decision between the two hypotheses. Up to the present, all the evidence is in favour of the neutron, while the quantum hypothesis can only be upheld if the conservation of energy and momentum be relinquished at some point.

J. CHADWICK.

Cavendish Laboratory,
Cambridge, Feb. 17.

71

THE PRODUCTION OF HIGH SPEED LIGHT IONS WITHOUT THE USE OF HIGH VOLTAGES

By Ernest O. Lawrence and M. Stanley Livingston
University of California

(Received February 20, 1932)

Abstract

The study of the nucleus would be greatly facilitated by the development of sources of high speed ions, particularly protons and helium ions, having kinetic energies in excess of 1,000,000 volt-electrons; for it appears that such swiftly moving particles are best suited to the task of nuclear excitation. The straightforward method of accelerating ions through the requisite differences of potential presents great experimental difficulties associated with the high electric fields necessarily involved. The present paper reports the development of a method that avoids these difficulties by means of the multiple acceleration of ions to high speeds without the use of high voltages. The method is as follows: Semi-circular hollow plates, not unlike duants of an electrometer, are mounted with their diametral edges adjacent, in a vacuum and in a uniform magnetic field that is normal to the plane of the plates. High frequency oscillations are applied to the plate electrodes producing an oscillating electric field over the diametral region between them. As a result during one half cycle the electric field accelerates ions, formed in the diametral region, into the interior of one of the electrodes, where they are bent around on circular paths by the magnetic field and eventually emerge again into the region between the electrodes. The magnetic field is adjusted so that the time required for traversal of a semi-circular path within the electrodes equals a half period of the oscillations. In consequence, when the ions return to the region between the electrodes, the electric field will have reversed direction, and the ions thus receive second increments of velocity on passing into the other electrode. Because the path radii within the electrodes are proportional to the velocities of the ions, the time required for a traversal of a semi-circular path is independent of their velocities. Hence if the ions take exactly one half cycle on their first semi-circles, they do likewise on all succeeding ones and therefore spiral around in resonance with the oscillating field until they reach the periphery of the apparatus. Their final kinetic energies are as many times greater than that corresponding to the voltage applied to the electrodes as the number of times they have crossed from one electrode to the other. This method is primarily designed for the acceleration of light ions and in the present experiments particular attention has been given to the production of high speed protons because of their presumably unique utility for experimental investigations of the atomic nucleus. Using a magnet with pole faces 11 inches in diameter, a current of 10^{-9} ampere of 1,220,000 volt-protons has been produced in a tube to which the maximum applied voltage was only 4000 volts. There are two features of the developed experimental method which have contributed largely to its success. First there is the focussing action of the electric and magnetic fields which prevents serious loss of ions as they are accelerated. In consequence of this, the magnitudes of the high speed ion currents obtainable in this indirect manner are comparable with those conceivably obtainable by direct high voltage methods. Moreover, the focussing action results in the generation of very narrow beams of ions—less than 1 mm cross-sectional diameter—which are ideal for experimental studies of collision processes. Of hardly less importance is the second feature of the method which is the simple and highly effective means for the correction of the magnetic field along the paths of the ions. This makes it possible, indeed easy, to operate the tube effectively with a very high amplification factor (i.e., ratio of final equivalent voltage of accelerated ions to applied voltage). In consequence, this method in its present stage of development constitutes a highly reliable and experimentally convenient source of high speed ions requiring relatively modest laboratory equipment. Moreover, the present experiments indicate that this indirect method of multiple acceleration now makes practicable the production in the laboratory of protons having kinetic energies in excess of 10,000,000 volt-electrons. With this in mind, a magnet having pole faces 114 cm in diameter is being installed in our laboratory.

Introduction

THE classical experiments of Rutherford and his associates[1] and Pose[2] on artificial disintegration, and of Bothe and Becker[3] on excitation of nuclear radiation, substantiate the view that the nucleus is susceptible to the same general methods of investigation that have been so successful in revealing the extra-nuclear properties of the atom. Especially do the results of their work point to the great fruitfulness of studies of nuclear transitions excited artificially in the laboratory. The development of methods of nuclear excitation on an extensive scale is thus a problem of great interest; its solution is probably the key to a new world of phenomena, the world of the nucleus.

But it is as difficult as it is interesting, for the nucleus resists such experimental attacks with a formidable wall of high binding energies. Nuclear energy levels are widely separated and, in consequence, processes of nuclear excitation involve enormous amounts of energy—millions of volt-electrons.

It is therefore of interest to inquire as to the most promising modes of nuclear excitation. Two general methods present themselves; excitation by absorption of radiation (gamma radiation), and excitation by intimate nuclear collisions of high speed particles.

Of the first it may be said that recent experimental studies [4,5] of the absorption of gamma radiation in matter show, for the heavier elements, variations with atomic number that indicate a quite appreciable nuclear effect. This suggests that nuclear excitation by absorption of radiation is perhaps a not infrequent process, and therefore that the development of an intense artificial source of gamma radiation of various wave-lengths would be of considerable value for nuclear studies. In our laboratory, as elsewhere, this being attempted.

But the collision method appears to be even more promising, in consequence of the researches of Rutherford and others cited above. Their pioneer investigations must always be regarded as really great experimental achievements, for they established definite and important information about nuclear processes of great rarity excited by exceedingly weak beams of bombarding particles—alpha-particles from radioactive sources. Moreover, and this is the point to be emphasized here, their work has shown strikingly the

[1] See Chapter 10 of Radiations from Radioactive Substances by Rutherford, Chadwick and Ellis.

[2] H. Pose, Zeits. f. Physik **64,** 1 (1930).

[3] W. Bothe and H. Becker, Zeits. f. Physik **66,** 1289 (1930).

[4] G. Beck, Naturwiss. **18,** 896 (1930).

[5] C. Y. Chao, Phys. Rev. **36,** 1519 (1930).

great fruitfulness of the kinetic collision method and the importance of the development of intense artificial sources of alpha-particles. Of course it cannot be inferred from their experiments that alpha-particles are the most effective nuclear projectiles: the question naturally arises whether lighter or heavier particles of given kinetic energy would be more effective in bringing about nuclear transitions.

A beginning has been made on the theoretical study of the nucleus and a partial answer to this question has been obtained. Gurney and Condon[6] and Gamow[7] have independently applied the ideas of the wave mechanics to radioactivity with considerable success. Gamow[8] has further considered along the same lines the penetration into the nucleus of swiftly moving charged particles (with excitation of nuclear transitions in mind) and has concluded that, for a given kinetic energy, the lighter the particle the greater is the probability that it will penetrate the nuclear potential wall. This result is not unconnected with the smaller momentum and consequent longer wavelength of the ligher particles; for it is well-known that transmission of matter waves through potential barriers becomes greater with increasing wavelengths.

If the probability of nuclear excitation by a charged particle were mainly dependent on its ability to penetrate the nuclear potential wall, electrons would be the most effective. However, there is considerable evidence that nuclear excitation by electrons is negligible. It suffices to mention here the current view that the average density of the extra-nuclear electrons is quite great in the region of the nucleus, i.e., that the nucleus is quite transparent to electrons; in other words, there are no available stable energy levels for them.

On the other hand, there is evidence that there are definite nuclear levels for protons as well as alpha-particles;[9] indeed, there is some justification for the view that the general principles of the quantum mechanics are applicable in the nucleus to protons and alpha particles. It is not possible at the present time to estimate the relative excitation probabilities of the protons and alpha particles that succeed in penetrating the nucleus. However, it does seem likely that the greater penetrability of the proton* is an advantage outweighing any differences in their excitation characteristics. Protons thus appear to be most suited to the task of nuclear excitation.

Though at present the relative efficacy of protons and alpha-particles
cannot be established with much certainty, it does seem safe to conclude at 75
least that the most efficacious nuclear projectiles will prove to be swiftly moving ions, probably of low atomic number. In consequence it is important to develop methods of accelerating ions to speeds much greater than have heretofore been produced in the laboratory.

[6] Gurney and Condon, Phys. Rev. **33,** 127 (1929).

[7] Gamow, Zeits. f. Physik **51,** 204 (1928).

[8] Gamow, Zeits. f. Physik **52,** 514 (1929).

[9] J. Chadwick, J. E. R. Constable, E. C. Pollard, Proc. Roy. Soc. **A130,** 463 (1930).

* According to Gamow's theory a one million volt-proton has as great a penetrating power as a sixteen million volt alpha-particle.

The importance of this is generally recognized and several laboratories are developing techniques of the production and the application to vacuum tubes of high voltages for the generation of high speed electrons and ions. Highly significant progress in this direction has been made by Coolidge,[10] Lauritsen,[11] Tuve, Breit, Hafstad, Dahl,[12] Brasch and Lange,[13] Cockroft and Walton,[14] Van de Graaff[15] and others, who have developed several distinct techniques which have been applied to voltages of the order of magnitude of one million.

These methods involving the direct utilization of high voltages are subject to certain practical limitations. The experimental difficulties go up rapidly with increasing voltage; there are the difficulties of corona and insulation and also there is the problem of design of suitable high voltage vacuum tubes.

Because of these difficulties we have thought it desirable to develop methods for the acceleration of charged particles that do not require the use of high voltages. Our objective is two fold: first, to make the production of particles having kinetic energies of the order of magnitude of one million volt-electrons a matter that can be carried through with quite modest laboratory equipment and with an experimental convenience that, it is hoped, will lead to a widespread attack on this highly important domain of physical phenomena; and second, to make practicable the production of particles having kinetic energies in excess of those producible by direct high voltage methods—perhaps in the range of 10,000,000 volt-electrons and above.

A method for the multiple acceleration of ions to high speeds, primarily designed for heavy ions, has recently been described in this journal.[16] The present paper is a report of the development of a method for the multiple acceleration of light ions.[17] Particular attention has been given to the acceleration of protons because of their apparent unique utility in nuclear studies. In the present work relatively large currents of 1,220,000 volt-protons have been generated and there is foreshadowed in the not distant future the production of 10,000,000 volt-protons.

The Experimental Method

In the method for the multiple acceleration of ions to high speeds, recently described,[16] the ions travel through a series of metal tubes in synchronism with an applied oscillating electric potential. It is so arranged that as an

[10] W. D. Collidge, Am. Inst. E. Eng. **47,** 212 (1928).

[11] C. C. Lauritsen and R. D. Bennett, Phys. Rev. **32,** 850 (1928).

[12] M. A. Tuve, G. Breit, L. R. Hafstad and O. Dahl, Phys. Rev. **35,** 66 (1930); M. A. Tuve, L. R. Hafstad, O. Dahl, Phys. Rev. **39,** 384, (1932).

[13] A. Brasch and J. Lange, Zeits. f. Physik **70,** 10 (1931).

[14] J. J. Cockroft and E. T. S. Walton, Proc. Roy. Soc. **A129,** 477 (1930).

[15] R. S. Van de Graaff, Schenectady Meeting American Physical Society, 1931.

[16] D. H. Sloan and E. O. Lawrence, Phys. Rev. **38,** 2021 (1931).

[17] This method was first described before the September, 1930, meeting of the National Academy of Sciences (Lawrence and Edlefsen, Science **72,** 376–377 (1930)). Later before the American Physical Society (Lawrence and Livingston, Phys. Rev. **37,** 1707, (1931)) results of a preliminary study of the practicability of the method were given. Further work was reported in a Letter to the Editor of the Physical Review (Lawrence and Livingston, Phys. Rev. **38,** 834 (1931).

ion travels from the interior of one tube to the interior of the next there is always an accelerating field, and the final velocity of the ion on emergence from the system corresponds approximately to a voltage as many times greater than the applied voltage between adjacent tubes as there are tubes. The method is most conveniently used for the acceleration of heavy ions; for light ions travel faster and hence require longer systems of tubes for any given frequency of applied oscillations.

The present experimental method makes use of the same principle of repeated acceleration of the ions by a similar sort of resonance with an oscillating electric field, but has overcome the difficulty of the cumbersomely long accelerating system by causing, with the aid of a magnetic field, the ions to circulate back and forth from the interior of one electrode to the interior of another.

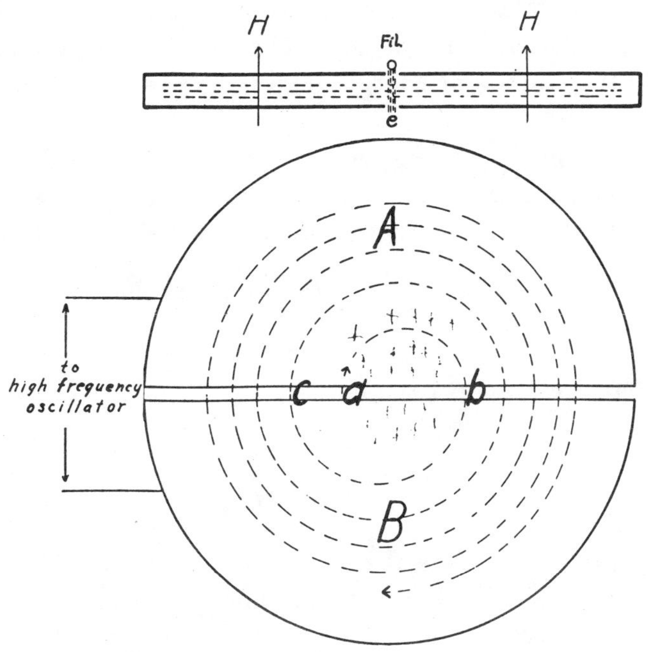

Fig. 1. Diagram of experimental method for multiple acceleration of ions.

This may be seen most readily by an outline of the experimental arrangement (Fig. 1). Two electrodes A, B in the form of semi-circular hollow plates are mounted in a vacuum tube in coplanar fashion with their diametral edges adjacent. By placing the system between the poles of a magnet, a magnetic field is introduced that is normal to the plane of the plates. High frequency electric oscillations are applied to the plates so that there results an oscillating electric field in the diametral region between them.

With this arrangement it is evident that, if at one moment there is an ion in the region between the electrodes, and electrode A is negative with respect to electrode B, then the ion will be accelerated to the interior of the former. Within the electrode the ion traverses a circular path because of the magnetic field, and ultimately emerges again between the electrodes; this is indicated in the diagram by the arc a .. b. If the time consumed by the ion in making the semi-circular path is equal to the half period of the electric oscillations, the electric field will have reversed and the ion will receive a second acceleration, passing into the interior of electrode B with a higher velocity. Again it travels on a semi-circular path (b .. c), but this time the radius of curvature is greater because of the greater velocity. For all velocities (neglecting variation of mass with velocity) the radius of the path is proportional to the velocity, so that the time required for traversal of a semi-circular path is independent of the ion's velocity. Therefore, if the ion travels its first half circle in a half cycle of the oscillations, it will do likewise on all succeeding paths. Hence it will circulate around on ever widening semi-circles from the interior of one electrode to the interior of the other, gaining an increment of energy on each crossing of the diametral region that corresponds to the momentary potential difference between the electrodes. Thus, if, as was done in the present experiments, high frequency oscillations having peak values of 4000 volts are applied to the electrodes, and protons are caused to spiral around in this way 150 times, they will receive 300 increments of energy, acquiring thereby a speed corresponding to 1,200,000 volts.

It is well to recapitulate these remarks in quantitative fashion. Along the circular paths within the electrodes the centrifugal force of an ion is balanced by the magnetic force on it, i.e., in customary notation,

$$\frac{mv^2}{r} = \frac{Hev}{c}. \tag{1}$$

It follows that the time for traversal of a semi-circular path is

$$t = \frac{\pi r}{v} = \frac{\pi mc}{He} \tag{2}$$

which is independent of the radius r of the path and the velocity v of the ion. The particle of mass m and charge e thus may be caused to travel in phase with the oscillating electric field by suitable adjustment of the magnetic field H: the relation between the wave-length λ of the oscillations and the corresponding synchronizing magnetic field H is in consequence

$$\lambda = \frac{2\pi mc^2}{He} \tag{3}$$

78 Thus for protons and a magnetic field of 10,000 gauss the corresponding wave-length is 19.4 meters; for heavier particles the proper wave-length is proportionately longer.*

It is easily shown also that the energy V in volt-electrons of the charged particles arriving at the periphery of the apparatus on a circle of radius r is

* It should be mentioned that, for a given wave-length, the ions resonate with the oscillations when magnetic fields of 1/3, 1/5, etc., of that given by Eq. (3) are used. Such types of resonance were observed in the earlier experimental studies. In the present experiments, however, the high speed ions resulting from the primary type of resonance only were able to pass through the slit system to the collector, because of the high deflecting voltages used.

$$V = 150 \frac{H^2 r^2}{c^2} \frac{e}{m} \cdot \tag{4}$$

Thus, the theoretical maximum producible energy varies as the square of the radius and the square of the magnetic field.

Experimental Arrangement

The experimental arrangement is shown diagrammatically in some detail in Fig. 2. Fig. 3 is a photograph of the brass vacuum tube with cover removed showing the filament, the accelerating electrode, the deflecting plates and slit system, the probe in front of the first slit mounted on a ground joint and the Faraday collector behind the last slit. An external view of the apparatus is shown in Fig. 4. Here the tube is shown between the magnet pole faces, connected with the oscillator, the vacuum system and hydrogen generator. This gives a good general idea of the modest extent of the equipment involved for the generation of protons having energies somewhat in excess of 1,000,000 volt-electrons. The control panel and electrometer, being on the other side, are not shown in the picture. The description of the apparatus follows.

The accelerating system. Though there are obvious advantages in applying the high frequency potentials with respect to ground to both accelerating electrodes, in the present experiments it was found convenient to apply the high frequency voltage to only one of the electrodes, as indicated in Fig. 2. This electrode was a semi-circular hollow brass plate 24 cm in diameter and 1 cm thick. The sides of the hollow plate were of thin brass so that the interior of the plate had approximately these dimensions. It was mounted on a water-cooled copper re-entrant tube which in turn passed through a copper to glass seal. The electrode insulated in this way was mounted in an evacuated brass box having internal dimensions 2.6 cm by 28.6 cm by 28.6 cm, there being thus a lateral clearance between the electrode and walls of the brass chamber of 8 mm.

The brass box itself constituted the other electrode of the accelerating system. Across the mid-section of the brass chamber parallel to the diametral edge of the electrode A was placed a brass dividing wall S with slits of the same dimensions as the opening of the nearby electrode. This arrangement gave rise to the same type of oscillating electric fields as would have been produced had there been used two insulated semi-circular electrodes with
their diametral edges adjacent and parallel. 79

The source of ions. An ideal source of ions is one that delivers to the diametral region between the electrodes large quantities of ions with low components of velocity normal to the plane of the accelerators. This requirement has most conveniently been met in the present experiments merely by having a filament placed above the diametral region from which a stream of electrons pass down along the magnetic lines of force, generating ions of gases in the tube. The ions so formed are pulled out sideways by the oscillating electric field. The electrons are not drawn out because of their very small radii of curvature in the magnetic field. Thus, the beam of electrons is col-

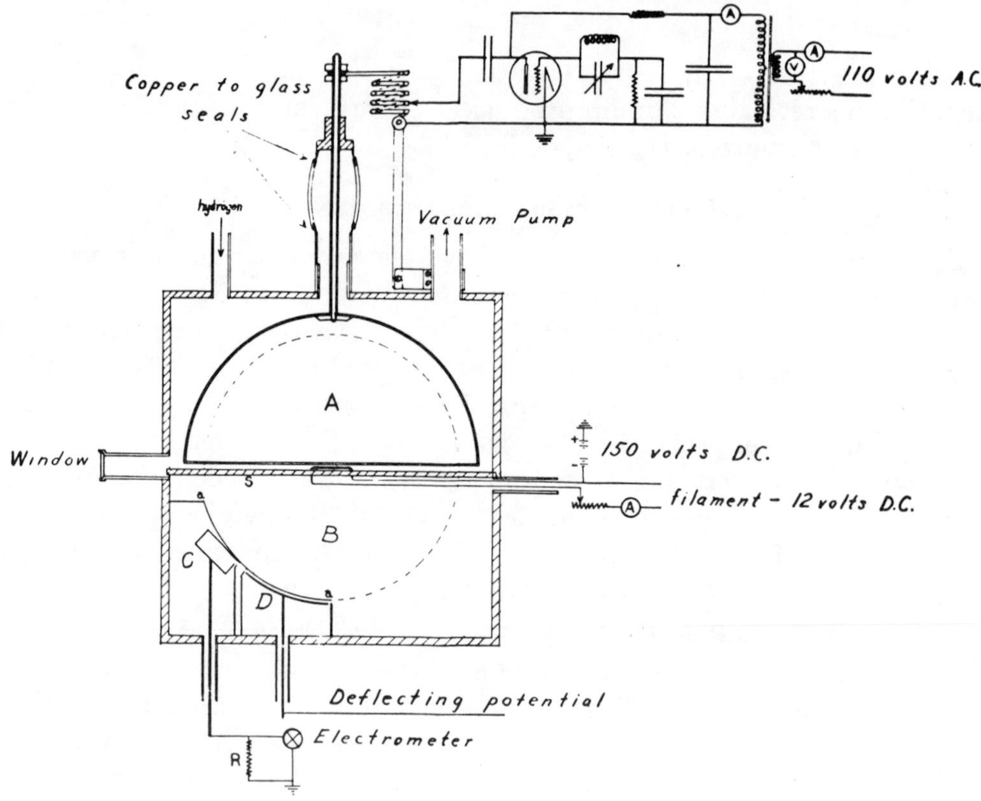

Fig. 2. Diagram of apparatus for the multiple acceleration of ions.

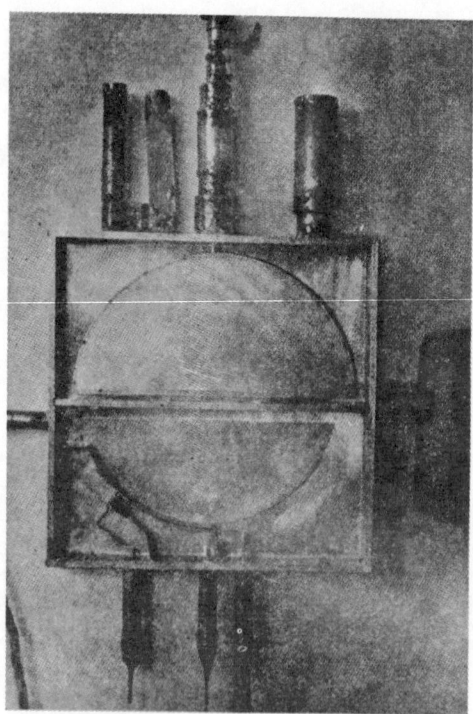

Fig. 3. Tube for the multiple acceleration of light ions—with cover removed.

limated and the ions are formed with negligible initial velocities right in the region where they are wanted. The oscillating electric field immediately draws them out and takes them on their spiral paths to the periphery. This arrangement is diagrammatically shown in the upper part of Fig. 1.

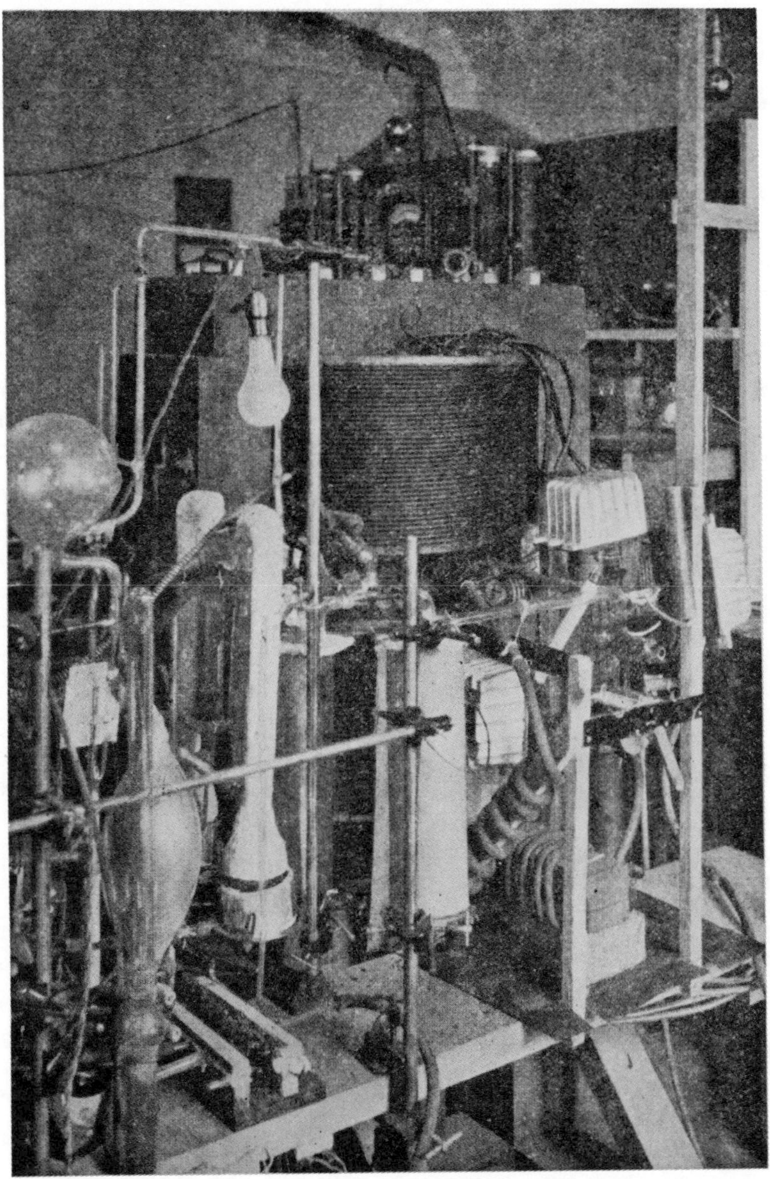

Fig. 4. External view of apparatus for generation of 1,220,000 volt protons.

The magnetic field. This experimental method requires a highly uniform magnetic field normal to the plane of the accelerating system. For example, if the ions are to circulate around 100 times, thereby gaining energy corresponding to 200 times the applied voltage, it is necessary that the magnetic field be uniform to a fraction of one percent. A general consideration of the matter leads one to the conclusion that, if possible, the magnetic field should be constant to about 0.1 percent from the center outward. Though this presumably difficult requirement has been met easily by an empirical method of field correction, the magnet used in the present experiments has pole faces machined as accurately as could be done conveniently. Its design was quite similar to that of Curtis.[18] The pole faces were 11 inches in diameter and the gap separation was $1\frac{1}{2}$ inches. Armco iron was used throughout the magnetic circuit. The magnetomotive force was provided by two coils of number 14 double cotton covered wire of 2,000 turns each. No water cooling was incorporated, for the magnet was not intended for high fields. In practice the magnet would give a field of 14,000 gauss for considerable periods without overheating. The pole faces were made parallel to about 0.2 percent and so it was to be expected that the magnetic field produced would be highly uniform. Exploration with a bismuth spiral confirmed this expectation, since it failed to show an appreciable variation of the magnetic field in the region between the poles, excepting within an inch of the periphery.

The collector system. In planning a suitable arrangement for collecting the high speed ions at the periphery of the apparatus, it was clearly desirable to devise something that would collect the high speed ions only and which would also measure their speeds. One might regard it as legitimate to suppose that the magnetic field itself and the distance of the collector from the center of the system would determine the speeds of the ions collected. This would be true provided there were no scattering and reflection of ions. To eliminate these extraneous effects a set of 1 mm slits was arranged on a circle a .. a, as shown in Fig. 2, of radius about 12 percent greater than the circle, indicated by the dotted line in the figure, having its center at the center of the tube and a radius of 11.5 cm. The two circles were tangent at the first slit as shown. The ions on arrival at the first slit would be traveling presumably on circles approximately like the dotted line, and hence would not be able to pass through the second and third slits to the Faraday collector C. Electrostatic deflecting plates D, separated by 2 mm, were placed between the first two slits, making possible the application of electrostatic fields to increase the radius of curvature of the paths of the high speed ions sufficiently to allow them to enter the collector. By applying suitable high potentials to the deflecting system in this way, only correspondingly high speed ions were registered.

The collector currents were measured by an electrometer shunted with a suitable high resistance leak.

82 **The oscillator.** The high frequency oscillations applied to the electrode were supplied by a 20 kilowatt Federal Telegraph water-cooled power tube in a "tuned plate tuned grid" circuit, for which the diagram of Fig. 2 is self-explanatory.

The Focussing Actions

When one considers the circulation of the ions around many times as they are accelerated to high speeds in this way, one wonders whether in practice an appreciable fraction of those starting out can ever be made to

[18] L. F. Curtis, Jour. Op. Soc. Am. 13, 73 (1926).

arrive at the periphery and to pass through a set of slits perhaps 1 mm wide and 1 cm long. The paths of the ions in the course of their acceleration would be several meters, and, because of the unavoidable spreading effects of space charge, thermal velocities and contact electromotive forces, as well as inhomogeneities of the applied fields, it would appear that the effective solid angle of the peripheral slit for the ions starting out would be exceedingly small.

Fortunately, however, this does not turn out to be the case. The electric and magnetic fields have been so arranged that they provide extremely strong focussing actions on the spiraling ions, which keep them circulating close to the median plane of the accelerating system.

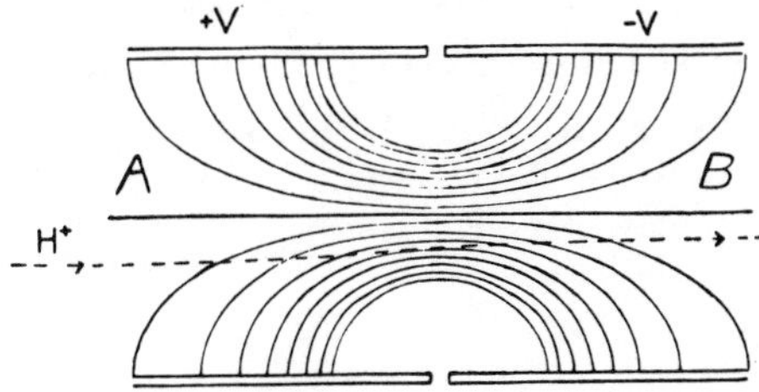

Fig. 5. Diagram indicating the focussing action of the electric field between the accelerating electrodes.

Fig. 5 shows the focussing action of the electric fields. There is depicted a cross-section of the diametral region between the accelerating electrodes with the nature of the field indicated by lines of force. There is shown also a dotted line which represents qualitatively the path of an ion as it passes from the interior of one electrode to the interior of the other. It is seen that, since it is off the median plane in electrode A, on crossing to B it receives an inward displacement towards the median plane. This is because of the existence of the curvature of the field, which over certain regions has an appreciable component normal to the plane, as indicated. If the velocity of the ion is very

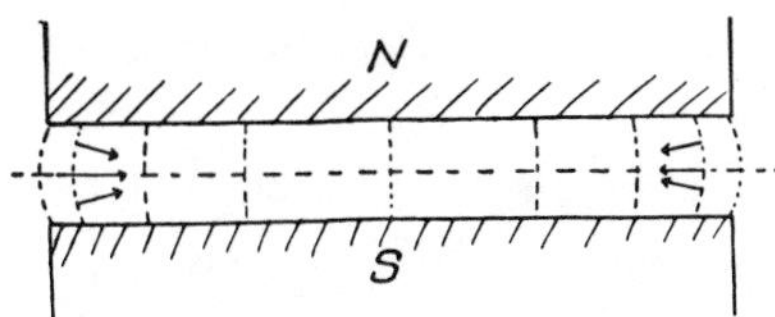

Fig. 6. Diagram indicating focussing action of magnetic field.

high in comparison to the increment of velocity gained in going from plate A to plate B, its displacement towards the center will be relatively small and,
to the first approximation, it may be described as due to the ion having been 83
accelerated inward on the first half of its path across and accelerated outward by an equal amount during the remainder of its journey, the net result being a displacement of the ion towards the center without acquiring a net transverse component of velocity. In general, however, the outward acceleration during the second half will not quite compensate the inward acceleration of the first, resulting in a gain of an inward component of velocity as well as an inward displacement. In any event, as the ion spirals around it will migrate back and forth across the median plane and will not be lost to the walls of the tube.

The magnetic field also has a focussing action. Fig. 6 shows diagrammatically the form of the field produced by the magnet. In the central region of the pole faces the magnetic field is quite uniform and normal to the plane of the faces; but out near the periphery the field has a curvature. Ions traveling on circles near the periphery experience thereby magnetic forces, indicated by the arrows. If the circular path is on the median plane then the magnetic force is towards the center in that plane. If the ion is traveling in a circle off the median plane, then there is a component of magnetic force that accelerates it towards the median plane, thereby giving effectively a focussing action.

We have experimentally examined these two focussing actions, using a probe in front of the first slit of the collector system that could be moved up and down across the beam by means of a ground joint (see Fig. 3). It was

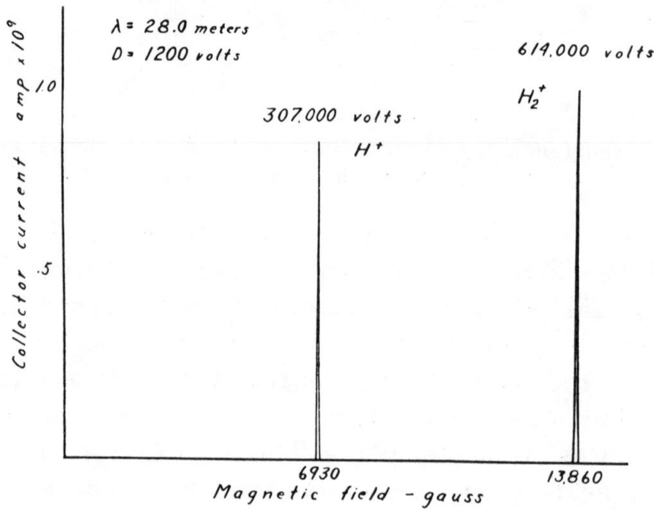

Fig. 7. Ion current to Faraday collector as a function of the magnetic field with oscillations of 28 meters wave-length applied to the accelerating electrodes.

found that the focussing actions were so powerful that *the beam of high speed ions had a width of less than one millimeter*. Such a narrow beam of ions of course is ideal for many experimental studies.

As a further test of the focussing action of the two fields, the median plane of the accelerating system was lowered 3 mm with respect to the plane of symmetry of the magnetic field. It was found that the high speed ion beam at the periphery traveled in a plane that was between the planes of symmetry of the two fields showing that both focussing actions were operative and at the periphery were of the same order of magnitude.

Letters to the Editor

[The Editor does not hold himself responsible for opinions expressed by his correspondents. He cannot undertake to return, or to correspond with the writers of, rejected manuscripts intended for this or any other part of NATURE. *No notice is taken of anonymous communications.*

NOTES ON POINTS IN SOME OF THIS WEEK'S LETTERS APPEAR ON P. 901.]

Elimination of Water from the Human Body

SHORTLY after the first application of radioactive isotopes as indicators, the late H. J. G. Moseley and one of the present writers discussed the prospect opened by the introduction of this method, when indulging in a cup of tea at the Manchester Physics Laboratory. The latter then expressed the wish that an indicator might be found which would allow one to determine the fate of the individual water molecules contained in the cup of tea consumed. Even a man of the vision and outlook of the late H. J. G. Moseley considered this hope to be a highly Utopian one.

The recent work of Urey and his collaborators brought, however, the above-mentioned wish within the range of realisation. Although diplogen and hydrogen, unlike the atoms of radioactive isotopes, are not practically inseparable by chemical means, yet if we add to a cup of tea a slight amount of heavy water and then find, for example, one per cent of the latter in the water which has left the body, we can assume that about one per cent of the 'normal' water molecules taken in with the cup of tea has shared the same fate.

TABLE 1.

Density of water prepared from urine after the intake of diluted heavy water.

Time elapsed since the intake of water started in hours	Urine (volume passed in c.c.)	Density difference between water prepared from urine and 'normal' (distilled) water
0·5	130	6×10^{-6}
0·8	190	10
1	230	15
1·2	210	21
1·5	230	23
1·8	290	25
2	160	21
2·5	80	20
4	120	18
8	130	20
10	290	18
17	320	20
23	140	19
24·5	210	18
42	820	19
67	1120	17
92	2100	17
244	—	10
340	—	8

That heavy water present in high dilution in the organism behaves like light water is borne out by the fact that the heavy water content of urine and other excreta is the same as that of ordinary tap water, within a limit of 1 : 100,000 as found by us and other experimenters[1]. If we slightly increase the heavy water content of the normal water we can assume that, with an accuracy sufficient for our purposes, the heavy water will show the same behaviour as the normal one. As a further argument in favour of this view, we may quote the results obtained when investigating the behaviour of highly diluted heavy water in the body of fishes[2].

Our first step was to investigate if water prepared from urine has the same density as the tap water drunk. The result was within $1 : 10^6$ in the affirmative. The preparation of water from urine was carried out by combined adsorption and distillation processes. 55 samples of urine and other excreta were investigated and more than 1000 distillation processes carried out. One of us took then in one experiment 150 c.c. and in another 250 c.c. water containing 0·46 per cent heavy water showing a density difference against normal water of 480×10^{-6}. As the increase in density of the urine obtained after the intake of these quantities was only a few units in a million, an experiment was made in which 2000 c.c. were taken. The increase in the density of the water obtained was then up to $25 : 10^6$. Some of the results are seen from Table 1.

From the above figures it follows that, after half an hour from the beginning of the intake of water, some of the water drunk is found in the urine, though only 0·2 per cent of the amount taken. The bulk of the water leaves the body at a slow rate and it takes 9 ± 1 days before half of the water taken has left the body.

We controlled the water balance during the experiments and found (in hot summer weather) that on an average 60 per cent of the water lost left the body through transpiration and evaporation. In the possession of these data, and as we find that the density of urine water and transpiration water is the same within the limits of our accuracy relevant for these considerations ($\pm$ 5 per cent of the density excess), we can calculate the time which elapses before half of the water taken left the body by an independent method. The result works out again as 9 ± 1 days. By dividing the last figure by $ln\ 2$ we get for the average time a water molecule spends in the body $13 \pm 1{\cdot}5$ days. To explain this comparatively long time, we have to assume that most of the water taken becomes completely mixed with the water content of the body. This assumption can be tested by calculating the water content of the body of the experimenter from the amount of diluted heavy water taken and the density of the water prepared from urine any day except the first one. We arrive at a water content of 43 ± 3 litres, namely,
63 ± 4 per cent in fair accordance with known data. 85

G. HEVESY.
E. HOFER.

Institut f. physikalische Chemie,
Universität, Freiburg i. Br.

[1] H. J. Emeléus, F. W. James, A. King, T. G. Pearson, R. H. Purcell and H. V. A. Briscoe, *J. Chem. Soc.*, August, p. 1207, 1934.

[2] G. v. Hevesy and E. Hofer, *Hoppe-Seylers Z.*, **225**, 28; 1934. cf. also G. N. Lewis, *Science*, **79**, 151; 1934. H. Erlenmeyer and H. Gärtner, *Helvet. chim. Acta*, **17**, 334; 1934.

Artificial Production of a New Kind of Radio-Element

By F. JOLIOT and I. CURIE, Institut du Radium, Paris

SOME months ago we discovered that certain light elements emit positrons under the action of α-particles[1]. Our latest experiments have shown a very striking fact: when an aluminium foil is irradiated on a polonium preparation, the emission of positrons does not cease immediately, when the active preparation is removed. The foil remains radioactive and the emission of radiation decays exponentially as for an ordinary radio-element. We observed the same phenomenon with boron and magnesium[2]. The half life period of the activity is 14 min. for boron, 2 min. 30 sec. for magnesium, 3 min. 15 sec. for aluminium.

We have observed no similar effect with hydrogen, lithium, beryllium, carbon, nitrogen, oxygen, fluorine, sodium, silicon, or phosphorus. Perhaps in some cases the life period is too short for easy observation.

The transmutation of beryllium, magnesium, and aluminium α-particles has given birth to new radio-elements emitting positrons. These radio-elements may be regarded as a known nucleus formed in a particular state of excitation; but it is much more probable that they are unknown isotopes which are always unstable.

For example, we propose for boron the following nuclear reaction:

$$ {}_5B^{10} + {}_2He^4 = {}_7N^{13} + {}_0n^1 $$

${}_7N^{13}$ being the radioactive nucleus that disintegrates with emission of positrons, giving a stable nucleus ${}_6C^{13}$. In the case of aluminium and magnesium, the radioactive nuclei would be ${}_{15}P^{30}$ and ${}_{14}Si^{27}$ respectively.

The positrons of aluminium seem to form a continuous spectrum similar to the β-ray spectrum. The maximum energy is about 3×10^6 e.v. As in the case of the continuous spectrum of β-rays, it will be perhaps necessary to admit the simultaneous emission of a neutrino (or of an antineutrino of Louis de Broglie) in order to satisfy the principle of the conservation of energy and of the conservation of the spin in the transmutation.

The transmutations that give birth to the new radio-elements are produced in the proportion of 10^{-7} or 10^{-6} of the number of α-particles, as for other transmutations. With a strong polonium preparation of 100 millicuries, one gets only about 100,000 atoms of the radioactive elements. Yet it is possible to determine their chemical properties, detecting their radiation with a counter or an ionisation chamber. Of course, the chemical reactions must be completed in a few minutes, before the activity has disappeared.

We have irradiated the compound boron nitride (BN). By heating boron nitride with caustic soda, gaseous ammonia is produced. The activity separates from the boron and is carried away with the ammonia. This agrees very well with the hypothesis that the radioactive nucleus is in this case an isotope of nitrogen.

When irradiated aluminium is dissolved in hydrochloric acid, the activity is carried away with the hydrogen in the gaseous state, and can be collected in a tube. The chemical reaction must be the formation of phosphine (PH_3) or silicon hydride (SiH_4). The precipitation of the activity with zirconium phosphate in acid solution seems to indicate that the radio-element is an isotope of phosphorus.

These experiments give the first chemical proof of artificial transmutation, and also the proof of the capture of the α-particle in these reactions[3].

We propose for the new radio-elements formed by transmutation of boron, magnesium and aluminium, the names *radionitrogen*, *radiosilicon*, *radiophosphorus*.

These elements and similar ones may possibly be formed in different nuclear reactions with other bombarding particles: protons, deutrons, neutrons For example, ${}_7N^{13}$ could perhaps be formed by the capture of a deutron in ${}_6C^{12}$, followed by the emission of a neutron.

[1] Irène Curie and F. Joliot, *J. Phys. et. Rad.*, **4**, 494; 1933.
[2] Irène Curie and F. Joliot, *C.R.*, **198**; 1934.
[3] Irène Curie et F. Joliot, *C.R.*, meeting of Feb. 29, 1934.

Letters to the Editor

[*The Editor does not hold himself responsible for opinions expressed by his correspondents. Neither can he undertake to return, nor to correspond with the writers of, rejected manuscripts intended for this or any other part of* NATURE. *No notice is taken of anonymous communications.*]

Radioactivity Induced by Neutron Bombardment

EXPERIMENTS have been carried out to ascertain whether neutron bombardment can produce an induced radioactivity, giving rise to unstable products which disintegrate with emission of β-particles. Preliminary results have been communicated in a letter to *La Ricerca Scientifica*, **5**, 282; 1934.

The source of neutrons is a sealed glass tube containing radium emanation and beryllium powder. The amount of radium emanation available varied in the different experiments from 30 to 630 millicuries. We are much indebted to Prof. G. C. Trabacchi, Laboratorio Fisico della Sanità Pubblica, for putting at our disposal such strong sources.

The elements, or in some cases compounds containing them, were used in the form of small cylinders. After irradiation with the source for a period which varied from a few minutes to several hours, they were put around a Geiger counter with walls of thin aluminium foil (about 0·2 mm. thickness) and the number of impulses per minute was registered.

So far, we have obtained an effect with the following elements:

Phosphorus—Strong effect. Half-period about 3 hours. The disintegration electrons could be photographed in the Wilson chamber. Chemical separation of the active product showed that the unstable element formed under the bombardment is probably silicon.

Iron—Period about 2 hours. As the result of chemical separation of the active product, this is probably manganese.

Silicon—Very strong effect. Period about 3 minutes. Electrons photographed in the Wilson chamber.

Aluminium—Strong effect. Period about 12 minutes. Electrons photographed in the Wilson chamber.

Chlorine—Gives an effect with a period much longer than that of any element investigated at present.

Vanadium—Period about 5 minutes.

Copper—Effect rather small. Period about 6 minutes.

Arsenic—Period about two days.

Silver—Strong effect. Period about 2 minutes.

Tellurium. Period about 1 hour.

Iodine—Intense effect. Period about 30 minutes.

Chromium—Intense effect. Period about 6 minutes. Electrons photographed in the Wilson chamber.

Barium—Small effect. Period about 2 minutes.

Fluorine—Period about 10 seconds.

The following elements have also given indication of an effect: sodium, magnesium, titanium, zirconium, zinc, strontium, antimony, selenium and bromine. Some elements give indication of having two or more periods, which may be partly due to several isotopic constituents and partly to successive radioactive transformations. The experiments are being continued in order to verify these results and to extend the research to other elements.

The nuclear reaction which causes these phenomena may be different in different cases. The chemical separation effected in the cases of iron and phosphorus seems to indicate that, at least in these two cases, the neutron is absorbed and a proton emitted. The unstable product, by the emission of a β-particle, returns to the original element.

The chemical separations have been carried out by Dr. O. D'Agostino. Dr. E. Amaldi and Dr. E. Segrè have collaborated in the physical research.

ENRICO FERMI.

Physical Institute,
Royal University, Rome.
April 10.

LETTERS TO THE EDITOR

Radioactive Iodine Isotopes

We have bombarded tellurium with 8 Mev deuterons and have found two new radioactive iodine isotopes, with half-lives of 13 hours and 8 days. The latter is created by two mechanisms: (1) by the decay of radio-tellurium and (2) by direct transmutation from stable tellurium. Process (1) is demonstrated by the fact that successive extractions of iodine, from the same solution of bombarded tellurium, show a growth of the 8-day period; this must therefore be associated with either I^{129} or I^{131}, as the second activity of a double decay: $Te^{128,\,130}(d,\,p)Te^{129,\,131}$; $Te^{129,\,131}\rightarrow I^{129,\,131}\rightarrow Xe^{129,\,131}$. Process (2), which is known to occur on the basis of relative intensities, is the usual type of reaction: $Te^{128,\,130}(d,\,n)I^{129,\,131}$. Conclusive proof of this identification and interpretation has been furnished by the extraction of the 8-day iodine from tellurium which has been bombarded with neutrons. We cannot as yet state the period of the radio-tellurium from which this iodine grows.

Absorption measurements on the negative electrons emitted by the 8-day iodine indicate a maximum energy of 0.9 Mev; a gamma-ray is also present.

We have irradiated iodine with the fast neutrons from a lithium plus deuterons source and confirm the 13-day period reported for the same bombardment by Tape and Cork,[1] who surmised it to be due to I^{126}. We have chemically identified this activity as an iodine isotope, so that the assignment to I^{126} appears to be definite. (The antimony fraction of this same bombardment was inactive, while the tellurium precipitate exhibited a 10-hour half-life which can be ascribed definitely to Te^{127}. This tellurium period has been reported previously,[1] following neutron and deuteron bombardment of tellurium, but without definite isotopic identification.)

The yield of the 8-day iodine from $Te(d,\,n)I$ is very much larger than that of the strongest 13-day iodine that we have been able to produce by the reaction $I^{127}(n,\,2n)I^{126}$.

This research has been aided by grants from the Research Corporation, The Chemical Foundation and the Josiah Macy Jr. Foundation.

J. J. Livingood
G. T. Seaborg

Radiation Laboratory, Physics Dept. (J. J. L.)
Chemistry Department (G. T. S.),
University of California,
Berkeley, California,
June 1, 1938.

[1] G. F. Tape and J. M. Cork, Phys. Rev. 53, 676 (1938).

Physical Review 54, 772, 1938

Nuclear Isomerism in Element 43

We wish to report briefly an interesting case of isomerism which has appeared during an investigation of the short-lived radioactive isotopes of element 43. The irradiation of molybdenum with deuterons or slow neutrons produces a radioactive molybdenum isotope with a half-life of 65 hours which emits electrons with an upper energy limit of approximately 1 Mev. (This molybdenum activity has also been reported recently by Sagane, Kojima, Miyamoto and Ikawa.)[1] This molybdenum decays into a second activity which has a half-life of 6 hours and which emits only a line spectrum of electrons. Since the molybdenum emits electrons, the daughter activity must be ascribed to element 43; chemical identification has been carried out and has confirmed this identification of the 6-hour activity. Absorption measurements in aluminum and measurements with a magnetic spectrograph[2] indicate an energy for the electrons of about 110 kev. This line spectrum must be due to the conversion electrons of a gamma-ray of about 130 kev energy. The 6-hour activity also emits x-radiation and γ-radiation. The absorption of the x-rays in molybdenum, columbium and zirconium shows a discontinuity that is consistent with the $K\alpha$ line of element 43, which is to be expected on the basis of the interpretation given below.

The simplest and most reasonable explanation for these facts is the existence of an excited state in this isotope of element 43 which reverts to the ground state by the emission of conversion electrons and gamma-rays with a half-life of 6 hours. A line of conversion electrons corresponding to a similar transition seems to have been detected by Pontecorvo[3] during a study of the nuclear isomerism in rhodium. A more complete discussion and a description of the experiments will be published later in the *Physical Review.*

We wish to thank Professor E. O. Lawrence for the privilege of working with the cyclotron and for his interest in this problem.

We wish also to express our appreciation to Mr. D. C. Kalbfell for the photographing of the line spectrum of electrons. This research has been aided by grants from the Research Corporation.

E. Segrè
G. T. Seaborg

Radiation Laboratory,
Department of Physics (E.S.),
Department of Chemistry (G.T.S.),
University of California,
Berkeley, California,
October 14, 1938.

[1] Sagane, Kojima, Mijamoto and Ikawa, Phys. Rev. **54**, 542 (1938).
[2] Kalbfell, Phys. Rev. **54**, 543 (1938).
[3] Pontecorvo, Phys. Rev. **54**, 542 (1938).

Proceedings
of the
Society
for
Experimental Biology and Medicine

Vol. 38. May, 1938. No. 4

9915 P

Radioactive Iodine as an Indicator in the Study of Thyroid Physiology.*

S. Hertz, A. Roberts and Robley D. Evans. (Introduced by Henry Jackson.)

From the Thyroid Clinic, Massachusetts General Hospital, Boston, and the Physics Department, Massachusetts Institute of Technology, Cambridge.

The known facts of thyroid physiology indicate that iodine is selectively taken up by the thyroid gland, and that in some measure that gland's function is regulated by its iodine content. Artificial radioactivity may be induced in a variety of elements by means of neutron bombardment. It seemed that the possibility of using "tagged" (radioactive) iodine as a physiologic indicator was one which demanded investigation.

Ethyl iodide (600-1000 cc) was irradiated in a paraffin-sur-
rounded bottle by immersing in it a neutron source consisting of
110 mg of radium mixed with beryllium in a sealed tube. The
radioactive iodine thus obtained was concentrated by a method
which has been described elsewhere.[1] This method gave a precipi- 95
tate of radioactive silver iodide, which was dissolved in a solution
of 0.5-1.0 g of sodium thiosulphate, and then diluted to 10-15 cc
for intravenous injection. In a series of 48 rabbits, no toxic effects
from the acute administration of such quantities were experienced.
Aliquot portions of the solution of radioactive iodine used for injection were withheld for measurement of radioactivity.

*This work was aided by a grant from the Milton Fund of Harvard University.

1 Roberts and Irvine, *Phys. Rev.*, 1938, **53**, 609.

A Geiger-Müller counter connected to a suitable vacuum tube amplifier and register to record the individual disintegrations of the radioactive atoms was used for detection of the radioactive iodine in various tissues. This apparatus is standardized and has been fully described elsewhere.[2-4] Since no gamma rays could be observed from radioactive iodine,[1] determinations had to be made from the beta radiations. The half-period of radioactive iodine is 26 minutes, so that accurate measurements could not be extended beyond about 40 minutes after injection, with the activities available to date.

Because of the low penetrating power of beta radiation it was necessary to sacrifice the animals to obtain the various tissues for measurement. The tissues were finely minced and spread on a flat surface and placed in direct contact with the Geiger-Müller counter.

The following tissues and body fluids, in addition to the thyroid, were examined: muscle, spleen, liver, pituitary, adrenals, frontal lobe of the brain, hypothalamus, salivary glands, ovaries, blood, urine, and cerebro-spinal fluid. The results in a typical case may be given as follows:

Rabbit No. 224: Thyroid previously rendered hyperplastic by the injection of anterior pituitary extract. 10 mg of I injected. 15 minutes elapsed between injection and killing of the rabbit.

TABLE I.

Organ	Radioactivity in arbitrary units (counts per min)	
Thyroid	38.5 ± 5	
Spleen (quantity equal to thyroid)	2 ± 5	
Liver (quantity equal to thyroid)	4 ± 5	
Pituitary	0	(5 units correspond to .008 mg of I)
Urine (residue after evaporation)	48 ± 5	(In other exp. 5 units may correspond to as little as .0007 mg of I)
Muscle (quantity equal to thyroid)	0	

96 In none of the tissues or fluids examined were quantities of iodine found which compared with that taken up by the thyroid, with the exception of the entire bladder urine residue after complete evaporation, and the blood, into which the radioactive iodine was directly injected. Quantities less than 0.05% of the injected iodine could not be detected in these samples. It must be stressed at this point that this method gives information only with regard to the injected

2 Langer and Whitaker, *Phys. Rev.*, 1937, **51**, 713.

3 Giarratana, *Rev. Sci. Instr.*, 1937, **8**, 390.

4 Gingrich, *Rev. Sci. Instr.*, 1936, **7**, 207.

iodine, and disregards any iodine previously present within the tissues.

Other measurements of the collection of iodine by the thyroid were performed, varying the dosage of iodine, the time elapsing between injection and sacrifices of the animals, and the functional state of the thyroid under conditions of thyrotropic stimulation, pregnancy, and spontaneous goiter. The results to date of these experiments are given in the accompanying graphs. They are being extended by further experiment.

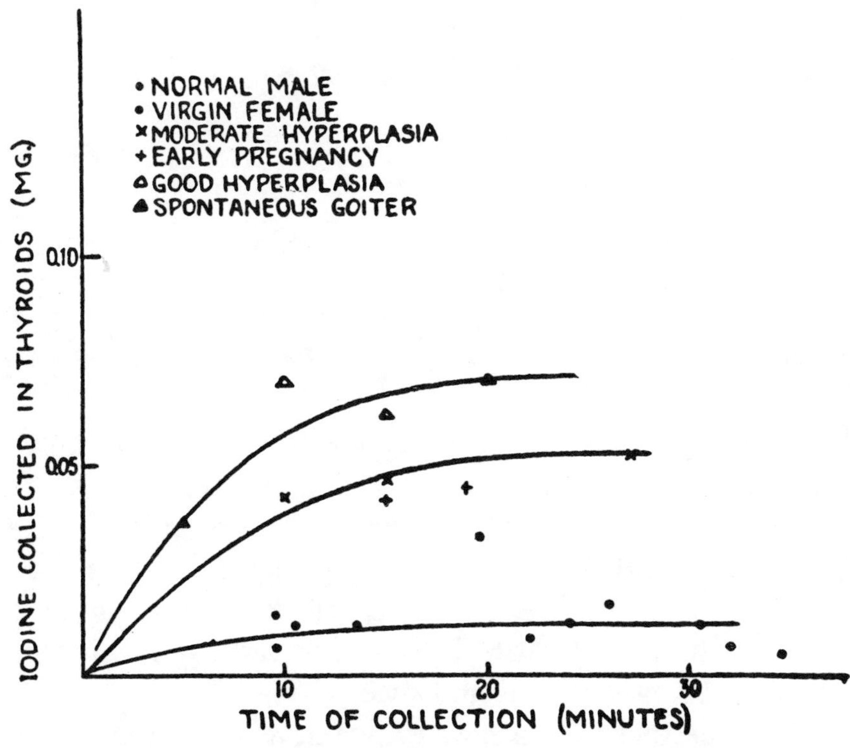

Fig. 1.

Comparison of the quantities of iodine collected by different types of rabbit thyroid glands when the time elapsing between injection and sacrifice is varied.

That the concentration of iodine in the thyroids is a biologically selective process is further attested by the uniformly negative results obtained when radioactive bromine was used, with a similar technic, in place of iodine.

The methods outlined above are established as giving useful information with regard to iodine distribution in the organism. Their accuracy can be expected to increase as sources of stronger radioactive iodine become available. The artificially radioactive material with which these experiments were performed is considered very weak, in comparison with that produced by means of the Van de Graaff electrostatic generator and the cyclotron. The data presented, however, do indicate that radioactive iodine is selectively

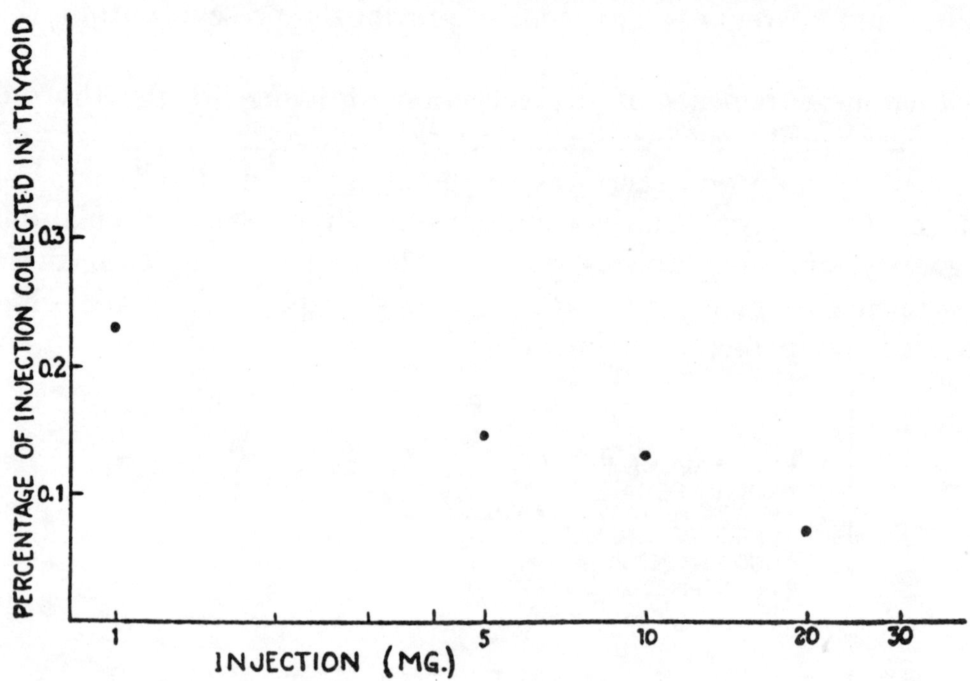

FIG. 2.

Comparison of the quantities of iodine collected by normal rabbit thyroid glands in the same time (15 minutes) when the amount injected is varied.

taken up by the thyroid under normal conditions in a definitely measurable amount. They further tend to show that under conditions of thyroid stimulation (hyperplasia), the collection in the same time is increased severalfold. It is therefore logical to suppose that when strongly active materials are available the concentrating power of the hyperplastic and neoplastic thyroid for radioactive iodine may be of clinical or therapeutic significance.

Recently the discovery of a new radioactive isotope of iodine has been announced.[5] This isotope has a half-period of 13 days. It is obvious that it will have many advantages over the 26-minute isotope for both indicator and therapeutic work. Such experiments as the above may now be extended over much longer time intervals fol-
98 lowing injection.

We are indebted to Professor J. H. Means of the Harvard Medical School for his stimulating interest in this work.

[5] Tape and Cork, *Phys. Rev.*, 1938, **53**, 676 A.

Disintegration of Uranium by Neutrons: a New Type of Nuclear Reaction

ON bombarding uranium with neutrons, Fermi and collaborators[1] found that at least four radioactive substances were produced, to two of which atomic numbers larger than 92 were ascribed. Further investigations[2] demonstrated the existence of at least nine radioactive periods, six of which were assigned to elements beyond uranium, and nuclear isomerism had to be assumed in order to account for their chemical behaviour together with their genetic relations.

In making chemical assignments, it was always assumed that these radioactive bodies had atomic numbers near that of the element bombarded, since only particles with one or two charges were known to be emitted from nuclei. A body, for example, with similar properties to those of osmium was assumed to be eka-osmium ($Z = 94$) rather than osmium ($Z = 76$) or ruthenium ($Z = 44$).

Following up an observation of Curie and Savitch[3], Hahn and Strassmann[4] found that a group of at least three radioactive bodies, formed from uranium under neutron bombardment, were chemically similar to barium and, therefore, presumably isotopic with radium. Further investigation[5], however, showed that it was impossible to separate these bodies from barium (although mesothorium, an isotope of radium, was readily separated in the same experiment), so that Hahn and Strassmann were forced to conclude that *isotopes of barium* ($Z = 56$) *are formed as a consequence of the bombardment of uranium* ($Z = 92$) *with neutrons*.

At first sight, this result seems very hard to understand. The formation of elements much below uranium has been considered before, but was always rejected for physical reasons, so long as the chemical evidence was not entirely clear cut. The emission, within a short time, of a large number of charged particles may be regarded as excluded by the small penetrability of the 'Coulomb barrier', indicated by Gamov's theory of alpha decay.

On the basis, however, of present ideas about the behaviour of heavy nuclei[6], an entirely different and essentially classical picture of these new disintegration processes suggests itself. On account of their close packing and strong energy exchange, the particles in a heavy nucleus would be expected to move in a collective way which has some resemblance to the movement of a liquid drop. If the movement is made sufficiently violent by adding energy, such a drop may divide itself into two smaller drops.

In the discussion of the energies involved in the deformation of nuclei, the concept of surface tension of nuclear matter has been used[7] and its value has been estimated from simple considerations regarding nuclear forces. It must be remembered, however, that the surface tension of a charged droplet is diminished by its charge, and a rough estimate shows that the surface tension of nuclei, decreasing with increasing nuclear charge, may become zero for atomic numbers of the order of 100.

It seems therefore possible that the uranium nucleus has only small stability of form, and may, after neutron capture, divide itself into two nuclei of roughly equal size (the precise ratio of sizes depending on finer structural features and perhaps partly on chance). These two nuclei will repel each other and should gain a total kinetic energy of *c.* 200 Mev., as calculated from nuclear radius and charge. This amount of energy may actually be expected to be available from the difference in packing fraction between uranium and the elements in the middle of the periodic system. The whole 'fission' process can thus be described in an essentially classical way, without having to consider quantum-mechanical 'tunnel effects', which would actually be extremely small, on account of the large masses involved.

After division, the high neutron/proton ratio of uranium will tend to readjust itself by beta decay to the lower value suitable for lighter elements. Probably each part will thus give rise to a chain of disintegrations. If one of the parts is an isotope of barium[5], the other will be krypton ($Z = 92 - 56$), which might decay through rubidium, strontium and yttrium to zirconium. Perhaps one or two of the supposed barium-lanthanum-cerium chains are then actually strontium-yttrium-zirconium chains.

It is possible[5], and seems to us rather probable, that the periods which have been ascribed to elements beyond uranium are also due to light elements. From the chemical evidence, the two short periods (10 sec. and 40 sec.) so far ascribed to ^{239}U might be masurium isotopes ($Z = 43$) decaying through ruthenium, rhodium, palladium and silver into cadmium.

In all these cases it might not be necessary to assume nuclear isomerism; but the different radioactive periods belonging to the same chemical element may then be attributed to different isotopes of this element, since varying proportions of neutrons may be given to the two parts of the uranium nucleus.

By bombarding thorium with neutrons, activities are obtained which have been ascribed to radium and actinium isotopes[8]. Some of these periods are approximately equal to periods of barium and lanthanum isotopes[5] resulting from the bombardment of uranium. We should therefore like to suggest that these periods are due to a 'fission' of thorium which is like that of uranium and results partly in the same products. Of course, it would be especially interesting if one could obtain one of these products from a light element, for example, by means of neutron capture.

It might be mentioned that the body with half-life 24 min.[2] which was chemically identified with uranium is probably really ^{239}U, and goes over into an eka-rhenium which appears inactive but may decay slowly, probably with emission of alpha particles. (From inspection of the natural radioactive elements, ^{239}U cannot be expected to give more than one or two beta decays; the long chain of observed decays has always puzzled us.) The formation of this body is a typical resonance process[9]; the compound state must have a life-time a million times longer than the time it would take the nucleus to divide itself. Perhaps this state corresponds to some highly symmetrical type of motion of nuclear matter which does not favour 'fission' of the nucleus.

LISE MEITNER.
Physical Institute,
Academy of Sciences,
Stockholm.

O. R. FRISCH.
Institute of Theoretical Physics,
University,
Copenhagen.
Jan. 16.

[1] Fermi, E., Amaldi, F., d'Agostino, O., Rasetti, F., and Segrè, E. *Proc. Roy. Soc.*, A, **146**, 483 (1934).
[2] See Meitner, L., Hahn, O., and Strassmann, F., *Z. Phys.*, **106**, 249 (1937).
[3] Curie, I., and Savitch, P., *C.R.*, **208**, 906, 1643 (1938).
[4] Hahn, O., and Strassmann, F., *Naturwiss.*, **26**, 756 (1938).
[5] Hahn, O., and Strassmann, F., *Naturwiss.*, **27**, 11 (1939).
[6] Bohr, N., NATURE, **137**, 344, 351 (1936).
[7] Bohr, N., and Kalckar, F., *Kgl. Danske Vid. Selskab, Math. Phys. Medd.*, **14**, Nr. 10 (1937).
[8] See Meitner, L., Strassmann, F., and Hahn, O., *Z. Phys.*, **109**, 538 (1938).
[9] Bethe, A. H., and Placzek, G., *Phys. Rev.*, **51**, 450 (1937).

SCIENCE

Vol. 103, No. 2685 | Friday, June 14, 1946

Availability of Radioactive Isotopes

Announcement From Headquarters, Manhattan Project, Washington, D.C.

PRODUCTION OF TRACER AND THERAPEUTIC RADIOISOTOPES has been heralded as one of the great peacetime contributions of the uranium chain-reacting pile. This use of the pile will unquestionably be rich in scientific, medical, and technological applications.

Manhattan Project scientific, technical, and administrative personnel have, since the inception of the pile, been cognizant of its peacetime potentialities and have, since the end of the war, been active in attempting to realize these opportunities. Since, however, war-built piles and wartime researches had other objectives, a considerable transition in researches, developments, and operations connected with piles must be effected before the supply of radioisotopes can begin to meet the demand.

Comments on Availability of Radioisotopes

(1) A pile cannot make the extensive variety of radioisotopes producible with the cyclotron because the cyclotron makes use of a much greater diversity in energy and type of nuclear bombarding projectiles. Present piles are copious sources of low-energy neutrons, which can give rise to large yields only of isotopes produced by (n,f) and (n,γ) processes.

(2) Although large numbers of radioisotopes are produced in abundance by the fission of uranium in the piles, their availability is limited by the difficulties encountered in isolating them. It has not yet been found feasible to remove individual fission products from waste solutions of the plutonium extraction process. Most of the fission products being made available are not salvaged by-products of the plutonium process but are in each case items requiring special production from unprocessed irradiated uranium.

(3) Most of the radioisotopes in greatest demand, such as C 14, S 35, and P 32, must be produced by the irradiation of materials foreign to the pile. Existing piles were not designed for this purpose.

(4) Although a pile is a copious source of neutrons, it is not a limitless source. It is possible to load a pile for nonfission product radioisotope production only up to the limit at which so many neutrons are absorbed in the introduced material that the chain reaction ceases even though the control rods are withdrawn as far as feasible. With available pile facilities, this limit does not permit the production of a sufficient quantity and quality of many radioisotopes to meet anticipated national demands. To accomplish this it would very likely be necessary to build piles especially designed for the purpose.

(5) Technical problems involved in the irradiation of some materials have been, and will continue to be, responsible for delays in making certain isotopes available by routine irradiation. Examples of such problems are: (a) proper canning of the material to prevent rupture of the container by its internal action or by the external action of the coolant, with consequent loss of the material and damage to the pile; (b) careful purification to prevent loss of neutrons by absorption in impurities as well as undesirable radioactivity in the irradiated material; and (c) proper distribution of the material throughout the pile to prevent local overheating or undesirable regulation characteristics of the pile.

Organization for Allocation and Distribution

In accordance with the established custom of the Manhattan Project of seeking competent outside advice and aid on vital scientific matters, such as nonproject distribution of isotopes, Maj. Gen. L. R. Groves asked the president of the National Academy of Sciences to nominate a representative committee of outstanding scientists to recommend policies and aid in establishing arrangements for a desirable distribution of those tracer and therapeutic isotopes available from Manhattan Project facilities. An interim Advisory Committee on Isotope Distribution Policy was formed, two representatives being chosen from each of the major fields of isotope application: Physics—Lee A. DuBridge (chairman), head, Physics Department, University of Rochester, and president-elect of California Institute of Technology, Pasadena; and Merle A. Tuve, head, Department of Terrestrial Magnetism, Carnegie Institution of Washington, Washington, D. C.; Chemistry—Linus Pauling, director, Gates and Crellin Chemistry Laboratories, California Institute of Technology; and Vincent du Vigneaud, head of the Department of Biochemistry, Cornell University Medical College, New York City; Medicine—Cornelius P. Rhoads, director of Memorial Hospital, New York City, and chairman of the Committee on Growth of the National Research Council; and Cecil J. Watson, head of the Department of Medicine, University of Minnesota Medical School, Minneapolis; Biology—Raymond E. Zirkle, professor of botany and director of the Institute for Biophysics and Radiobiology, University of Chicago, Chicago, Illinois; and A. Baird Hastings, head of the Department of Biological Chemistry, Harvard University Medical School, Cambridge; Applied Science—Zay Jeffries, vice-president and manager of Chemicals Department, General Electric Company, Pittsfield, Massachusetts; and L. F. Curtiss, chief of the Radioactivity Section, National Bureau of Standards, Washington, D. C. Paul C. Aebersold, chief of the Isotopes Branch, Research Division, Manhattan District, was chosen acting secretary to coordinate the efforts of the Committee and to effect liaison with the Project.

The recommendations of this Committee on a suitable interim mechanism for allocation and distribution have been adopted without modification. This mechanism is as follows:

(1) All requests will be submitted to the Isotopes Branch, Research Division, Manhattan District, where each request will be reviewed with regard to all technical questions affecting the requester and the Project. This initial review will be made by a group of scientists in the Project who have had much experience in the production of radioisotopes and in technical matters concerned with their use.

(2) Nonproject requests will then be referred to an Advisory Subcommittee on Allocation and Distribution, which has been appointed by Gen. Groves on the nominations of the Distribution Policy Committee. This Subcommittee will have the responsibility of advising on the allocation and distribution of isotopes according to the scientific value of the intended application and the qualifications of the requester. It will operate under the supervision of the Distribution Policy Committee and in conformity with its approved policies. Its members are: K. T. Bainbridge (physics), Harvard University, chairman; J. W. Kennedy (chemistry), Washington University, St. Louis; J. G. Hamilton (biology and medicine), University of California; P. C. Aebersold (biophysics), Manhattan District, secretary.

(3) Each request for material for use in human beings will be referred by the Subcommittee on Allocation and Distribution to a Subcommittee on Human Application, which was similarly nominated and appointed. This Subcommittee will have final veto power on any distribution suggested for human application. Its members, chosen from among radiologists and clinicians experienced in radioisotope uses, are: Andrew H. Dowdy, University of Rochester, chairman; H. L. Friedell, Western Reserve University; G. Failla, Columbia University.

(4) Small Panels of Consultants, nominated by the Policy Committee from a number of specialized fields of possible isotope application and from various regions of the Nation, will be available as advisers on scientific matters connected with requests.

(5) Manhattan Project personnel have not been excluded from membership in any of the nonproject advisory groups. In many cases their membership has been strongly advocated by the Distribution Policy Committee.

(6) Effective liaison will be maintained between the Isotopes Branch of the Manhattan District Research Division, which initially receives and finally effects distribution on nonproject isotope requests, and the associated advisory groups whose functions are set forth above.

Principles of Allocation and Distribution

In establishing initial policies on the distribution of scarce materials, the criterion used has been the maximum benefit to the national welfare, due consideration being given to the limited amount of available material. The initial policies adopted are:

(1) Isotopes will be made available to individuals only through qualified institutions. The administration of the institution will make the necessary financial and legal arrangements, but the material will be allotted for the uses specified in the request.

(2) Secondary distribution of isotopes will not be sanctioned unless indicated and authorized under the original request or subsequently in writing through the accepted channels for requests.

(3) The initial order of priority adopted for the allocation of materials and of production effort is established according to intended use of the material, as follows: (a) publishable researches in the fundamental sciences, including human tracer applications, requiring relatively small samples; (b) therapeutic, diagnostic, and tracer applications in human beings and publishable researches in the fundamental sciences requiring larger samples; (c) training and education by accredited institutions in the techniques and applications of radioisotopes; and (d) publishable researches in the applied sciences. Allocation of material for researches which are not to be published or for routine commercial applications was considered by the Distribution Policy Committee not to fall within its responsibilities. Allocation for routine commercial

applications will be deferred until experience is gained with supplying the research needs previously mentioned. Special groups may then be established to advise on such allocation.

Production and Distribution Arrangements Within the Project

As indicated in the section on availability, none of the separate purified radioisotopes is in routine operational production. In some cases research groups have progressed only to the point of investigating how irradiations can best be performed to create a given isotope and how to isolate the isotope in small amounts. In other cases methods are under investigation in development groups for increasing the scale of irradiation and chemical processing. In a few cases it has now become possible to start placing irradiations and chemical processing into the hands of technical operations groups for routine "production."

Research into methods of small-scale creation of most of the isotopes took place widely before the establishment of the Project; since then, it has been carried on extensively by project laboratories engaged in nuclear research. Thus, credit for the results of research on radioisotopes is shared by many nonproject and project personnel. Most of the research within the Project in this regard has been done by nuclear physics and radiochemistry groups at Clinton Laboratories at Oak Ridge, at the Radiation Laboratory of the University of California, and at the Metallurgical and Argonne Laboratories of the University of Chicago.

The present "experimental-lot production" has been carried on largely by the Clinton Laboratories, which since July 1945 have been administered by the Monsanto Chemical Company. In the case of several isotopes in great demand, the Argonne Laboratory has cooperated in preparing materials in proper form for irradiation at Hanford and in testing the results. The Du Pont Company, operators of the Hanford Plant, has cooperated in making irradiations of materials possible at Hanford. The Monsanto Chemical Company has agreed to initiate the routine production of nationally demanded radioisotopes and to distribute them from the Clinton Laboratories under District Administration.

A Manhattan Project Technical Advisory Committee on Isotopes has been active in maintaining liaison between major laboratories of the Project on (1) production and distribution matters concerned with the national distribution program and (2) developments in radioisotope techniques and applications. This Committee is composed as follows: J. R. Coe, W. E. Cohn, R. McCullough, A. H. Snell, and K. Z. Morgan, of the Clinton Laboratories; W. H. Zinn, W. F. Libby, and R. E. Zirkle, of the Argonne and Metallurgical Laboratories; J. G. Hamilton, B. J. Moyer, and R. E. Connick, of the University of California Radiation Laboratory; J. H. Manley and R. Taschek, of the Los Alamos Scientific Laboratories; and, in regard to concentrated stable isotopes, H. L. Hull and C. E. Larson, of the Tennessee Eastman Corporation, Oak Ridge.

Details of Radioisotope Availability[1]

Pile-produced Radioisotopes

Radioactive isotopes are created in chain-reacting piles by two processes: (1) the fission of U 235 nuclei, which maintains the chain reaction, and (2) neutron absorption by nonfissionable nuclei placed in the pile for the purpose. The former—the so-called "fission products"—exist as a mixture of many radioactive species, each free of significant amounts of stable (carrier) isotopes, in a large amount of the parent substance, uranium. The desired radioisotope must subsequently be separated from uranium and from the other fission products, as well as from any neptunium and plutonium formed by neutron capture in U 238. In the chemical process actually used, the fission products are separated from the mixture either as individual radioactive species or as groups of species (Col. 1, Table 1).

The Fission Products

The methods now in operation for the preparation of fission-product radioisotopes were developed to meet certain definite specifications, which in turn were set by the biological work in which the radioactive materials were to be used. These specifications called for 0.1–1.0 curie[2] amounts of each of the major fission products in carrier-free, essentially solid-free (<10 mg./curie) form, and radiochemically pure (>90–98 per cent, depending on the species); smaller or less pure amounts of minor species were also required. The radiation intensities involved in working with mixtures of fission products at the curie level required the invention and use of chemical processes which were remotely controlled from behind specially constructed lead and concrete barriers and were economical of material. For these reasons the existing processes and equipment are not suited to isolate fission products in forms radically different from those listed. However, since these methods permit the isolation without carrier of nearly every fission product of half-life from 1 week to 30 years and occurring in significant amount, this inflexibility is not considered to be a handicap.

[1] Only those radioisotopes of half-life greater than 12 hours are considered.

[2] The curie is here defined as 3.7×10^{10} disintegrations second. [See statement by Condon and Curtis, p. 712. Ed.]

Those fission-product radioisotopes which can now be isolated[3] from pile uranium in moderate quantity and good quality without added carrier are listed in Tables 1, 2, and 3. In Table 1 are given also the latest data on half-life and radiation energies for each radioelement involved and also the properties of daughter radioisotopes which will be present. The values in the columns headed *"Approximate maximum unit quantity which may be made available" give essentially the amount which may be supplied at one time; requests for more than this amount may be temporarily or indefinitely delayed in fulfillment.* The activity stated in this column is related to the figures giving volume and other characteristics of the preparations.

TABLE 1*

FISSION PRODUCTS†

Group	Radioisotope	Half-life	Energies β Mev	Energies γ Mev	Radioactive daughters: Isotope	Radioactive daughters: Half-life	Radioactive daughters: Energies β Mev	Radioactive daughters: Energies γ Mev	Probable contaminants	Approx. max. unit quantity which may be made available (Curies)	Carrier added (Mg.)	Solids present (nonvol.) (Mg.)	Solvent	Volume (Ml.)	Class
I‡	Zr 95	65 d	1.0§ / 0.39§	0.73	Cb 95	35 d	0.15	0.75	.....	1	0	∼ 0	½% − $H_2C_2O_4$	50	A
	Cb 95	35 d	0.15	0.75	None										
II	Y 91	57 d	1.8	....	None				61	1	0	∼ 0	HCl	< 25	A
III‡	Ce 141	28 d	0.6	0.22	None				Pr	1	0	∼ 0	"	"	A
	Ce 144	275 d	0.35	....	Pr 144	17 m	3.1	....							
IV	Ba 140	12.8 d	1.05 / 0.4	0.5	La 140	40 h	1.4, 2.2	1.63‖	Sr	1	0	∼ 0	"	"	B
V‡	Sr 89	53 d	1.5	....	None				Ba	1	0	∼ 0	"	"	A
	Sr 90	25 y	0.6	....	Y 90	65 h	2.2	....							
VI‡	Pr 143	13.8 d	1.0	....	None				Ce, Y	0.1	0	∼ 0	"	"	B–C
	Nd 147	11 d	0.17 / 0.85	0.6	61 147	∼ 4 y	0.2	....							
	61 147	∼ 4 y	0.2	....	None										
	Eu 156	15.4 d	0.5 / 2.5	2	None										
	Eu 155	2–3 y	0.2	0.084	None										
VII	Cs 137	33 y	0.5 / 0.8	0.75	None				.....	0.01	0	∼ 0			A
VIII‡	Ru 103	42 d	0.2 / 0.8	0.56					.....	0.1 – 0.1	0	∼ 0	"	< 25	A–B
	Ru 106	1 y	< 0.005	....	Rh 106	30 s	3.9	....							
	Te 127	90 d	0.7	0.086											
	Te 129	32 d	1.8	0.1 / 0.3 / 0.8											

* Most data in this table are hitherto unpublished M.E.D. work.

† For I 131, see Tables 3 and 6.

‡ Specific composition depends on age.

§ Two per cent 1.0 Mev and 98 per cent 0.39 Mev.

‖ Complex spectrum.

The letters in the column headed "Class" are an attempt to indicate approximate availability and have the following meanings: A: usually on hand (long half-life permits stock-piling); B: often on hand (shorter half-life does not permit stock-piling); C: seldom on hand; produced on experimental basis only; D: not on hand; can be done but with difficulty.

Inasmuch as a routine production system, with attendant control and standards, does not exist, *no*

[3] It must be emphasized that no routine production system yet exists. The radioisotopes being made available at this time are the results of research and development proceedings.

guarantees of radiochemical or chemical purity or other such characteristic of any entry in any table may be made, although every effort will be made to turn out as high a quality of material as possible. Information relating to the known characteristics of any preparation will be furnished.

To obtain an isotope of this kind involves the insertion of the element, in a suitable form,[4] into the pile and its subsequent removal. Even though in some cases (n,p) radiocontaminants are produced along with the desired (n,γ)-induced radioisotope, no chemical separation process on the active material will be done prior to shipping (hence the term "service irradiation" to describe such an activation). In order to utilize the available facilities most efficiently, these materials will be exposed in the same containers in which they will be shipped, and only certain quantities will be irradiated. Therefore, *those radioelements supplied without processing will be available only in units which are 1, 0.1, 0.01, and (sometimes) 0.001 part of the quantities listed under "Approximate maximum unit quantity which may be made available."*

TABLE 2

FISSION PRODUCTS

(Derived from products in Table 1)

Source (Group in Table 1)	Radio-isotope	Probable radioactive contaminants	Approx. max. unit quantity which may be made available	Carrier added	Solids present (nonvol.)	Solvent	Volume	Class
			Curies		Mg.			
I	Cb 95	Zr	0.05	0		½% = $H_2C_2O_4$	< 25 ml.	C
VIII	Ru 103 Ru 106		0.05	0	~ 0	HCl	"	C
VIII	Te 127 Te 129		0.05	0	~ 0	"	"	C
VI	Pr 143*	Nd, 61	0.02	0	~ 0	"	"	C–D†
VI	Nd 147	Pr, 61	0.02	0	~ 0	"	"	C–D†
VI	61 147	Pr, Nd	10^{-4}	0	~ 0	"	"	C–D†

* See Table 6. † Depends on purity required and age.

Nonfission Radioisotopes

In Tables 4–6 are listed those neutron-induced radioisotopes of half-life greater than 12 hours which are known or believed to be producible in the pile.

(1) *Non-carrier-free radioisotopes; simple (n,γ) reactions* (Table 4). The most prominent reaction is simple neutron absorption, yielding a radioactive element isotopic with the parent element. This is the (n,γ) reaction (Table 4), which differs from transmutation and fission reactions in that carrier-free material is *not* produced (except in those few cases where a radioactive chain is begun).

TABLE 3

FISSION PRODUCTS

(By-products usually on hand in impure form)

Radio-isotope	Quantity usually available	Carrier added	Solids (nonvol.)	Solvent	Volume	Class
	Curies	Mg.	Mg.			
Sr 89 Sr 90 *	1	0	~ 0	N/2 HCl	< 25 ml.	A
I 131†	0.1	0	~ 0	N/10 HNO_3	< 25 ml.	B
Ba 140*	1	> 0	> 0	N/2 HCl	< 25 ml.	B

* See Table 1 for radiation characteristics of isotopes and daughters.

† See Table 6.

(2) *Carrier-free radioisotopes* (Tables 5 and 6). Transmutation reactions yield radioisotopes which differ chemically from their parents and hence exist *without*[5] stable isotopic "carrier." Only a small number of elements are known to undergo (n,p), (n,α), etc. reactions to any appreciable degree in the pile; however, the few which do yield some of the most important radioelements (Table 5). In addition to these types, in which transmutations are effected, there is a group of (n,γ)-induced decay chains which can be utilized to yield carrier-free material (Table 6). In this case a radioisotope produced by a (n,γ) re-

[4] In many cases it is advisable to irradiate elements in the form of a compound. The particular compound selected must be such as to lend itself to irradiation under the expected pile conditions. Undesirable radioactive species and unsatisfactory containers must be avoided. For these and other reasons, the materials to be exposed in the pile for radioisotope production will usually be supplied and packaged by the Project.

[5] Except for impurities below detectable levels.

TABLE 4

LONG-LIVED RADIOACTIVE ISOTOPES PRODUCIBLE IN PILE BY (n,γ) REACTIONS

(Items in italics—Manhattan Project data)

Active isotope	Half-life	Radiation Mev β	Radiation Mev γ	Approx. specific activity (mc./gram element)*	Approx. max. unit quantity which may be made available*	Class
Na 24	14.8 h	1.4	1.4, 2.8	250	100 mc.	A
P 32	14.3 d	1.69		72	500 mc.‖	A
S 35†	87.1 d	*0.17*		1.0	1 mc.‖	D
Cl 36†	*10^6 y*	*0.66*		~ 0.002	10 μc.	D
K 42	12.4 h	3.5	?	20	1 c.	D
Ca 41	8.5 d	K	1.1	0.34	10 mc.	D
Ca 45	180 d	*0.3*		3.8	100 mc.‖	C
Sc 46†	85 d	0.26, 1.5	1.25	125	1 mc.	C
Ti 51	72 d	0.36	1.0	0.13	1 mc.	D
Cr 51	26.5 d	K	*0.32*	70	100 mc.	C
Fe 55	~ 4 y	K		0.07	100 μc.	C
Fe 59	*44 d*	0.26, 0.46	1.1, 1.3	0.15	1 mc.	C
Co 60	5.3 y	0.3	1.1, 1.3	48	100 mc.	B
Ni 59	*15 y*	*0.05* β^+			10 μc.	D
Cu 64	12.8 h	0.58 β^+, 0.66 β^-		440	10 mc.	C
Zn 65	250 d	0.4 β^+, K, e-	1.14	3.6	100 mc.	D
Zn 69	13.8 h	I.T., 1.0	0.439	10	100 mc.	D
Ga 72	14.1 h	*3.4*, 0.8	0.84, *2.25*	230	100 mc.	C
Ge 71 ‡	11 d	*0.6*	0.5	14	100 mc.	D
Ge 77 ‡	12 h	1.9		0.9	10 mc.	D
As 76	26.8 h	1.1, 1.7, 2.7	0.57, *1.25*	770	100 mc.	C
Se 75	*125 d*	K, e-	*0.18, 0.35*	5.6	100 mc.	D
Br 82	34 h	0.465	0.547, 0.787, 1.35	170	100 mc.	C
Rb 86	19.5 d	1.60		52	100 mc.	D
Sr 89	53 d	1.5		0.2	10 mc.¶	D
Y 90	65 h	2.5		150	100 mc.¶	C
Zr 95‡	*65 d*	1.0, 0.39[z]	*0.73*	0.32	¶	D
Mo 99‡	67 h	1.3	0.24, *0.75*	12	100 mc.	D
Ru 103	*42 d*	0.2, *0.8*	0.56	6.4	10 mc.	D
Ag 108, 110	225 d	*1.3*	0.6, 0.9	10	100 mc.**	D
Cd 115 ‡	*2.8 d*	1.11	0.65	33.2	10 mc.	D
Cd 115 ‡	*43 d*	1.5		1.6	1 mc.	D
In 114	48 d	I.T., e-, 2.0	0.19	200	100 mc.	C
Sn 113	< 100 d	K, e-	0.085	0.26	1 mc.	D
Sb 122	2.8 d	0.81, 1.64	0.8	400	100 mc.	C
Sb 124	60 d	0.74, 2.45	1.72	33	100 mc.	C
106 Te 127 ‡	90 d	I.T., e-, *0.7*	0.086	0.3	10 mc.¶	C
Te 129 ‡	32 d	I.T., e-, 1.8	0.102, *0.3, 0.8*	0.3	10 mc.¶	C
Te 131 ‡	30 h	I.T. β^-	0.177	0.3	10 mc.¶	C
Cs 134	2 y	*0.75*	*0.8*	200	·1 c.¶ **	C
Ba 131‡	12 d	K, e-	*1.2* (?)	0.44	10 mc.¶	C
La 140	40 h	1.4, 2.2	1.63§	760	100 mc.¶	D

[z] Two per cent 1.0 Mev and 98 per cent 0.39 Mev particles.

TABLE 4—(*Continued*)

(Items in italics—Manhattan Project data)

Active isotope	Half-life	Radiation Mev β	Radiation Mev γ	Approx. specific activity (mc./gram element)*	Approx. max. unit quantity which may be made available*	Class
Ce 141 } ‡	28 d	0.6	0.22	90	100 mc.¶	C
Ce 143 }	33 h	*1.36*	*0.5*	22	100 mc.¶	C
Pr 142	19.3 h	2.14	1.9	750	100 mc.**	C
Eu 154	6.5 y	0.9	Present	250	100 mc.	D
Ta 182	97 d	*0.53*	1.22, *1.13*§	300	100 mc.	C
W 185	77 d	0.6	†	10	100 mc.	C
Os 191 }	32 h	1.5	Present	44	100 mc.	D
Os 193 }	17 d	0.35	Present	103	100 mc.	D
Ir 192, 194	{ 19 h { 70 d	2.2 Present	{ 1.35 { 0.3, 0.4	~ 250	100 mc.	C
Au 198	2.7 d	0.8	0.12, 0.44	6,000	100 mc.**	C
Hg 197 }	{ 64 h { 25 h	{ K, e- { K, e-	{ 0.075 { 0.13, 0.16	11	100 mc.	D
Hg 203, 205 }	51.5 d	*0.3*	0.28	16	100 mc.	D
Tl 206	3.5 y	0.87		2	10 mc.	D
Bi 210‡	5.0 d	1.17		9	10 mc.	C

* May be raised in special circumstances.
† Radioactive contaminant will be present from (n,p) reaction.
‡ Radioactive (nonisotopic) daughter will be present.
§ Complex.
‖ See Table 5.
¶ See Tables 1–3.
** See Table 6.

action decays to a radioactive daughter which is nonisotopic with its parent and with the source material.

A separation of the desired active species from the stable parent and from any (n,γ)-induced radioisotopes of this parent must usually be made before use. Since the parent exists in bulk and there is often formed a large amount of radioactive material which is isotopic with the parent, the processing is not always a simple matter. The same considerations hold in the case of daughters of neutron-induced decay chains.

Again, because of the desire to make available the greatest number of radioisotopes, *such carrier-free species will usually be supplied in the irradiated material, unseparated from the parent and radioisotopes of the parent.* In these cases, as in all others, any

TABLE 5

RADIOACTIVE ISOTOPES FROM TRANSMUTATION REACTIONS

(Items in italics—Manhattan Project data)

Method of formation	Active isotope	Half-life	Radiation Mev β	Target material	Yield mc./gram element irradiated	Conditions for shipment (C.F. = carrier-free)	Approx. max. unit quantity which may be made available	Class
(n,p)	C 14	~ 25,000 y	0.145	$Ca(NO_3)_2$		$BaCO_3$	1 mc.	A
	P 32	14.3 d	1.69	S	0.5*	{ In S { C.F. in 0.1 *N* HCl	500 mc.†, ‡	B B
	S 35	87.1 d	*0.17*	KCl or other chloride	1.5*	{ In KCl { C.F.	10 mc.†	B D
	Ca 45	180 d	*0.3*	Sc_2O_3	0.57*	{ In Sc { C.F. in conc. HCl	100 μc.†, ‡	C C
(n,α)	H 3	~ 31 y	0.015	Li salt		Unavailable at present		

* Experimental data.
† See Table 4.
‡ May be raised in special circumstances.

pertinent experience in a particular separation will be made available. In a few cases, where the element is rare or where the separation is too hazardous to be accomplished without special facilities, only separated material will be supplied.

The symbols in the "Class" column of Tables 4, 5, and 6 have essentially the same meaning as those in Tables 1, 2, and 3 except for "D," which here indicates a reaction which has been reported but has not yet been checked by present personnel.

Pile Irradiation Services for Other Than Radioisotope Production

Materials to be exposed in the pile for radioisotope production will usually be supplied and packaged by the Project. The reasons for this are: (1) to insure that materials and containers introduced into the pile for the desired radioisotope production have minimal parasitic neutron absorption and minimal subsequent radioactivity, and (2) to avoid the possibility of loss of the irradiated material or of danger to the operation of the pile.

Requests for special irradiations, in which the requester desires to furnish the material, may arise because of: (1) other intended purposes than radioisotope production or (2) especially prepared or very rare materials. Such irradiations may require special
108 handling which will be difficult to arrange during the inauguration period of the radioisotope distribution program. When sufficient experience has been gained in handling the normal irradiations and when a scale of charges is determined, special irradiation services may be announced.

Availability of Concentrated Stable Isotopes

In answer to numerous inquiries some brief comments are in order regarding the Project's ability to furnish concentrated stable isotopes. Arrangements have been completed thus far for the production, allocation, and sale of radioisotopes only. It may require considerable time to arrange these matters for such concentrated stable isotopes as may become available in excess of project needs.

The situation in regard to availability is now as follows:

(1) *Deuterium.* There is no heavy water or H 2 available.

(2) *Boron 10.* Small amounts of highly concentrated B 10 may be available for special neutron counter purposes. Prices and distribution mechanism are yet to be determined. These will be announced when arranged.

(3) *Carbon 13.* This isotope is mentioned separately only because of the wide interest in it for tracer purposes, particularly in organic chemistry and biology. There are no project facilities which can at present be converted to concentrate C 13 in production amounts without great expense both in the conversion of equipment and in operation. The cost of C 13 based on operational expenses alone would be considerably higher than costs quoted for C 13 concentrated by chemical exchange methods.

(4) *Isotopes of elements 3 to 82.* Small experimental lots of isotopes of nongaseous elements have been concentrated for project nuclear researches using electromagnetic pilot plant facilities of the Tennessee Eastman Corporation at Oak Ridge.

TABLE 6

Radioactive Isotopes From (n,γ)-produced Chains

(Items in italics—Manhattan Project data)

Active daughter isotope	Half-life	Radiation Mev β	Radiation Mev γ	Target material	Half-life of parent	Yield mc./gram element irradiated	Conditions for shipment	Approx. max. unit quantity which may be made available	Class
As 77	*40 h*	*0.8*		GeO_2	12.0 h	0.9	In GeO_2	1 mc.†	D
Rh 105	36 h	0.5		RuO_2	4.0 h	7.2	In RuO_2	10 mc.	D
Ag 111	7.5 d	0.8		Pd	26 m	9.7	In Pd	10 mc.	C
I 131	8.0 d	0.6	{ 0.367 0.080	Te	30 h	2.5*	{ In Te C.F. in 0.5 *N* H_2SO_4	100 mc.	B C
Cs 131	*10.2 d*	*K*		*$BaCO_3$*	*12 d*	~ 0.4*	{ In $BaCO_3$ C.F. in 0.1 *N* HCl	100 μc.†	B C
Pr 143	13.8 d	1.0		CeO_2	33 h	9.1*	{ In Ce C.F. in 0.1 *N* HCl	10 mc.†	B C
Au 199	3.3 d	1.01	0.45	Pt	31 m	19.3	In Pt	†	D

* Experimental data. † See Table 4.

Studies have only recently begun on production costs and on the obtainable quality and quantity of concentrated materials. In general, production is quite expensive, and it is difficult to achieve the high isotopic purity desired for many nuclear studies. Arrangements may be formulated for nonproject distribution of experimental lots after more experience has been gained with concentration and assay methods and after project needs become more clear.

As the situation warrants, announcements will be made concerning the availability of concentrated stable isotopes.

Charges

Charges will be made for irradiated materials and processed isotopes, as is the case for many widely useful products resulting from other research efforts. Pending experience, a reasonable charge is considered to be one based on the "out-of-pocket" operational expenses necessitated by the nonproject production and service program. Charges will not include costs of rental, or construction of plant and major facilities or of research and development directed toward the supplying of isotopes in general. The Project will supply the major facilities and develop the production methods, but will assess a charge for the additional running expenses of man power and materials incurred by the filling of nonproject requests. Shipping expenses will be paid by the requester. Details of these arrangements and the prices to be charged may be obtained upon request from the Isotopes Branch of the Manhattan District Research Division.

Mechanism for Making Requests

As explained in the section on "Principles of Allocation and Distribution," radioactive materials will not initially be distributed directly to private individuals but only to accredited institutions or organizations. However, materials will be allocated to an individual or a department for the specific uses proposed in the request.

A request may be initiated by a responsible applicant in an accredited institution by a short letter to the Isotopes Branch, Research Division, Manhattan District, P. O. Box E, Oak Ridge, Tennessee. This letter should request application forms, price quotations, and any essential information not contained in this notice. It should indicate briefly the radioisotopes desired, the approximate quantities needed, and the use to be made of the materials. If the desired material can be produced or made available and the intended use is one for which the isotope is suited, application forms will be furnished the applicant. These forms will permit applicants to supply in a concise and uniform manner the necessary detailed information on the basis of which the reviewers and the nonproject Advisory Subcommittee on Allocation and Distribution will be able to recommend action.

Action on an initial formal application cannot be initiated unless it has been indicated on the application that, when material is allotted, an "Agreement for Order and Receipt of Radioactive Materials" will be negotiated by the business administration of the requesting institution. This agreement relates to business and legal responsibilities in connection with the ordering, receipt, application, and disposal of radioactive materials by the applicant. The honoring of subsequent applications from the same individual or department can be arranged on a continuing basis by the indication of authorization for this in the originally negotiated agreement. All correspondence concerning requests and all forms should be addressed to the Isotopes Branch, as indicated above.

RADIOACTIVE IODINE THERAPY

Effect on Functioning Metastases of Adenocarcinoma of the Thyroid

S. M. SEIDLIN, M.D.
L. D. MARINELLI, M.A.
and
ELEANOR OSHRY, B.S.
New York

Therapy of neoplastic disease usually consists of two phases: first, the treatment of the primary focus and, second, that of metastases. Specifically, in adenocarcinoma of the thyroid, the primary site together with its immediate extensions is conventionally treated by surgery, radiation or both. Distant metastases, if treated, are usually subjected to palliative external irradiation. This paper is a report of successful therapy of a case of metastatic adenocarcinoma of the thyroid treated by the principle of specific internal irradiation with radioactive iodine.

The earliest study of the uptake of radioactive iodine in 2 cases of carcinoma was reported by Hamilton and his associates [1] in 1940. In 1942 he described 2 more cases [2] in which tracer doses of radioactive iodine had been given to the patients prior to the removal of carcinomatous thyroids. Radioautographs of the excised glands showed no significant deposition of the radioactive iodine in malignant areas in any of these cases.

In April 1942, Keston, Ball, Frantz and Palmer [3] reported the first positive evidence of pickup of the radioactive iodine by a metastasis from a carcinoma of the thyroid. In a patient with multiple lesions, Geiger counter measurements showed appreciable uptake of radioactive iodine in only one of the metastases. Subsequently, from the autopsy, these authors [4] reported that "the bulk of the metastatic tissue was undifferentiated. The metastasis which showed consistent uptake of iodine was the only one which grossly resembled thyroid tissue and which, microscopically, showed chiefly well differentiated tumor."

Leiter, Seidlin, Marinelli and Baumann [5] in a report of 2 cases (1 of which is the subject of the present paper) of hyperthyroidism due to adenocarcinoma of the thyroid and to functioning metastases showed that the effect of thiouracil on the basal metabolic rate, plasma cholesterol, blood iodine and excretion of radioactive iodine in these patients was in every respect

---

From the Medical Division and Department of Medical Physics of the Montefiore Hospital and the Physics Department of the Memorial Hospital.

A preliminary report of this work was presented at the Clinical Research Meeting of the New York Academy of Medicine on May 16, 1945.

Aided by grants from the Dazian Foundation for Medical Research and from the Lederle Laboratories to Dr. S. M. Seidlin at Montefiore Hospital.

The cooperation of the staffs of the Massachusetts Institute of Technology and Washington University cyclotrons and of Dr. R. D. Evans made this work possible.

Dr. Louis Leiter, Chief of the Medical Division of Montefiore Hospital, gave valuable assistance throughout this work, as did Dr. David Marine and Dr. S. H. Rosen in the field of thyroid pathology and Dr. E. J. Baumann in iodine chemistry. Dr. Solomon Fineman reviewed the roentgenograms. Valuable technical assistance was rendered by Elizabeth F. Focht, Ruth Hill, George Ross, Louella Tulip and Dr. A. A. Yalow.

1. Hamilton, J. G.; Soley, M. H., and Eichorn, K. B.: Deposition of Radioactive Iodine in Human Thyroid Tissue, Univ. California Publ., Pharmacol. **1:** 339-368, 1940.

2. Hamilton, J. G.: The Use of Radioactive Tracers in Biology and Medicine, Radiology **39:** 541-572 (Nov.) 1942.

3. Keston, A. S.; Ball, R. P.; Frantz, V. K., and Palmer, W. W.: Storage of Radioactive Iodine in a Metastasis from Thyroid Carcinoma, Science **95:** 362-363 (April 3) 1942.

4. Frantz, V. K.; Ball, R. P.; Keston, A. S., and Palmer, W. W.: Thyroid Carcinoma with Metastases: Studied with Radioactive Iodine, Ann. Surg. **119:** 668-669 (May) 1944.

5. Leiter, L.; Seidlin, S. M.; Marinelli, L. D., and Baumann, E. J.: Adenocarcinoma of the Thyroid with Hyperthyroidism and Functional Metastases: I. Studies with Thiouracil and Radio-Iodine, J. Clin. Endocrinol. **6:** 247-261 (March) 1946.

similar to the response already described [6] in the literature on ordinary thyrotoxicosis or hyperthyroidism. This indicates that thiouracil suppresses hormone production by functioning metastases from adenocarcinoma of the thyroid as readily as it inhibits this process in the hyperplastic thyroid of ordinary hyperthyroidism.

Since physiologically the thyroid cell, normal or malignant, cannot distinguish between inert and radioactive iodine, we are utilizing the normal affinity of this cell for iodine as a method of "selective irradiation" of a type of carcinoma of the thyroid. We now report the results of three years' study of the therapeutic effect of radioactive iodine in 1 case of metastatic carcinoma of the thyroid, in which all demonstrable metastases were shown to pick up radioactive iodine.

Radioactive iodine, as used in this and similar studies, consists of a mixture, in varying proportions, of two isotopes, I^{131}, half life 12.6 hours, and I^{131}, half life 8.0 days, prepared in a cyclotron by the bombardment of tellurium with deuterons. These two isotopes are chemically identical with stable iodine and cannot be separated by ordinary chemical or physiologic methods and processes. Both I^{130} and I^{131} emit beta rays (high speed electrons) which cause intense ionization within a few millimeters of tissue, as well as gamma rays which cause a negligible amount of ionization within the body and are sufficiently penetrating to be detected readily by an external Geiger counter.

REPORT OF CASE

Observations Prior to Radioactive Iodine Therapy.—Thyroidectomy: B. B., a man aged 51, had in 1923, at the age of 30, undergone a thyroidectomy because of substernal goiter and pressure symptoms on the trachea. He had no thyrotoxicosis. The histologic diagnosis was "malignant adenoma."

Pathologic Report: The pathologic report gave a gross description of three pieces of tissue received. The first one measured 5 by 5 by 3 cm. It was firm in consistency, and the cut section showed a fairly dense central core of connective tissue. No cystic or hemorrhagic areas were observed. The outer portion of the section disclosed a brownish yellow semipurulent material. The remaining two pieces of tissue were relatively the same in general structure but averaged about 2.5 cm. in thickness.

On microscopic examination, sections of the goiter showed no normal structures. Sections of tissue revealed definite fibrous change and there was an abundant pinkish hyaline-like stroma manifesting cell formation. There was a definite, highly atypical epithelial overgrowth which showed abundant growth and a tendency toward cord formation. In these areas no acini resembling the normal were seen. The nuclei of the cells took a rich blue stain. The growth showed no definite capsule surrounding it. Areas showing cartilage formation were present. No hemorrhage or infection was observed.

Recurrence and Laminectomy: Postoperatively there were no symptoms of hypothyroidism. The patient was in apparent good health for fifteen years. Then there developed palpitation, nervousness, loss of weight and signs typical of hyperthyroidism. In addition, severe pains developed in the lower back and radiated down the legs. On examination at another hospital in October 1939, a small pulsating tumor was found in the midline of the back at the level of the twelfth thoracic vertebra. Visualization by injection of diodrast showed the tumor to be extradural and extraosseous. Roentgenograms of the skeleton revealed no osseous lesions. The basal metabolic rate was + 40 per cent. A laminectomy was performed in November 1939. The tumor proved to be a metastatic carcinoma of the thyroid (fig. 1).

The histologic report revealed that the slide [7] showed several large ragged fragments of tissue, one of which contained spicules of bone and consisted of irregular cellular areas formed by broad hyalinized stroma bands. The general pattern was the same in all portions and consisted of irregular, often elongated, closely packed follicles with infoldings of the lining epithelium which varied from cuboidal to low columnar. There was no well formed stroma. Traces of granular colloid-like material were present in some follicles. In some areas the follicles appeared to have atrophied leaving the hyalinized-like bands previously mentioned. There were large areas of necrosis and some foci of hemorrhage. No mitosis was seen.

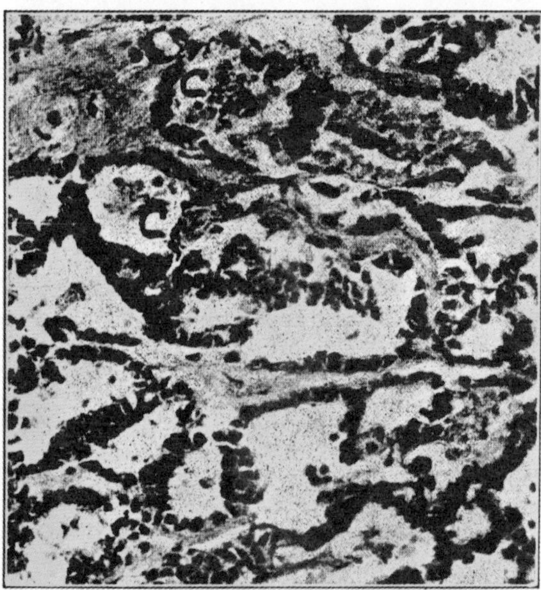

Fig. 1.—Photomicrograph of metastatic tumor in the twelfth thoracic vertebra magnified 400 times. Note follicular architecture and traces of granular colloid-like material (*c*) in some follicles.

The nuclei were fairly regular, dark and vesicular. The diagnosis was metastatic adenocarcinoma of the thyroid.[8]

Treatment and Course: A thyroid crisis developed postoperatively. A few weeks later an exploratory operation was performed in the region of the thyroid and no thyroid tissue, normal or malignant, was found. Because of continuing pain, physiotherapy was given to the patient. In the next two years the symptoms and signs of hyperthyroidism increased. In December 1941 the basal metabolic rate was + 45 per cent. In addition, roentgen ray films of the lungs revealed "numerous circular deposits in the lower lobe on the left side and in the cardiohepatic angle on the right side, strongly suspicious of metastatic lesions." There was also radiographic evidence of destruction of the right upper femur (1.0 by 2.0 cm.) and the second rib on the left side. A gastrointestinal roentgenologic series was negative. A film of the pelvis taken at this time was reported negative for metastases, but our subsequent review (1946) of the plate revealed a small area (0.6 by 1.8 cm.) of early destructive changes in the inner border of the left ileum, above the acetabulum, just below the incisura ischiadica major. From December 1941 to February 1942 high voltage

6. Mackenzie, C. G., and Mackenzie, J. B.: Effect of Sulfonamides and Thioureas on the Thyroid Gland and Basal Metabolism, Endocrinology **32:** 185-209 (Feb.) 1943. Astwood, E. B.: The Chemical Nature of Compounds Which Inhibit the Function of the Thyroid Gland, J. Pharmacol. & Exper. Therap. **78:** 79-89 (May) 1943. Williams, R. H., and Bissell, G. W.: Thiouracil in the Treatment of Thyrotoxicosis, New England J. Med. **229:** 97-108 (July 15) 1943. Williams, R. H., and Clute, H. M.: Thiouracil in the Treatment of Thyrotoxicosis, ibid. **230:** 657-667 (June 1) 1944. Rawson, R. W.; Evans, R. D.; Means, J. H.; Peacock, W. C.; Lerman, J., and Cortell, R. R.: The Effect of Thiouracil on the Thyroid Glands of Patients with Graves' Disease, J. Clin. Endocrinol. **4:** 1-11 (Jan.) 1944. Franklin, A. L.; Chaikoff, I. L., and Lerner, S. R.: The Influence of Goitrogenic Substances on the Conversion in Vitro of Inorganic Iodine to Thyroxine and Diiodotyrosine by Thyroid Tissue with Radioactive Iodine as Indicator, J. Biol. Chem. **153:** 151-162 (April) 1944. Rawson, R. W.; Tannheimer, J. F., and Peacock, W. C.: The Uptake of Radioactive Iodine by the Thyroids of Rats Made Goitrous by Potassium Thiocyanate and by Thiouracil, Endocrinology **34:** 245-253 (April) 1944.

7. Courtesy of Dr. H. L. Jaffe, Hospital for Joint Diseases.

8. The slide was reviewed by Dr. David Marine.

roentgen therapy was administered[9] as follows: dorsolumbar spine, 4,060 r; right upper femur, 3,180 r delivered through three fields. This course of therapy did not produce any symptomatic improvement.

Radioactive Iodine Therapy.—Observations at Hospitalization: On admission to Montefiore Hospital on April 20, 1942, the patient still had symptoms of pain in the lower part of the spine, in addition to the previously mentioned symptoms of hyperthyroidism.

The physical examination showed a rather small, emaciated, poorly developed man, aged 48, weight 38 Kg. and height 146 cm.; he was hyperkinetic, his blood pressure was 128 mm. of mercury systolic and 50 diastolic; his pulse rate was 100 to 110. There were no eye signs. There was a thyroidectomy scar in the neck, and no thyroid tissue was palpable. The heart was normal except for tachycardia. The lungs were clear. There was a laminectomy scar and tenderness over the dorsolumbar spine. The eye grounds were normal. The skin was warm, and there was a coarse tremor of the hands. The basal metabolic rate on May 7, 1942 was + 36 per cent. The plasma cholesterol about this time was 114 mg. per hundred cubic centimeters and the blood iodine[10] soon thereafter was 11.9 micrograms per hundred cubic centimeters.

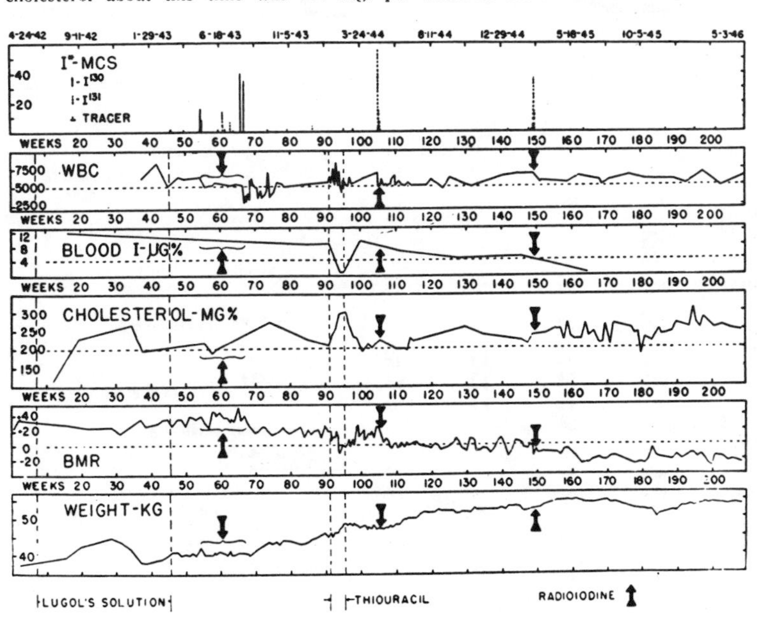

Fig. 2.—Response of clinical criteria to the administration of I^*.

Other laboratory examinations revealed nothing of special significance. The blood chemistry tests showed calcium, 10.3 mg., and phosphorus, 3.9 mg. per hundred cubic centimeters; phosphatase (alkaline) 12.2 Bodansky units; total serum protein, 6.7 Gm.; serum albumin, 3.2 Gm.; serum globulin, 3.5 Gm., and uric acid, 3.9 mg. per hundred cubic centimeters. The Wassermann and Kahn tests were negative; the blood count was within normal limits. Urinalysis was negative. The Ewald test showed free hydrochloric acid, none; combined acid 20 per cent.

A roentgenologic examination of the chest on April 25, 1942 revealed several rounded shadows suggestive of metastases in the lower lobe of the left lung; an extensive destructive lesion (5 cm. long) which involved the lateral and posterior aspect of the second rib on the left side; a circumscribed shadow (3.2 by 1.1 cm.) in the left infraclavicular region, which seemingly arose from the involved rib and represented a soft tissue mass. A picture of the dorsolumbar spine on Nov. 10, 1942 disclosed evidence of laminectomy; the spinous processes of the eleventh and twelfth thoracic vertebrae and the first lumbar vertebra were missing, and osteoporosis involved all the vertebrae. The pelvis on April 25, 1942 showed a small area of bone absorption (0.6 by 2.3 cm.) along the medial aspect of the left ileum above the acetabulum. The femurs on Oct. 29, 1942 presented a small area (larger than in films of December 1941) of bone absorption in the cortex of the right femur just below the lesser trochanter.

In view of the evident hyperthyroidism, iodine as Lugol's solution was administered every day in doses varying from 1 to 6 cc., from June 13, 1942 to March 8, 1943.[5]

As shown in figure 2, a mild remission in the hyperthyroidism occurred in response to the iodine therapy. By January 1943, iodine given as Lugol's solution in doses of 3 to 4 cc. a day lost its effectiveness even in regard to the hyperthyroidism itself, and its continued administration produced little further improvement.

The lesions of the bone continued to grow, and pain persisted. Another course of roentgen therapy was instituted as follows: right upper femur 3,260 r through two fields, and left pelvis 1,985 r through two fields. There was no relief of pain.

Administration of Radioactive Iodine: In March 1943 a tracer dose of radioactive iodine was given orally in the form of sodium iodide in water. This method of administration has been used for all doses. Geiger counter measurements revealed iodine retention by all the known lesions plus two previously unsuspected ones (fig. 3); one in the skull and one, not evident in the roentgenograms, located in the region of the ischium. During the taking of Geiger counter measurements, the patient asked that the counter be placed on the right parietal part of his head, for, he stated, there is a pain there which "is not a headache." Surprisingly, the counter registered the uptake of radioactive iodine. A subsequent roentgenogram (May 18, 1943) of the skull was reported as disclosing a fairly sharply circumscribed area of bone rarefaction (3.7 by 3.5 cm.) in the right posterior parietal region. At this time an exhaustive study of radioactive iodine uptake in the neck was made, and no evidence of residual functioning thyroid tissue could be established (see later comment). Due to technical difficulties, no attempt was made to study the radioactive iodine content of the lung metastases reported by the roentgen ray diagnostic department.

Measurements on urine after several tracer doses revealed that the patient excreted a relatively small amount (30 per cent to 40 per cent) of the tracer dose over a seventy-two to ninety-six hour period. The first course of radioactive iodine therapy, a total of 102 millicuries of the 12.6 hour isotope (I^{130}) and 20.5 millicures of the 8 day isotope (I^{131}), was administered between May and August, 1943 (see the accompanying table). The estimated radiation dose[11] to the tumors was 10,600 equivalent r,[12] whereas that for the blood was 70 equivalent r.

Since this course was administered in fractions of varying potency, it was possible to determine the effect of the different radiation doses on the leukocyte count. The I^{131} had no

9. Radiation dosages in this paper refer to tumor doses exclusively. Tumor depths were estimated from roentgenograms. Data used here were obtained from Rosh, R., and Raider, L.: Radiation Therapy of Carcinoma of the Thyroid, Radiology **44:** 556-564 (June) 1945 and a personal communication from Dr. Rosh.

10. Baumann, E. J., and Metzger, N.: On the Amount of Iodine in the Blood, J. Biol. Chem. **121:** 231-234 (Oct.) 1937.

11. This dose and the following therapeutic doses are calculated on the basis of an effective tumor volume of 312 cc. (vide infra) and on the basis of I^* (I^* refers to radioactive iodine without specifying the isotope) retained; that is, that administered minus that excreted in the urine. The possible change in effective tumor volume with time has been neglected. It would have been preferable, and is planned in the future to estimate tumor dose by actual measurements in vivo.

12. Equivalent roentgens as used herein are defined and discussed in Marinelli, L. D.: Dosage Determinations with Radioactive Isotopes, Am. J. Roentgenol. **47:** 210-216 (Feb.) 1942.

significant effect while the I 130 had a considerable, though temporary, depressing influence (fig. 2). The expanded curve, figure 4, shows that after one dose of 40 millicuries of I 130 the white blood cell count dropped from 5,150 to 2,900 in one week. The blood count returned to normal in ten days even though another dose of 35 millicuries of I 130 was given while the count was low.

The resulting improvement in the patient's clinical picture was definite in the course of the next few months. By November 1943 the pains diminished, the basal metabolic rate dropped from an average level of above + 35 per cent to about + 20 per cent, the patient gained about 7 Kg. in weight and roentgenologically there was no demonstrable growth of the metastases.

Biopsy: On Nov. 6, 1943, a dissection biopsy of the metastasis in the second rib on the left side was performed by Dr. A. H. Aufses. In order to obtain a radioautograph of this lesion and to ascertain the radioactive iodine concentration in the tumor tissue, a large tracer dose of I 131 (5 millicuries) was administered eight days before the operation. To remove the tumor on the second rib on the left side it was necessary to perform a scapula-mobilizing incision, with

From these figures and from the total urinary excretion up to the time of the biopsy it is possible to calculate the apparent tumor weight in the patient, assuming that the iodine concentration is uniform throughout the metastases and that no appreciable radioactive iodine is present in nontumorous tissues. This value is 312 Gm. It is interesting to note at this point that an independent calculation of the tumor volume based on the contour of the metastases in the roentgen ray films agrees with the above value.

A comparison of the biopsy tissue (figs. 5 and 9) with a section of the tissue removed on laminectomy in October 1939 (fig. 1) revealed close similarity.

Pathologic Report: The pathologic report was as follows: On macroscopic examination the fresh specimen was an oval mass measuring 7.5 by 4.3 by 2.5 cm. and weighing 41.9 Gm. It was enclosed in a grayish white capsule about 0.5 cm. thick on the surface of which there were, in places, some fibrofatty tissue and muscle. Attached to the capsule on one surface there was a piece of rib measuring 3.5 cm. in length to which was attached some fragments of muscle and fascia. The mass was moderately soft, rather rubbery in consistency. On section, the tissue presented a mottled appearance, predomi-

Complete Tabulation of I Administered*

Date	Week	Iodine: Carrier (Mg.)	Iodine: Radioactive (Mc.)	Isotope	Excretion, per Cent per 24 Hours: 1	2	3	4	Remarks
3/11/43	45	0.15	Tr.‡	....	60.0	7.5	1.8	0.5	Iodine as lugol's solution 6/13/42 to 3/8/43
4/ 6/43	49	?	Tr.	....	25.0	15.0	...	...	
5/11/43	54	<0.5	17	I^{130}	11.7	...	...	...	
5/12/43	54	?	7.6	I^{130}	....	...	...	...	
6/15/43	59	0.3	2	I^{130}	14.1	3.0	...	...	
6/23/43	60	Neg.	13.5	I^{131}	26.8	2.6	...	...	
6/26/43	61	?	Tr.	....	....	...	...	...	
7/ 9/43	63	?	7.0	I^{131}	19.5	3.3	2.7	2.5	
7/15/43	63	?	Tr.	....	....	...	...	...	
7/29/43	65	<0.5	40.0 †	I^{130}	20.3	4.1	3.4	3.1	
8/ 5/43	66	<0.5	35.0 †	I^{130}	39.3	5.3	4.1	3.7	3 day stool, 2.3 per cent
9/22/43	73	Tr.	Tr.	....	15.1	1.6	2.3	2.8	
10/30/43	79	Tr.	2.0	I^{131}	27.4	4.4	2.9	2.8	
12/19/43	86	0.3	5.0	I^{131}	33.6	3.6	1.2	2.1	
2/21/44	95	0.03	Tr.	....	79.2	3.7	1.7	1.4	Pre-biopsy
3/10/44	98	0.1	Tr.	....	82.0	2.6	2.2	1.8	Thiouracil 1/23/44 to 2/21/44
4/28/44	105	2.5	{ 55.4 † / 3.2 †	{ I^{131} / I^{130} }	45.9	...	...	...	Blood curve taken
4/29/44	105	?	13.8	I^{131}	....	...	...	...	Refeeding
4/30/44	105	?	6.3	I^{131}	....	...	...	...	Refeeding
8/ 2/44	118	0.25	Tr.	....	26.0	2.8	1.3	1.0	
1/13/45	142	<0.2	Tr.	....	45.4	3.5	1.4	1.0	
2/23/45	148	<0.5	Tr.	....	?	?	?	?	
3/ 2/45	149	0.01	Tr.	....	34.1	...	...	...	Thyrotropic hormone 2/8/45 to 2/25/45
3/ 3/45	149	1.0	{ 41.6 † / 6.0 †	{ I^{131} / I^{130} }	54.3	7.7	1.6	...	Blood curve taken
3/ 6/45	149	?	13.4	I^{131}	....	...	...	...	Refeeding
6/11/45	163	0.3	Tr.	....	59.0	8.2	1.9	1.7	
11/24/45	187	<0.002	Tr.	....	59.8	0.6	0.9	...	
1/21/46	195	<0.04	Tr.	....	54.9	8.1	1.8	1.2	
3/ 6/46	201	14.0	Tr.	....	74.7	12.4	1.9	0.4	Large amount of carrier iodine

* I* refers to radioactive iodine without specifying the isotope.[11]
‡ Tr. indicates a tracer dose.
† Measurements of initial activity in millicuries carefully carried out.

incision through the muscles of the posterior chest wall. The postoperative course was uneventful, and the patient made an excellent recovery.

Several radioautographs of the biopsy specimen were obtained by following in general the technic already described by Hamilton.[2] Figure 6 shows a representative radioautograph and figure 7 is the eosin and hematoxylin stained section from which it was made. A superimposition[13] of these two photo-
114 graphs is shown in figure 8. A detailed comparison between radioautograph and photomicrograph shows specific localization of the radioactive iodine within the regions of viable thyroid tumor cells.

The total iodine content per gram of dry tissue of the biopsy specimen was 0.192 mg. with a thyroxin fraction of 17.4 per cent. The radioactive iodine content of the tumor tissue at the time of the biopsy was determined on four separate fresh specimens, weighing 0.28, 0.17, 1.49 and 2.05 Gm., respectively. The results were 0.18, 0.16, 0.19 and 0.20 per cent of the administered dose per gram of wet tissue.[14]

13. This composite photograph was made by John M. Walke of the Physics Department of Memorial Hospital.
14. Dr. Albert Keston made an independent determination on two of the specimens.

nantly pale brownish with small and larger irregular dark red areas of congestion and hemorrhage, small translucent gray and yellowish foci and a few small, opaque, yellowish areas, probably of necrosis. Some thin grayish white strands of fibrous tissue could be seen running through the mass. The portion of rib attached to the mass was invaded on its adherent surface by tumor similar to and continuous with that of the mass, and fine bony spicules could be palpated in the latter for a distance of 1 cm. or more from the rib.

Microscopic examination revealed that the specimen consisted of sections of the tumor fixed in solution of formaldehyde and in Orth's solution and of decalcified portions of the tumor which included invaded rib. The tumor was surrounded by a thick capsule of dense fibrous tissue covered by fibrofatty tissue containing striated muscle fibers as well as some nerves and thickened arteries. The muscle fibers showed considerable atrophy and degeneration. Occasional focal infiltrations of small round cells were seen. The rather extensive hemorrhage in the capsule and surrounding tissue was probably largely traumatic. There was slight invasion of the capsule by tumor in a few places. In all sections the central two thirds or more of the tumor showed extensive necrosis, hemorrhage and edema. This portion of the tumor consisted largely of fibrinous material which in areas was loose and fibrillar and in other places, dense and hyaline-like. Mixed with this in varying amounts were edema fluid, red blood corpuscles and in a few foci, necrotic and disintegrating polymorphonuclear leukocytes. Small and larger foci of viable tumor, frequently compressed, distorted and

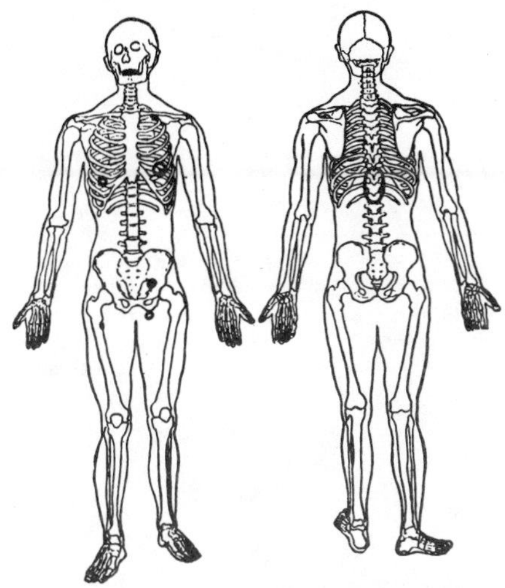

Fig. 3.—Location of metastases; solid black areas indicate osseous lesions, open circles indicate extraosseous lesions.

degenerating, were also seen in this central area. In places bands of edematous and hyaline-like stroma covered by flattened cells separated islands of fibrinous material, and in other places spindle cells growing in this material suggested organization. The peripheral, viable portion of the tumor disclosed little variation in architecture. It consisted of well differentiated follicles which disclosed considerable variation in size and shape but were predominantly small. The larger ones frequently showed infoldings and occasionally buds of new follicles in the walls. Some were widely dilated and others, compressed and slitlike. The follicles were lined for the most part by fairly uniform large cuboidal cells and in many instances by columnar cells. These cells had abundant acidophilic cytoplasm and fairly large, round, usually central but frequently basal, vesicular and hyperchromatic nuclei with

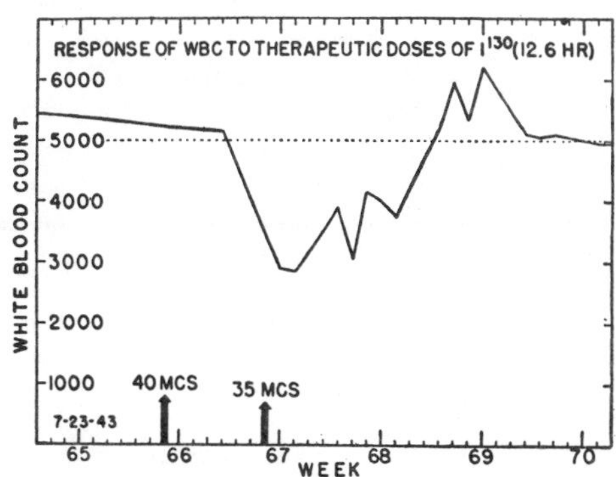

Fig. 4.—Effect of large amounts of I^{130} on the white blood cell count.

fairly large nucleoli. No mitotic figures were seen. The nuclei on the whole were uniform, but an occasional large hyperchromatic nucleus was seen as well as occasional small pyknotic ones. In large areas the abundant cytoplasm was deeply acidophilic, and the cells resembled the so-called Hürthle cell. In some areas distended follicles were lined by low cuboidal or flattened epithelium. Although most of the follicles were empty or contained some red blood corpuscles and fibrin-like material, a considerable number contained a homogeneous colloid-like material which took a pale pink stain. In some areas the follicles were closely packed and separated only by narrow strands of connective tissue which contained many thin-walled sinusoid-like vascular channels, frequently engorged. In other areas the connective tissue septums were widened by edema and hemorrhage so that the follicles became widely separated. In still other areas there was appreciable fibrosis with atrophy of follicles; the fibrous tissue was cellular in some foci and partly hyalinized in others. Numerous hematoidin crystals were present in areas of recent hemorrhage. A few spicules of bone, some of them necrotic, were seen deep within the tumor.

Sections taken through rib and adjacent tumor showed invasion of the bone by tumor with replacement of the marrow by a loose connective tissue. There was active formation of new bone, usually by apposition on old trabeculae, together with a lesser degree of osseous destruction. Spicules of bone

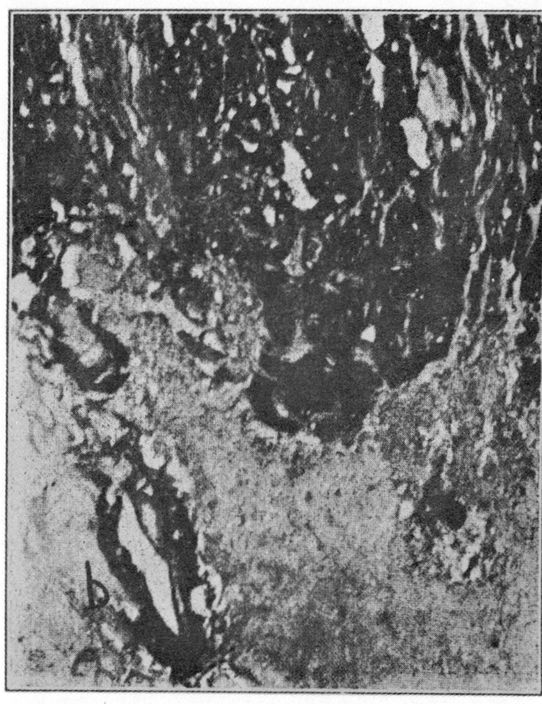

Fig. 5.—Circled area in figure 7 slightly reduced from a low power magnification of 25 times. Note narrow zone of viable tumor around blood vessel (*b*) which showed uptake of radioactive iodine in figure 6.

were seen deep within the tumor itself; some of them were new bone arising from connective tissue septums. Similar new bone formation from connective tissue was seen in one place in the capsule.

The diagnosis was metastatic thyroid adenocarcinoma of the differentiated small follicle type.[15]

Subsequent Treatment and Course: From Jan. 23 to Feb. 21, 1944, the patient was submitted to a course of treatment with thiouracil. This was done to check further on the functional nature of the metastases. The thiouracil therapy produced a striking remission of the hyperthyroidism, which, however, promptly recurred after the treatment was discontinued. The effect of thiouracil on the objective criteria of hyperthyroidism is shown in figure 2.

By the end of April 1944 the patient's condition had reached what might be called a state of equilibrium. His weight remained unchanged for two months at the level of 48 Kg., with basal metabolic rate at about + 10 per cent and the

15. Dr. S. H. Rosen and Dr. David Marine.

plasma cholesterol level between 200 and 214 mg. per hundred cubic centimeters. The blood iodine on March 24 was 9.4 micrograms per hundred cubic centimeters. Roentgenograms taken on April 21, 1944, showed no detectable changes in the various metastases. The second therapeutic dose of radioactive iodine, 55.4 millicuries of the eight day isotope, was administered on April 28, 1944. Twenty-seven per cent of this dose (13.8 millicuries) was extracted from a twenty-one hour urine collection [16] and readministered on April 29. A second fraction from urine was obtained later (6.3 millicuries) and readministered on April 30. Thus a total of 75.5 millicuries was administered within three days, giving a radiation dose of 18,200 equivalent r to the tumor and 64 equivalent r to the blood. The white blood cell count showed only a slight temporary fall from 6,000 to 4,500, which, in our opinion, was not significant. The basal metabolic rate dropped to zero in about three weeks and remained at about this level until March 1945. The plasma cholesterol fluctuated from a level of about 200 mg. per hundred cubic centimeters to a somewhat higher level. The blood iodine level dropped to 6.5 micrograms on June 10, 1944, to 4.7 micrograms on Oct. 7, 1944 and to 5.1 micrograms per hundred cubic centimeters on Feb. 8, 1945. The patient's weight began to rise about three weeks after the administration of the therapeutic dose of radioactive iodine and continued to rise steadily from 48 Kg. in April 1944 to 53 Kg. in January 1945. Shortly after this second therapeutic dose of radioactive iodine a temporary sharply circumscribed alopecia appeared over the area corresponding to the skull metastasis. The patient's general well-being improved, his pains diminished, his locomotion improved, and he complained of getting fat. Roentgenograms on Aug. 19, 1944 and Feb. 6, 1945 showed no change.

From Feb. 8 to 25, 1945, the patient was given intramuscular injections of thyrotropic factor (Armour's; Rowlands-Parkes' units per cubic centimeter). The injections were given in divided doses every one or two days for a total of 33 cc. in eighteen days. During this interval of treatment there was no rise in the basal metabolic rate, no significant change in plasma cholesterol and a slight fall in blood iodine (from 5.1 to 4.1 micrograms per hundred cubic centimeters). Bioassays of the urine for thyrotropic hormone [17] both before and during the interval of this treatment were negative, indicating that the patient's own thyrotropic hormone was inactivated by the tumor tissue.[18]

On March 3, 1945, the third therapeutic dose of radioactive iodine was given. It consisted of 41.6 millicures of I^{131} plus 16.0 millicuries recovered from the urine and fed three days later. The total of 57.6 millicuries gave a tumor dose of 11,600 equivalent r, a blood dose of 41 equivalent r. The patient's weight increased and the basal metabolic rate, which was in the normal range immediately before the treatment, dropped to —27 per cent in about three months and has remained consistently low. The plasma cholesterol increased slightly and has remained above the pretreatment level. The blood iodine dropped from 4.1 micrograms per hundred cubic centimeters immediately before this third therapeutic dose to 0.8 microgram per hundred cubic centimeters three months later.

The patient's general condition is good. He moves freely about the hospital and is engaged in occupational therapy.

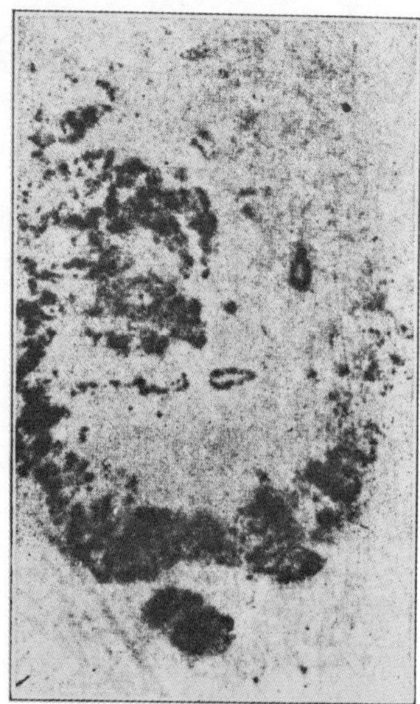

Fig. 6.—Radioautograph of an entire unstained section of metastatic tumor in second rib on the left side with magnification slightly reduced from 8 times, showing distribution of radioactive iodine in the viable tissue.

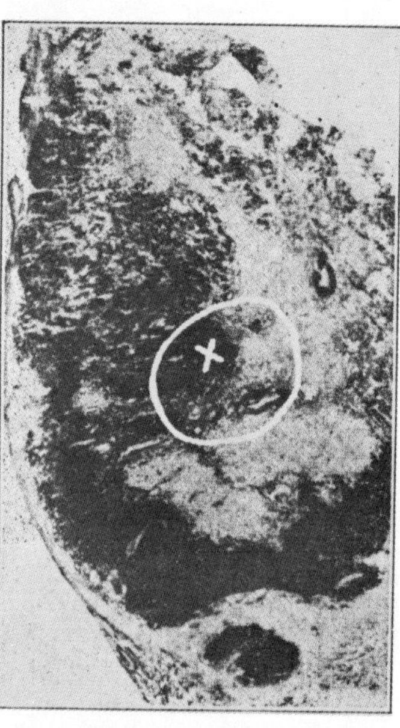

Fig. 7.—Photomicrograph of section used for figure 6 stained with eosin and hematoxylin, same magnification. Note viable (dark) and necrotic (light) areas.

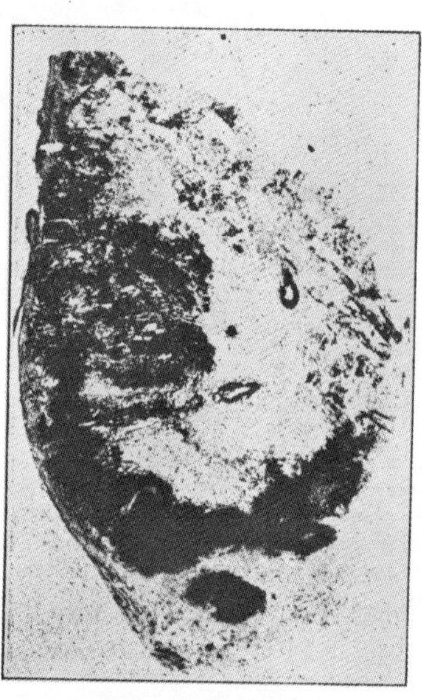

Fig. 8.—photograph of figures 6 and 7 superimposed, showing coincidence of radioactive iodine distribution with the viable tumor.

COMMENT

Adenocarcinoma of the thyroid is generally considered highly radioresistant. H. F. Hare [19] specifically stated that alveolar carcinoma of the thyroid is not changed histologically by 6,000 r (x-ray). For a successfully treated patient (his case 2) Hare gives the dimensions of the tumor and the interstitial radon dose employed. Calculations show the gamma ray dose to be close to 20,000 r, a value well beyond the reach of external radiation.

16. Dr. E. J. Baumann, Chemistry Department, Montefiore Hospital, developed a procedure for extracting iodine from urine so that it could be refed to the patient in the form of sodium iodide. This technic was utilized whenever the amount of I * involved warranted it. The efficiency of recovery was consistently high, 80 to 95 per cent.

17. Determinations were made on young guinea pigs weighing 200 Gm., using total weight of thyroid gland and degree of hyperplasia as criteria. Extraction of thyrotropic hormone from the urine followed the method described by Jones, M. S.: Study of Thyrotropic Hormone in Clinical States, Endocrinology **24**: 665-671 (May) 1939.

18. Seidlin, S. M.: The Metabolism of the Thyrotrophic and Gonadotrophic Hormones, Endocrinology **26**: 696-702 (April) 1940. Rawson, R. W.; Sterne, G. D., and Aub, J. C.: Physiological Reactions of the Thyroid-Stimulating Hormone of the Pituitary: I. Its Inactivation by Exposure to Thyroid Tissue in Vitro, ibid. **30**: 240-245 (Feb.) 1942.

19. Hare, H. F.: Radiation Treatment of Carcinoma of the Thyroid, Am. J. Roentgenol. **46**: 451-453 (Oct.) 1941.

Since 1 microcurie of 8 day iodine destroyed per gram of tissue gives approximately 150 equivalent r,[20] to achieve comparable dosage we must concentrate at least 133 microcuries in each cubic centimeter of tumor, if turnover is assumed to be zero. For our patient, with approximately 300 cc. of tumor tissue, such a dose would require that 40 millicures of I^{131} be fixed in the tumors. The actual amount to be fed, however, may be several times this amount, because of the loss of iodine by excretion and by deposition in other tissues, especially if normal thyroid tissue is present.

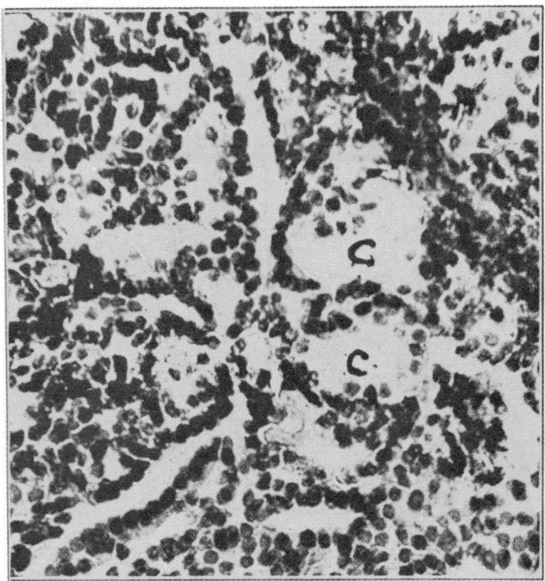

Fig. 9.—Higher magnification (400 times) of section taken at X in figure 7. Note follicular structure and colloid-like material (*c*) in a few follicles.

In addition to these rough quantitative considerations, criteria of a biologic nature, such as the time factor and lack of irradiation of the tumor bed beyond a few millimeters, must be considered in comparing the results of 8 day iodine beta ray therapy with those of 3.82 day radon gamma ray therapy. These remain to be assessed on the basis of additional experience.

Over a period of three years, our patient has received nearly 40,000 equivalent r to each of his tumors. In spite of the remarkable clinical improvement, it cannot be concluded that the functioning tumors have been completely destroyed because recent tracer studies, although showing a marked increase in excretion, still show localization of radioactive iodine in the lesions. Further therapy is indicated and is being planned, the limiting factor being the availability of the isotope in sufficient quantity. The criterion for completion of I * therapy will be the lack of radioactive iodine pickup by any of the known metastases, although the possibility remains that the tumors, even in the absence of any uptake, will not be completely destroyed.

20. A complete description of experimental methods and calculations will be given in a companion paper now in preparation.

All available roentgenograms taken of this patient since July 1939 were reviewed recently in order to evaluate as precisely as possible the progress of the various skeletal lesions. Between July and October of 1939, films were made of the spine, pelvis, skull, arms, legs and left femur. At this time all the regions were negative for metastases. In November 1939, the extraosseous metastatic tumor in the back was removed. By 1941 there were early lesions in the right femur, right ileum and chest as described in the case history. These lesions increased in size, and the one in the skull was discovered in 1943. Frequent plates were taken of all these regions from 1942 until the present, and they show that there was no increase in the area of bone destruction in any region after the first therapeutic dose of I * was administered in 1943. Representative films showing the progress of three of the lesions are shown in figures 10, 11 and 12.

The urinary excretion of radioactive iodine was followed after almost every dose, tracer or therapeutic; on several occasions the collection period was longer than a month. As an illustration, the data obtained after the dose of Aug. 5, 1943, is shown in figure 13. Plotted on semilogarithmic paper, the curve shows two distinct, consecutive rates of change in daily excretion, the break occurring three days after administration. In the same figure a second curve is shown which represents the daily excretion of radioactive iodine by this patient soon after the cessation of thiouracil therapy. The data as a whole seem consistent with the hypothesis that in both instances the excretion of radioactive iodine within three days of administration is governed by a mechanism different from the one which governs its excretion thereafter.

The concentration of radioactive iodine in the blood as a function of time was studied in order to gain information of physiologic and radiologic significance. Shown in figure 14 is a composite curve obtained after the administration of the last two therapeutic doses of radioactive iodine (April 28, 1944; March 3, 1945). The individual determinations pertaining to each study are shown in detail. The data of Frantz and her associates[4] are also shown for comparison. From the curve it is seen that the level of I * in the blood

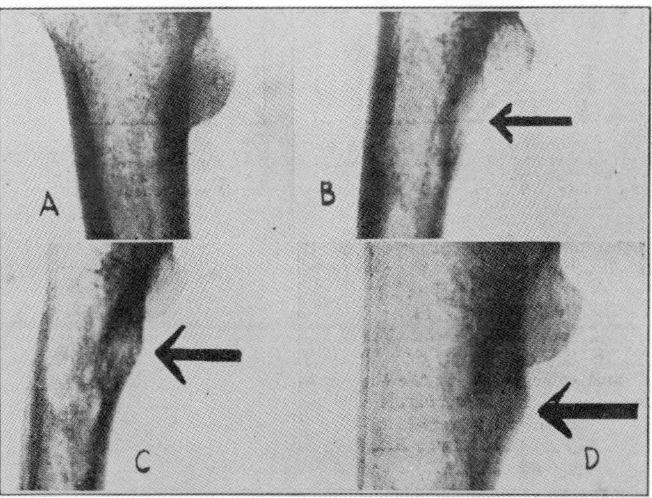

Fig. 10.—Roentgenologic appearance of lesion of the femur on *A*, Oct. 30, 1939; *B*, Oct. 29, 1942; *C*, June 22, 1944, and *D* (a higher magnification), May 22, 1946.

remains essentially constant for a considerable period after the first day. An analysis of the detailed data obtained on this particular patient indicates that the curve represents three different phases; a rapid initial turnover (about twenty-four hours) which is succeeded by a stabilized level of one week's duration, and finally, a slow but steady decline.

Many authors have reported significant drops in the white blood count after the administration of radioactive isotopes other than iodine. Our experience with large doses of radioactive iodine shows that with this element the effects on the white blood cells are not pronounced and are short-lived. A drop in total leukocytes with no significant variation in the differential was observed after the administration of large amounts of I^{130} but not after the use of I^{131}, although the total blood dosages were comparable in magnitude. However, since radiation from the 12.6 hour isotope is delivered almost entirely within two days, whereas from the 8 day isotope nearly the same proportion is delivered within thirty-two days, we must infer that the time factor is mainly responsible for the previously stated results. This is analogous to many other radiobiologic phenomena such as erythema production with single and fractional roentgen therapy, in which time is an important factor.

It is logical to assume that the effect of this factor on tumor tissue will be in the same direction as it is on the blood. Therefore, consideration of the time factor alone might seem to contraindicate the use of I^{131} in the treatment of tumors because higher doses would be required to obtain a given effect. The value of radiation treatment, however, must be based on the differential effect on both tumor and normal tissue. It can be shown for oral administration of the isotope that the ratio of the tumor dose [21] to the blood dose is about 80 when I^{130} is used and about 300 when I^{131} is used. Thus, the use of I^{131} would be approximately four times as effective as the use of I^{130} if there were no time factor involved. To offset this advantage the differential time factor would have to render the 12.6 hour isotope more than four times as effective for a given blood dose as the 8 day isotope before there could be a question about the advisability of the use of I^{131} in preference to I^{130}. This remains to be determined.

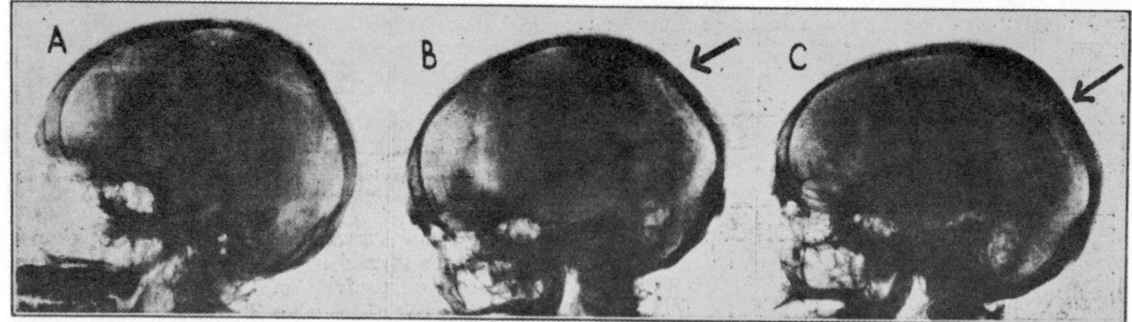

Fig. 11.—Roentgenologic appearance of lesion of the skull on *A*, Oct. 30, 1939; *B*, May 18, 1943, and *C*, Feb. 4, 1946.

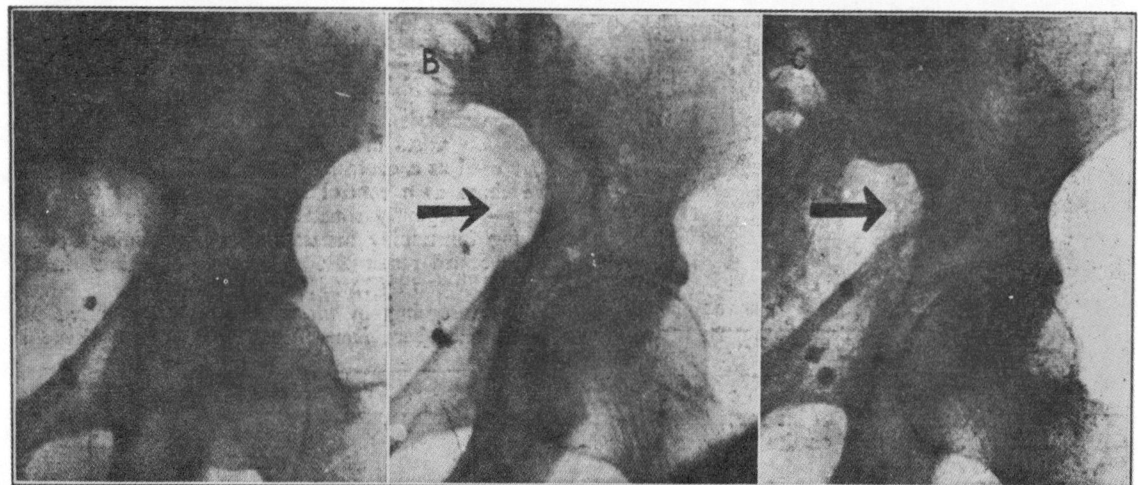

Fig. 12.—Roentgenologic appearance of lesion of ilium on *A*, July 17, 1939; *B*, Nov. 10, 1942, and *C*, May 22, 1946.

118

In earlier studies [22] of thyroid–iodine metabolism by the use of I * it was shown that irrespective of the total amount of iodine administered, the hyperactive gland initially retains more I * than the normal gland but loses it faster. The rate of loss seems to increase with larger amounts of carrier iodine.

With this in mind as well as with the purpose of determining ultimately the actual radiation dose deliv-

21. Calculated on the basis of the experimental curve of concentration of the I * in the blood and a net tumor elimination rate of 0.5 per cent per day.

22. Hertz, S.; Roberts, A., and Salter, W. T.: Radioactive Iodine as an Indicator in Thyroid Physiology: IV. The Metabolism of Iodine in Graves' Disease, J. Clin. Investigation **21**: 25-32 (Jan.) 1942. Hamilton.[3]

ered to the tumors, the I * turnover in the lesions was studied by means of suitable Geiger-Mueller counters under reproducible geometric conditions. This was done several times between May and August 1943, as well as ten months and one year after the third therapeutic dose. Unfortunately, the 1943 measurements—due to circumstances partially beyond our control—cannot be interpreted without making some assumptions. The only thing that can be said is that several days after the administration of a tracer dose of I^{131} the activity of all the lesions, when corrected for decay of 8 day iodine, disclosed the elimination of about 0.5 per cent of the dose per day. This observation per se cannot be interpreted as a demonstration that the tumor tissue metabolized I * at the rate of normal thyroid tissue, although this was our impression. The latest data (1946), figures 15 and 16, taken much more accurately, show a rapid loss of I * in the two lesions studied when 40 micrograms of carrier iodine was administered. With the larger amount of carrier iodine, the rate of loss was not as great, in

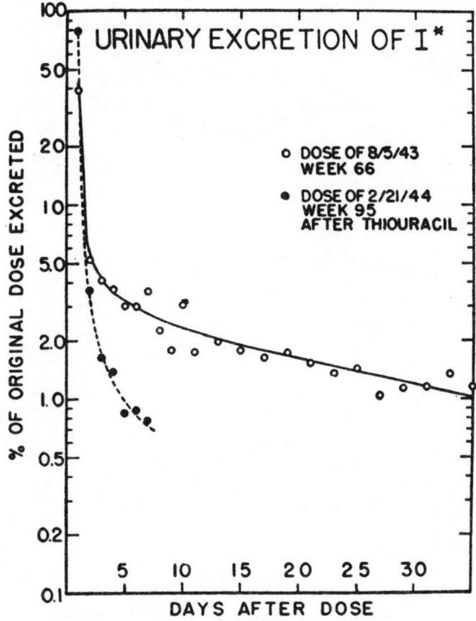

Fig. 13.—Typical trend of urinary excretion of I *.

proportion. We are unable to interpret these data in the light of published works on the turnover of I * in the thyroid itself.

Owing to the unusual nature of this case, that is, hyperthyroidism despite total thyroidectomy, the procedure and results of our studies of radioactivity over the region of the original thyroid as well as over the metastases may be of interest.

The experimental setup and the theoretic considerations will be described in detail in another paper. It suffices to state here that the Geiger counter is shielded with a ¾ inch (1.91 cm.) thickness of lead and provided with a suitable window. The activity of any lesion or region is obtained by taking the difference between readings with the window open and those with the window plugged with a ¾ inch (1.91 cm.) thickness of lead. This method greatly facilitates the localization of radioactive iodine in contiguous lesions.

The counter readings over the thyroid area were on the average only 5 per cent of the readings obtained over the metastasis of the skull. This percentage did not change materially throughout the course of the study. The readings over the thyroid region were two to three times the readings taken over the lateral surface of the right calf but consistently less than readings obtained over the apex of the right lung, although both regions were free from metastases. A comparison with 2 nonthyroidectomized patients under similar conditions

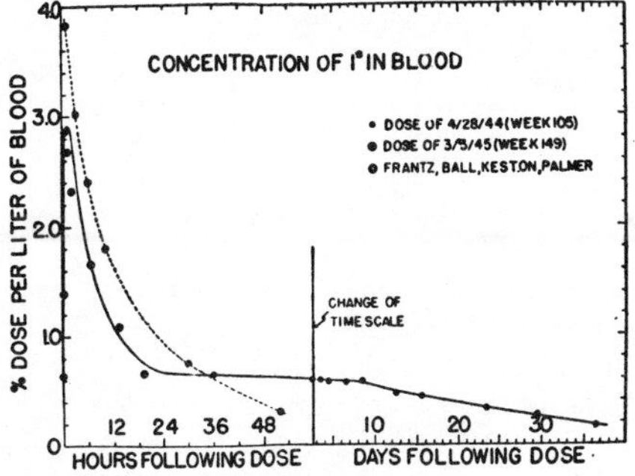

Fig. 14.—Concentration of I * in the blood (corrected for decay) after oral administration of the radioactive element.

of dosage and excretion showed that iodine pickup in this patient's thyroid region was only 4 per cent and 6 per cent, respectively, of the iodine pickup in the thyroid regions of the other 2 patients.

While the evidence presented herein shows clearly that there was little activity over the thyroid region, it might be argued that since this activity was greater than that obtained over the calf, the existence of some residual thyroid tissue cannot be ruled out. However, the presence of functioning metastases in the neighborhood of the thyroid region will cause some scattered gamma radiation to enter the instrument. No similar condition exists in the region of the calf, which was first used as a control. But when, with this in mind, we chose as a control region the apex of the right lung—analogously situated with respect to the neighboring functioning metastases, but containing none—we obtained readings even greater than those in the thyroid region by 15 to 30 per cent.

The foregoing, in our opinion, is presumptive evidence that there is no functioning thyroid tissue in

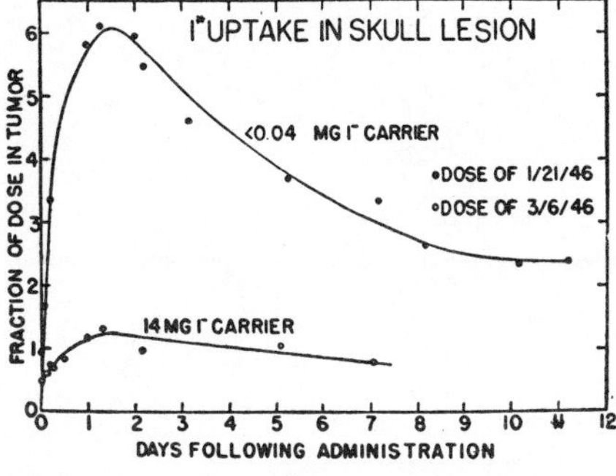

Fig. 15.—I * uptake in a representative lesion of the skull subsequent to the administration of doses containing different amounts of carrier iodine.

the neck and confirms the previous surgical observations.

It is pertinent to mention that 4 cases of metastatic carcinoma of the thyroid without clinical hyperthyroidism have been studied with radioactive iodine and have shown selective localization in the lesions. Two of these are now under treatment with I.*

SUMMARY

A case of metastatic adenocarcinoma of the thyroid is reported in which treatment by means of radioactive iodine has been successful. The patient was completely thyroidectomized for "malignant adenoma" in 1923, with neither thyrotoxicosis then nor hypothyroidism postoperatively; fifteen years later there developed classic symptoms of hyperthyroidism and severe pain in the lower back. In October 1939 a pulsating tumor removed from the level of the twelfth thoracic vertebra proved to be metastatic thyroid adenocarcinoma (histologically well differentiated, with small follicles and colloid). In the next two years hyperthyroidism increased and roentgenograms revealed new metastases in the lungs, upper part of the right femur, second rib on the left side, left ileum and skull. Roentgenologic irradiation of the metastases proved ineffectual.

In March 1943 a tracer dose of radioactive iodine revealed iodine retention by all the known lesions and no evidence of residual thyroid tissue in the neck. Therapeutic amounts of radioactive iodine were administered orally between May and October 1943. Definite and lasting clinical improvement followed. In April 1944 and March 1945 additional I* was administered with a resultant disappearance of pain, increase in weight and progressive change in all clinical criteria in the direction of hypothyroidism. Roentgenographic evidence pointed to an arrest if not a regression of the disease. No untoward effects followed this therapy.

Radioactive iodine seems to be an effective therapeutic agent in the control of this type of tumor.

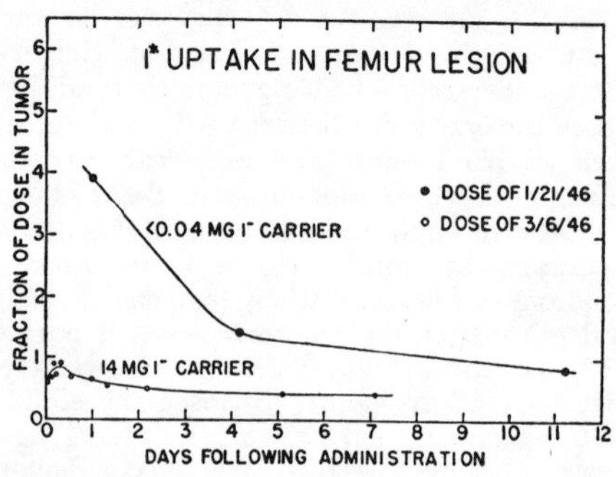

Fig. 16.—I* uptake in a representative lesion of the femur subsequent to the administration of doses containing different amounts of carrier iodine. The fraction of dose in the tumor is proportional to the ratio of counts obtained over the given lesion under fixed geometric conditions to counts obtained at the same time on an aliquot part of the administered I*. Thus, figures 15 and 16 represent correctly the time change in concentration in any one lesion, but because of the geometric differences involved in the measurements they do not permit direct comparison of the I* concentration in the two lesions.

Use of Radioactive Diiodofluorescein in the Diagnosis and Localization of Brain Tumors [1]

GEORGE E. MOORE[2]

Department of Surgery,
University of Minnesota Medical School, Minneapolis

The use of fluorescein has recently been suggested as an aid in the diagnosis of malignancy (*1*). In the initial report it was observed that brain tumors appeared to exhibit a consistent special affinity for the absorption of previously injected fluorescein.

In an attempt to extend the clinical usefulness of the fluorescein technique, radioactive derivatives of the dye have been prepared. Since it is considered safe to use, for clinical purposes, only those isotopes with a short half-life, and since the detection of deep-seated intracranial lesions requires the emission of gamma radiation, diiodofluorescein was synthesized to contain I^{131}. The amount of I^{131} added was adjusted to give 1 mc of radioactivity/10 cc of a 2% solution of the final product, sodium diiodofluorescein. An amount of dye calculated to contain 500–600 μc of radioactivity was injected intravenously in each case. In order to give a comparable dose of radioactivity to patients on subsequent days, increasing volumes of the dye were injected as the I^{131} decayed. Previous toxicity studies have shown that the ML/50 of diiodofluorescein is comparable to that of eosin; no toxic reactions have been encountered from the small amount of dye administered.

All counts were obtained by means of a beta-gamma Geiger-Müller tube protected from background radiation by a 2-cm-thick lead shield, provided with a lead cone to reduce the area being counted, and mounted on a portable X-ray unit. Thin lead foils were placed over the counter window to filter out beta radiation. A quenching circuit attached directly to the Geiger-Müller tube from the scaler allowed easy manipulation of the detection unit over the patient. Counts were taken for 3- to 5-min intervals at each of several positions on the skull with the cone of the detection unit directly on the skin. An attempt was made to obtain counts over symmetrical positions on the right and left sides of the head, as well as counts along the midline. After a complete survey, an examination of sites of higher activity was repeated in order to localize more definitely the suspected lesion. At times uncooperativeness of a patient due to the intracranial lesion made an adequate survey impossible.

Although counting was begun soon after dye was injected, differential readings between areas over the suspected tumor and symmetrical control areas did not become evident until an interval of 2–4 hrs had elapsed. This interval, required for the development of maximal differences in concentration of dye by the normal and tumor tissue, corresponds closely to the time lag prior to the appearance of maximal fluorescence noted in the earlier study (*1*) of brain tumors. Soon after the dye is injected, higher counts are obtained over the large venous sinuses; then, as the dye is removed from the blood stream, the counts tend to equalize over all parts of the brain with the exception of the area over the tumor, where the highest counts are recorded. In cases in which the tumor is accompanied by a large amount of edema, somewhat higher counts may be obtained over the entire affected hemisphere. As experience with the technique increased, a single series of counts at the proper interval was found satisfactory to localize the tumor. A majority of the tests were carried out without knowledge of the neurological findings, roentgen examination, and staff opinion. Only cases with questionable intracranial neoplasms were examined by this method.

To date 15 patients suspected of harboring intracranial neoplasms have been subjected to this technique. The last 12 cases are summarized in Table 1. Three previous cases with known site of recurrence, following previous partial operative excision, were studied by the radioactive dye method before the diagnosis of new cases was attempted.

Correct diagnoses of negative findings (Cases 1 and 9), as well as positive, have been made. Case 12 is of special interest. From the results of the counts obtained with the radioactive dye technique, a definite area was outlined on the skull over the site of the tumor. This outline coincided closely to the extent of the superficially situated meningeoma found at operation.

The limitations of this technique are as yet unknown, and its clinical usefulness is still to be determined. Further studies of the differential concentration of the radioactive dye in normal and edematous brain tissue as well as various tumors, clinical and experimental, are in progress. Preliminary experiments utilizing induced brain tumors in mice have revealed the concentration of dye in the tumor tissue to be as high as 80 times that found in the adjacent normal brain. Measurements of various concentrations of radioactive diiodofluorescein under physical conditions simulating those found clinically have verified the feasibility of the technique and will be reported upon later.

Reference

1. MOORE, G. E. *Science*, 1947, **106**, 130–131.

[1] This research was supported by a grant from the National Cancer Institute and the U. S. Public Health Service, the Malignant Disease Research Fund, and the Flora L. Rosenblatt Fund for Cancer Research.

The author wishes to express his appreciation to W. T. Peyton and his staff for making the clinical cases available and to J. F. Marvin, of the Department of Biophysics, for much helpful advice.

[2] Senior Research Fellow, U. S. Public Health Service.

TABLE 1

		Clinical preoperative diagnosis	Conclusions from radioactive dye technique	Operative findings
(1)	K.W.	Meningeoma of right sphenoid ridge	No tumor	Aneurysm of right internal carotid
(2)	E.S.	(?)Tumor of right temporal or parietal lobe	Tumor of right parietal occipital area	Ependymal blastoma, right occipital lobe
(3)	T.B.	Tumor of right temporal lobe	(?)Tumor of right temporal area	Meningeoma of right middle fossa
(4)	P.K.	Metastatic tumor of right parietal lobe	Tumor in right parietal area	Metastatic tumor of right parietal lobe
(5)	L.S.	(?)Metastatic tumor of right motor cortex	No tumor on right; (?) tumor of left frontal lobe	No tumor on right, left side not explored
(6)	H.L.	(?)Tumor	Tumor of posterior frontal lobe on right	Glioblastoma of right temporal lobe
(7)	J.H.	Tumor of right frontal lobe	Tumor of right frontal lobe	Ependymal blastoma of right frontal lobe
(8)	J.B.	(?)Tumor	Tumor to left of the midline, posterior frontal area	Meningeoma of left posterior frontal area
(9)	G.H.	(?)Tumor	No tumor	Normal ventriculogram, no operation
(10)	E.J.	Large tumor of right parietal lobe	Tumor of right parietal area	Right parietal tumor by ventriculogram and biopsy
(11)	L.W.	Right acoustic neuroma	No significant counts	Right acoustic neuroma
(12)	A.B.	Subdural hematoma, right side	Tumor of right frontal lobe near midline	Meningeoma of right frontal lobe near midline

Alkali Halide Scintillation Counters

ROBERT HOFSTADTER
Princeton University, Princeton, New Jersey
May 20, 1948

It has been shown by J. W. Coltman, H. Kallman, M. Deutsch, and G. B. Collins[1] that beta-particles and gamma-rays can be detected by the scintillations which these ionizing radiations produce in certain crystals. Among the most successful for practical applications are naphthalene and perhaps anthracene.[2] Such crystals are not particularly suitable for many purposes since their densities are small (about 1 g/cc), their atomic numbers low, and their light flashes are small, so that the photo-multiplier detector must be cooled to reduce background noise pulses.

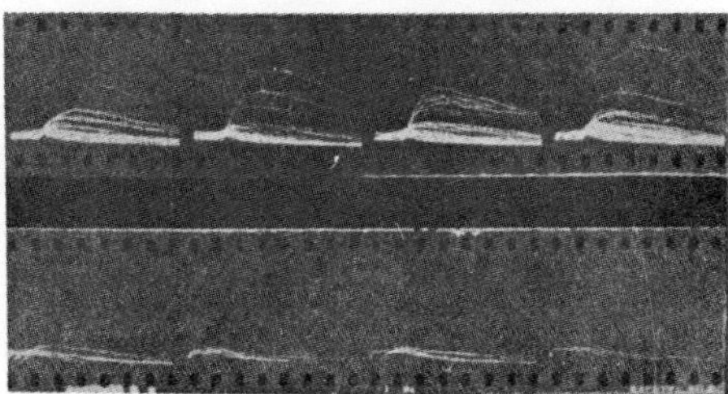

FIG. 1. Oscilloscope screen photographs taken at random for 1/30 second. Above, pulses due to NaI(Tl) and below, pulses due to naphthalene under identical circumstances. Sweep calibration: total length of sweep equals 4.3 microseconds.

From the known properties of the alkali halide phosphors[3] it occurred to the author that these materials, of moderate density (2.0 to 4.5 g/cc), medium atomic numbers, great transparency, and beautiful form, might be very suitable for scintillation counters. The time during which light flashes are emitted is also known to be small, although phosphorescence is observed in some specimens.[4]

The author had in his possession a crystal of potassium iodide with a small thallium impurity (probably 0.1 percent or so) which was kindly provided him a year ago by Mr. Frank B. Quinlan of the General Electric Company. This crystal had been grown in 1938 by Dr. Frederick Seitz and Mr. Quinlan. Accordingly, the author, with the help of Mr. J. C. D. Milton, made an attempt to detect gamma-rays with this crystal and a 931A type photo-multiplier. The attempt was successful and will be described at a later time.

Since potassium is radioactive and, moreover, since the pulses observed in KI were somewhat smaller than those observed with naphthalene samples, the author prepared some powder samples of NaI plus thallium. The results were very encouraging, for pulses caused by alpha-particles were equal, if not greater, than those observed with ZnS (silver), which is known to be a very efficient phosphor. The powder sample proved to be hydroscopic when exexposed to air and, in addition, a yellow film formed on the surface. In a few hours the pulses due to alpha-particles were considerably smaller than the original ones.

Another NaI sample was made in vacuum in a 0.5-inch quartz tube with the result that a mass ($\sim$8.0 g) of extremely luminescent small crystals was produced. The crystals are about one or two millimeters on a side. When the quartz tube containing the crystals was placed close to a photo-multiplier, very large pulses were observed from radium gamma-rays. These pulses were larger than those observed with a clear piece of naphthalene (5.8 g) of comparable size. Of course, this NaI sample is completely unaffected by atmospheric conditions and is quite convenient for normal handling. A comparison of results is shown in Figs. 1 and 2. Figure 1 shows oscilloscope pictures of 1/30-second random exposures taken under identical circumstances with the NaI sample and with naphthalene. The source was 0.1-millicurie radium at 16 cm, filtered by 3/32-inch brass. Figure 2 shows a differential bias curve taken under identical conditions for the two materials. From the rise times of the pulses in NaI there is some evidence that the light flashes are emitted in about one microsecond or less. All work reported has been carried on at room temperature.

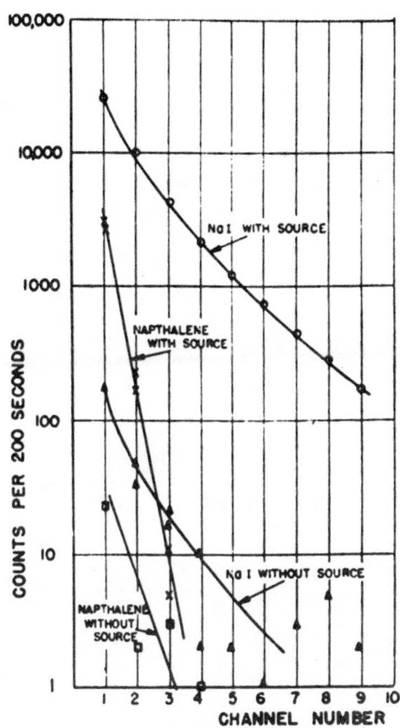

FIG. 2. Differential bias curves for pulses from NaI(Tl) and naphthalene. Channel 1 records pulses in the range 5-10 volts. Channel 2, 10-15 volts, etc.

Further work in progress is designed to produce large single crystals of this and other alkali halides with thallium impurities. A neutron counter using a lithium halide seems to be a reasonable possibility.

In tests made by placing crystals of NaI, KI, and naphthalene on photographic plates (Eastman 103-O) much greater light output was observed from NaI and KI than from naphthalene samples of comparable size. Apparently, naphthalene is not an efficient phosphor.

A sample of NaI in a quartz tube gave measurable 123
blackening of a photographic plate when the combination was exposed for thirty minutes to the gamma-rays of 1.8 millicuries of radium at a meter distance.

A more complete description of these results is being prepared.

The author wishes to thank Professors J. A. Wheeler and R. Sherr for interesting discussions, and Professors M. G. White and H. W. Fulbright for loan of equipment used in these tests.

[1] J. W. Coltman and F. H. Marshall, Phys. Rev. **72**, 528 (1947); H. Kallman, Natur und Technik (July 1947); M. Deutsch, Nucleonics 2, 58 (1948); G. B. Collins and Rosalie C. Hoyt, Phys. Rev. **73**, 1259 (1948).
[2] P. R. Belland R. C. Davis, Bull. Am. Phys. Soc. **23**, No. 3, 52 (1948). X12.
[3] R. Hilsch, Zeits. f. Physik **44**, 860 (1927); W. von Meyeren, Zeits. f. Physik **61**, 329 (1930).
[4] E. H. Hutten and P. Pringsheim, J. Chem. Phys. **16**, 241 (1948).

SURGERY
GYNECOLOGY AND OBSTETRICS

VOLUME 91 OCTOBER, 1950 NUMBER 4

THE USE OF RADIOACTIVE IODINATED PLASMA PROTEIN IN THE STUDY OF BLOOD VOLUME

JOHN P. STORAASLI, M.D., HARVEY KRIEGER, M.D., HYMER L. FRIEDELL, M.D., and WILLIAM D. HOLDEN, M.D., F.A.C.S., Cleveland, Ohio

IN recent years the importance of the circulating blood volume and its relationship to disease has become more evident. The direct method for determining blood volume, which is of importance clinically, depends upon the dilution of a test substance injected into the blood stream. The requirements of an ideal test substance are that: (1) it remains in the vascular system for a relatively long period; (2) it mixes readily with the normal constituents of blood; (3) it is easily identified and measured; and (4) it is nontoxic.

The azo dyes have been the chief source of these test substances. The extensive investigations of one of these dyes, T-1824, by Gibson, Gregerson, and others (3, 4, 1) have led to its widespread clinical and experimental use for the determination of blood volumes. These investigators have shown that, under the proper conditions, relatively accurate results can be obtained by this method.

More recently, with the availability of radioactive isotopes, easier and more accurate means of estimating blood volumes have evolved. Hevesy first utilized radioactive phosphorus for labeling erythrocytes to study total circulating erythrocyte mass. Hahn, by feeding radioactive iron to donors, devised an excellent alternative method for determining red cell volume. Although these methods have given satisfactory results, both present practical disadvantages. The latter method requires a donor with the appropriate blood type. With the radioactive phosphorus method, there is an undesirable delay required in the preparation of the labeled red cells before the determination can be performed.

Fine and Seligman devised a method by which they could label plasma protein with radioactive iodine, and with this material study plasma volumes in experimental animals. This method was selected by us and its efficacy in the study of blood volumes in humans was investigated. Iodinated protein appears to satisfy the requirements listed and has the significant feature of being derived from a normal constituent of plasma.

Blood volume studies on 76 human subjects will be reported here. The subjects were ambulatory hospital patients in normal fluid and protein balance. In 30 of the individuals, the disappearance of the iodinated protein from the vascular system was studied over an 8 hour period. In 31 patients, plasma volume studies were determined under basal conditions. In 15 patients, a comparison of plasma volumes determined with both T-1824 and iodinated protein was made.

Since the iodinated albumin disappears from the blood stream, as will be shown subsequently, experimental procedures were undertaken, in animals and humans, to determine the fate of the injected material.

FATE OF THE IODINATED PROTEIN IN VIVO

The distribution of iodinated rat plasma protein after intravenous injection was obtained in a group of 16 albino rats for various intervals up to and including 24 hours. Various organs and tissues were assayed and their radioactivity was compared to that of the plasma. The thyroid gland was the only organ showing significant amounts of radioactivity. During the 24 hour period of this experiment, the radioactivity in this organ increased with time so that approximately 5 per cent of the total activity was found in the thyroid gland at the end of 24 hours. The radioactivity of the other tissues and organs was negligible and appeared to depend upon the vascularity of the tissue. Figure 1 shows the gross distribution of iodinated protein by means of radio-

From the Departments of Radiology and Surgery, University Hospitals of Cleveland, Western Reserve University.
Supported in part under A.E.C. contract No. W-31-109-eng-78 with Western Reserve University.
Presented before the Clinical Congress of the American College of Surgeons, Chicago, October 17 to 21, 1949.

autographs, made from transections of rats. There appears to be little difference in the distribution of the injected material at 6 and 24 hours. The vascular channels are well outlined in each radioautograph.

The urine and body tissues of 2 dogs were assayed for activity 12 and 24 hours after the intravenous injection of iodinated protein. Urine was collected continuously throughout the periods of observation. The tissues examined for radioactivity consisted of thyroid, spleen, liver, kidney, muscle, fat, and intestine. The radioactivity measured in these tissues, when compared to that of blood, was found to be negligible and for practical purposes could be accounted for by the presence of the blood in the vascular channels contained within the examined tissues. At the end of 12 and 24 hours, the urine contained respectively 3.2 and 7.6 per cent of the injected radioactive iodine.

Experimental studies have been conducted and reported elsewhere (8) on the rate of appearance of radioactive protein in thoracic duct lymph after an intravenous injection. The details of these experiments will not be presented here except to state that 10 minutes following the injection of the radioactive protein a negligible amount (under 2 per cent) was found in the lymph. This was sufficiently small to be disregarded in the determination of the plasma volume. As time progressed, however, the radioactivity of the plasma and lymph approached equilibrium. It was also determined by dialysis that the radioiodine remained bound to protein.

Twelve patients who were to receive spinal anesthesia were given radioactive iodinated protein at various intervals preceding the administration of the anesthesia. In no instance could any radioactivity be detected in the spinal fluid. In 6 of these patients, biopsies of muscle and fat obtained during the course of the operation showed very little radioactivity. In 1 patient, bile was obtained 45 minutes after intravenous injection of iodinated protein and no significant activity was found. Studies on patients confined to bed have shown that an average of 8 to 12 per cent of the injected radioactive iodine is found in the urine in 24 hours.

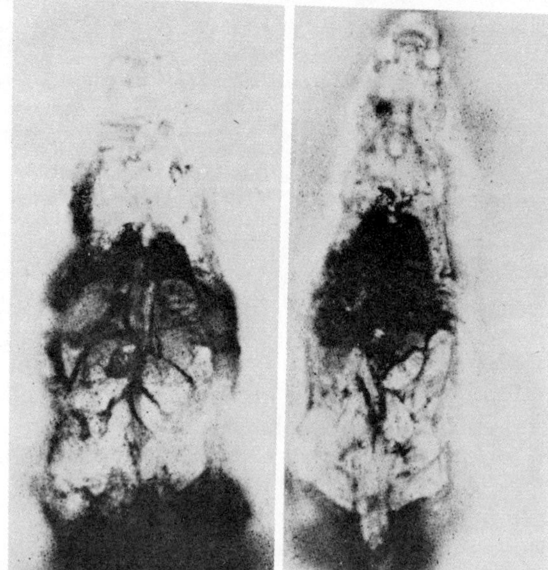

Fig. 1. Radioautographs of rats made at 6 and 24 hour intervals. The dark shadows represent the distribution of iodinated protein. The vascular channels are well outlined.

From these studies it was observed that the disappearance of iodinated protein from the vascular system probably occurs in two ways.

The first is due to the liberation of radioactive iodine from the protein. This is manifested by the excretion of iodine in the urine as well as by the increased radioactivity over the thyroid gland. The second is due to the diffusion of iodinated protein from the vascular bed to the extravascular spaces, as demonstrated in the studies of thoracic lymph.

METHOD

The studies on human subjects were performed while they were in a fasting state. The subjects were confined to bed until the experiment was completed, with the exceptions to be noted. During the earlier part of this work, careful records of the blood pressure, pulse, respiratory rate, urinary output, and emotional state of the patients were made. When no perceptible change was observed, these measurements were discontinued. In studies designed to determine the disappearance rate of iodinated protein from the plasma, fasting conditions and confinement to bed were maintained for 6 hours. (The effect on the contour

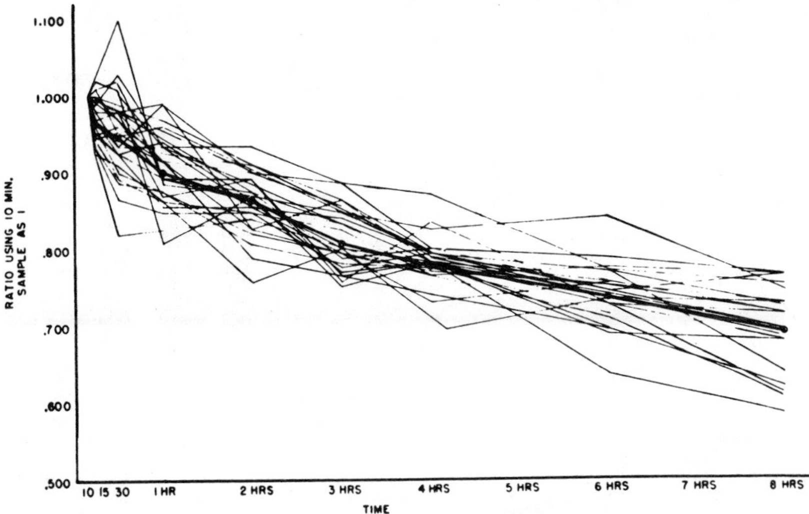

Fig. 2. This graph shows the disappearance of iodinated protein from the blood in 30 patients. The 10 minute sample was used as a reference point. The "heavy line" is the composite curve of the group.

of the disappearance curve when these restrictions were eliminated will be discussed.) The height and weight of each patient were recorded.

The radioactive iodine used in this work was a fission product obtained from the Isotope Division of the Atomic Energy Commission at Oak Ridge, Tennessee. The isotope was radioactive iodine with a half life of 8 days. Radioactive iodine decays by emitting both beta particles and gamma rays. Measurements of the radioactivity were made by utilizing the beta particles of radioactive iodine. Gamma counting of samples of plasma was not attempted because of the low efficiency with the conventional methods. Gamma counting was employed only when the patients were surveyed with a portable Geiger-Mueller counter. (In these circumstances, only the gamma rays will be detected by the counter since the beta particles are readily absorbed in a few millimeters of tissue.)

As noted previously, the iodinated protein was prepared according to the method originally described by Fine and Seligman. In this method of fixing the radioactive iodine to the protein, about 15 to 30 per cent of the iodine is bound to the albumin fraction[1]. The iodinated protein solution is then diluted with a sufficient quantity of 0.9 per cent saline solution so that there are approximately 2 to 3 microcuries of radioactive iodine per cubic centimeter of solution to be injected. There is less than 1 gram of protein in the quantity of solution to be injected for each determination. During the initial part of this work, human plasma was used as a source of protein, but for the past year human serum albumin has been used.

For each determination exactly 20 cubic centimeters of the iodinated protein solution were injected intravenously. This was used to minimize the error of injection[2]. At the desired time intervals after injection, 6 to 8 cubic centimeters of whole blood were withdrawn without stasis from a vein and placed in a calibrated test tube containing a few particles of crystalline heparin. The blood was centrifuged at 3,500 revolutions per minute for 20 minutes and exactly 1 cubic centimeter of the supernatant plasma was pipetted into a porcelain crucible and allowed to dry in air. The radioactivity was measured with a 127
Geiger-Mueller counter. The conventional bell-shaped end window Geiger tube, placed at a fixed distance, was used. Exactly 1 cubic

[1]At the present time, iodinated human serum albumin is being prepared in which yields have been obtained with 70 to 80 per cent of radioactive iodine bound to the albumin.

[2]Smaller volumes can be used. We find, however, that larger volumes are easier to handle. With 20 cubic centimeters volumes, the error of injection could be kept within ± 1 per cent.

TABLE I.—THE AVERAGE RATIO OF DISAPPEARANCE RATES OF IODINATED PROTEIN FROM BLOOD IN 30 PATIENTS FOR VARIOUS INTERVALS UP TO 8 HOURS

Time	Average ratio*	Standard deviation	Coefficient of variation
5 min.	1.055	± .036	± 3.4
10 min.	1.000		
15 min.	.963	± .027	± 2.8
30 min.	.947	± .047	± 5.0
60 min.	.900	± .041	± 4.5
2 hr.	.862	± .041	± 4.7
3 hr.	.808	± .040	± 4.9
4 hr.	.778	± .030	± 3.8
6 hr.	.737	± .035	± 4.7
8 hr.	.689	± .059	± 8.5

*The average ratio is the value of each point on the heavy line (composite curve) in Figure 2.

centimeter of the original iodinated protein solution, diluted 1 to 100 with plasma, was used as a standard. Use of the latter rendered calculation of the plasma volume simple, by obviating the necessity of considering decay and the geometry of the counting system. The porcelain crucibles were constructed so that 1 cubic centimeter of solution just covered the bottom. The plasma samples and the standard preparations were dried in air for 24 hours before the counting was performed. This was necessary because many samples were being counted simultaneously. (The plasma volume, however, can be determined by counting the wet plasma specimen without loss of accuracy.) Each sample was counted for a long enough period of time to reduce the counting error to less than 2 per cent. Total counts per sample were usually around 5,000. Hematocrits and plasma protein concentrations were obtained from specific gravities measured by the copper sulfate method. Reference was made to the charts provided by Phillips and co-workers. At the present time, protein determinations are being performed by the use of a photoelectric colorimeter (7). The plasma volume was calculated from the following formula:

$$\frac{\text{Counts in standard per c.c.} \times \text{volume injected} \times \text{dilution of standard}}{\text{Counts in sample per c.c.}} = \text{Plasma volume}$$

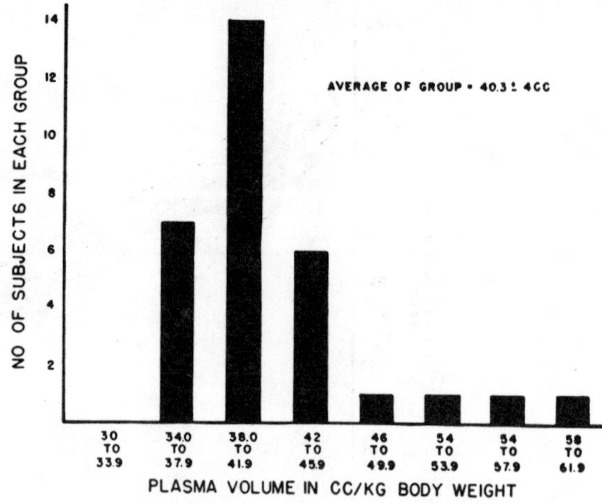

Fig. 3. This graph shows the distribution of plasma volumes, determined with iodinated protein, in cubic centimeters per kilogram body weight in 31 normal subjects.

The total blood volume was calculated as follows:

$$\frac{\text{Plasma volume}}{100 - \text{hematocrit}} = \text{Blood volume}$$

RESULTS AND DISCUSSION

To determine the rate at which the iodinated protein disappeared from the blood stream, 30 patients were studied. These patients were healthy individuals who had been admitted to the hospital for hernioplasties or plastic repairs. In order to measure the disappearance rate, the plasma specimen obtained 10 minutes after injection was used as a reference point and designated as unity. We assumed this to be the time of maximum mixing and minimum loss from the blood stream. The 10 minute interval may not represent the optimum time. Other time intervals following injection may be desirable, when cardiovascular dynamics and capillary permeability in localized areas of the body are altered. Experiments are being performed at the present time in an attempt to arrive at a more satisfactory solution of this problem.

By dividing the counts of successive samples of plasma over a 24 hour period by the count of the 10 minute sample, ratios were obtained which indicated the rate of disappearance of the radioactive protein. The ratios obtained at various intervals were plotted as noted in Figure 2. The composite curve (heavy line) was obtained by plotting the

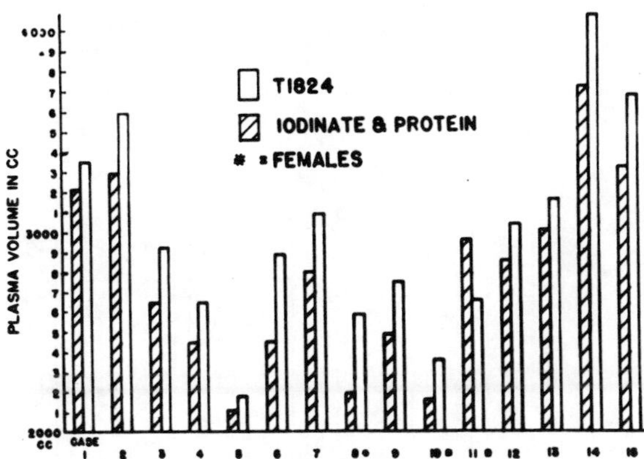

Fig. 4. This graph compares plasma volume determinations performed simultaneously using T-1824 and iodinated protein. In only 1 instance (Case 11) was the volume obtained by T-1824 less than that by the iodinated protein.

averages of the ratios at each interval for all the patients. Table I demonstrates the average disappearance ratio at each time interval with standard deviations and coefficient of variation.

It may be seen that the iodinated protein leaves the blood stream at a slow rate. At the end of 1 hour, 90 per cent of the injected protein is still present in the blood; at the end of 4 hours, 78 per cent remains; and 24 hours following the injection, 55 per cent remains although this is not shown in Figure 2 or Table I.

The narrow percentage of deviation or coefficient of variation for each curve gives considerable significance to the composite disappearance curve. Up to and including the 6 hour specimens, the percentage of deviation was under ± 5 (Table I). This is well within the range of error suitable for biological measurement. At the end of 8 hours, the percentage of deviation attains ± 8.5 and at 24 hours it is greater. This increase in the coefficient of variation after 6 hours may, in part, be explained by the abolition of controlled conditions. After 6 hours the patients were allowed out of bed and fluid intake was unrestricted.

Since the iodinated protein disappears from the blood stream at a reasonably fixed slow rate, it should be possible to calculate the plasma volume by determining any point on the disappearance curve from 10 minutes to 6 hours after the injection of the radioactive iodinated protein. Large deviations from the normal disappearance curve should be easily detectable if there is no significant loss of protein from the blood stream as a result of blood loss or localized change in capillary permeability during the course of the study.

TABLE II.—NORMAL BLOOD VOLUME STUDIES IN HEALTHY MALES

Name	Age years	Weight in kgm.	Plasma volume c.c.	Plasma volume c.c./kgm.	Hematocrit	Total blood volume	Total blood volume c.c./kgm.
1. R.W.	20	68	3865	56.8*	34.9	5946	87.4
2. J.M.	26	77	3162	41.1	45.3	5749	74.6
3. W.F.	25	82	2972	36.2	48.2	5715	70.5
4. W.W.†	28	80	3422	42.7	41.9	5900	73.7
5. A.A.	54	76	3417	44.9	43.8	6101	80.2
6. I.A.	38	73	2921	40.0	48.7	5727	78.4
7. W.R.	27	64	2564	40.0	40.3	4240	66.3
8. A.M.	40	58	2251	38.8	48.0	4328	74.6
9. H.C.	24	73	2451	33.6	46.2	4724	64.7
10. H.M.	37	75	2856	38.0	45.0	5129	68.4
11. J.B.	31	73	2695	37.0	39.3	4418	60.5
12. S.C.	29	66	2773	42.0	45.0	5041	76.3
13. D.M.	38	74	2903	39.2	46.0	5375	72.6
14. G.K.	25	65	2378	36.6	39.0	3898	60.0
15. P.N.	30	68	2738	40.3	48.0	5265	77.4
16. J.W.	34	74	2521	34.0	42.4	4518	61.0
17. W.W.†	28	88	3305	37.5	37.8	5331	61.0
18. R.R.	38	88	3720	42.3	48.7	6888	78.3
19. J.G.	27	88	3110	35.3	45.9	6100	69.3
20. R.M.	26	74	2884	39.0	47.7	5546	75.0
21. G.P.	29	63	3894	61.8*	36.3	6048	96.0
22. F.N.	28	82	4010	48.9	42.1	6913	84.3
23. H.B.	30	59	3125	52.9	38.1	5040	85.4
24. W.H.	29	60	2530	42.2	40.5	4300	71.6
25. R.N.	24	100	3420	34.2	46.3	6340	63.4
26. T.T.	18	58	2580	44.5	43.1	4550	78.5
27. J.K.	40	90	3380	37.5	46.0	6450	71.6
28. P.W.	21	56.5	2260	40.0	47.0	4280	75.7
29. F.S.	30	66	2710	41.0	49.0	5350	81.0
30. N.P.	29	77	3500	45.0	47.0	6650	86.5
31. A.G.	35	67.5	2740	40.6	48.0	5270	78.5

Average plasma volume in c.c./kgm. 40.3 ± 4.2.
*Patients excluded from calculation of average value since their plasma volumes in c.c./kgm. were greater than 3 standard deviations from the mean.
†Patients No. 4 and 17 are the same patient. Plasma volumes were done 1 month apart.

Plasma and blood volumes were determined on 31 male patients (Table II). Their ages ranged from 18 to 54 years, although the majority of them were between 25 and 35 years of age. Their weights ranged from 56.5 to 100 kilograms. Plasma volumes ranged from 34.0 to 61.8 cubic centimeters per kilogram.

Correlation of plasma or blood volume with any readily determined biologic measurement such as height, weight, or surface area, is not entirely satisfactory. Figure 3 demonstrates the distribution of patients according to cubic centimeters of plasma volume per kilogram of body weight. Fourteen of the 31 patients fall between 38 and 42 cubic centimeters per kilogram, whereas 27 of the 31 patients fall between 34 and 46 cubic centimeters per kilogram. The mean plasma volume per kilogram of body weight is 40.3 ± 4.2 cubic centimeters. The correlation coefficient of plasma volume with weight was found to be .47 in our series of 31 patients. Since weight is obviously an unsatisfactory biologic measurement for predicting plasma volumes, it is essential that predetermined normal plasma volume measurements be obtained in each individual to be studied. This will permit estimation of subsequent deviations from the normal when physiological alterations occur.

An important biological measurement which may be used as a basis for estimating plasma volume is the specific gravity of the whole body. Such a measurement involves the total weight and volume of the individual. The latter can be done only by water displacement. This procedure is not one to which a sick patient could be subjected. Furthermore, it would be of little value in physical conditions associated with marked water deficit or excess. Studies are in progress to determine if the relationship between body specific gravity and plasma volume is of practical value.

Figure 4 demonstrates a comparison of plasma volumes determined simultaneously with radioactive iodinated protein and T-1824 in 15 individuals. Blood specimens were drawn 10 minutes after the injection of both the dye and iodinated protein. The most significant feature of this study is that the plasma volumes determined with the use of the radioactive protein were, with 1 exception,

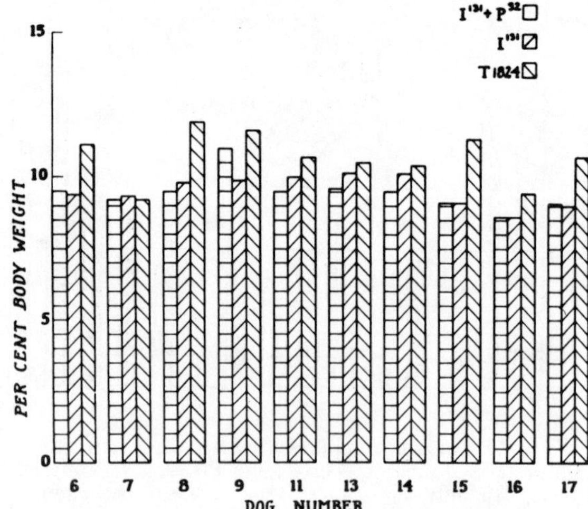

Fig. 5. This graph gives a comparison of total blood volumes (expressed as per cent body weight) in dogs using iodinated protein and radioactive phosphorus labeled red cells, iodinated protein and hematocrit, and T-1824 and hematocrit. In only 1 instance (dog 7) was the blood volume determined with T-1824 less than by the other two methods. Published with permission of *Proceedings of the Society for Experimental Biology and Medicine.*

smaller than those obtained with the dye T-1824. This was found to be true also in the case of work in dogs in which we compared the volume by using T-1824, iodinated protein, and red cells labeled with radioactive phosphorus (9). Figure 5 gives the results of this study. These results show that at the 10 minute interval there is a greater dilution of T-1824 than of iodinated protein. Since the determinations were done simultaneously, the greater dilution of the dye must present a greater loss of the dye from the vascular spaces. The minimum time required for complete mixing of an intravenously injected material within the blood stream is not known accurately. There is, indeed, some reason to believe that it varies in different physiological and pathological states. It may be that, as more information is obtained concerning the mixing time, the 10 minute interval between the injection and the withdrawal of blood will have to be revised.

Rawson has proved that the successful use of T-1824 depends upon its rapid and complete binding to the albumin fraction of plasma. However, during the first few minutes following the injection of T-1824, a certain amount of the dye escapes from the vascular system. This will vary from one individual to another and will also depend upon the protein status of the patient.

A far greater advantage of the use of iodinated protein in determination of blood volume is the fact that repeated blood volume determinations after short intervals of time can be carried out on the same individual. This is not true of T-1824. Rawson has found by electrophoresis that the dye is completely bound to albumin when the concentration is .004 per cent or less. Any further injection of T-1824 into the blood stream will be rapidly and effectively taken out by the reticuloendothelial system.

SUMMARY

A method of determining the plasma volume of patients has been presented. It involves the measurement of the dilution of protein tagged with radioactive iodine after intravenous injection. Dilution is determined by measuring iodinated protein labeled with radioactive iodine before the injection and plasma periodically after the injection.

The technique of the procedure is simple and subject to small error. Repeated determinations can be performed within a short time.

The stability of the iodinated protein and its relatively secure retention within the vascular system permit a more accurate estimate of the plasma volume than has hitherto been possible. This method is probably of no more value than others when there is marked disturbance of normal physiology, as in profoun shock, or other conditions effecting capillar permeability.

REFERENCES

1. Davis, L. J. Determination of blood volume in ma with "Evans" blue (T-1824). Edinburgh M. J 1942, 49: 465.
2. Fine, J., and Seligman, A. M. Traumatic shock study of problem of "lost plasma" in hemorrhagi shock by use of radioactive plasma protein. J. Clir Invest., 1943, 22: 285.
3. Gibson, J. G. II, and Evans, W. A. Jr. Clinica studies of the blood volume—I, clinical applicatio of a method employing the azo dye "Evans blue' and the spectrophotometer. J. Clin. Invest., 1937 16: 301.
4. Gregerson, M. J. A practical method for the determination of blood volume with the dye T-1824 J. Laborat. Clin. M., 1944, 29: 1266.
5. Hahn, P. F., Balfour, W. M., Ross, J. R., Bale, W. F., and Whipple, G. H. Red cell volume, circulating and total, as determined by radio iron. Science, 1941, 93: 87.
6. Hevesy, G., and Zerahn, K. Determination of the red corpuscle content. Acta physiol. scand., 1942, 4: 376.
7. Kingsley, G. R. Direct biuret method for determination of serum proteins as applied to photoelectric and visual colorimetry. J. Laborat. Clin. M., 1942, 27: 840.
8. Krieger, H., Holden, W. D., Hubay, C. A., Scott, M. W., Storaasli, J. P., and Friedell, H. L. Appearance of protein tagged with radioactive iodine in thoracic duct lymph. Proc. Soc. Exp. Biol., N.Y., 1950, 73: 124.
9. Krieger, H., Storaasli, J. P., Friedell, H. L., and Holden, W. D. A comparative study of blood volume in dogs. Proc. Soc. Exp. Biol., N.Y., 1948, 68: 511.
10. Phillips, R. A. et al. Copper sulfate method for measuring specific gravities of whole blood and plasma. Bull. U. S. Army M. Dep., 1943, 71: 66.
11. Rawson, R. A. Binding of T-1824 and structurally related diazo dyes by plasma proteins. Am. J. Physiol., 1943, 138: 708.

Instrumentation for I^{131} Use in Medical Studies*

By Benedict Cassen,† Lawrence Curtis,† Clifton Reed‡ and Raymond Libby§

Scintillation counters have proved useful for the detection of gamma radiation from tissue. Several types of such counters have been designed at this laboratory to detect the gammas from I^{131}. The success of one of these for delineation of thyroid glands has led to the construction of a device for automatic scanning of the gland area and recording of the result

1. Localizing Counter

A scintillation counter specially designed in this laboratory for the localization of radioiodine in biological systems has been reported.¶ Further tests have shown that the intrinsic sesitivity of this counter is, in practice, greater than that reported.

Several improvements have been made, notable among them being the use of a better cement (Hyrax) for making optical contact between the calcium tungstate and the phototube envelope. With this counter it is easy to detect, with ¼-in. resolution, the boundary of a region containing only 0.2 μc of radioiodine per cm².

It has been shown possible‖ to delineate with fair accuracy the thyroid glands of patients given a dose of about 150 μc of radioiodine. (With this type of counter it is also possible to localize, readily and exactly, metastasized thyroid tissue in lymph nodes.) The procedure described here for delineating the thyroid glands is tedious but has been greatly improved by mounting the tube on a rack so that it can be moved in either of two directions at right angles to each other. This is done with lead screws turned by small hand cranks.

The outlines thus obtained were compared with the shape of the gland after removal by operation, or on autopsy, and were surprisingly accurate. The results indicated the desirability of an automatic scanning and recording device. Such a device has been built and is described in the last part of this paper.

2. Hand-Held Localizing Counter

A hand-held localizing counter that can be used for rapid determination of the boundaries of a thyroid gland, or other active tissue, by marking the outline on the patient's neck with a skin pencil, has been developed. This method is not as accurate as the point by point or scanning procedure, but is much less tedious and makes possible very rapid clinical location and classification of abnormalities and metastases.

* The information presented is based on work performed under Contract AT-04-1-GEN-12 between the Atomic Energy Commission and the University of California at Los Angeles. Section 5 of this paper has been reviewed in the Veterans Administration and published with approval of the Chief Medical Director. The statements and conclusions of the authors are the result of their own study and do not necessarily reflect the opinion or policy of the Veterans Administration.

Mr. Reed is co-author for Sections 1–4: Dr. Libby is co-author for Section 5.

† School of Medicine, University of California at Los Angeles.

‡ Formerly at the School of Medicine. University of California at Los Angeles. Now at the R. C. Scientific Instrument Co., Playa del Rey, California.

§ Radioisotope Laboratory, Wadsworth General Hospital, Veterans Administration Center, Los Angeles.

¶ B. Cassen, L. Curtis, C. Reed, NUCLEONICS **6,** No. 2, 78 (1950); UCLA-49 (1949).

‖ H. Allen, Jr., R. Libby, B. Cassen, *J. Clin. Endocrinol.* **11,** 492 (1950).

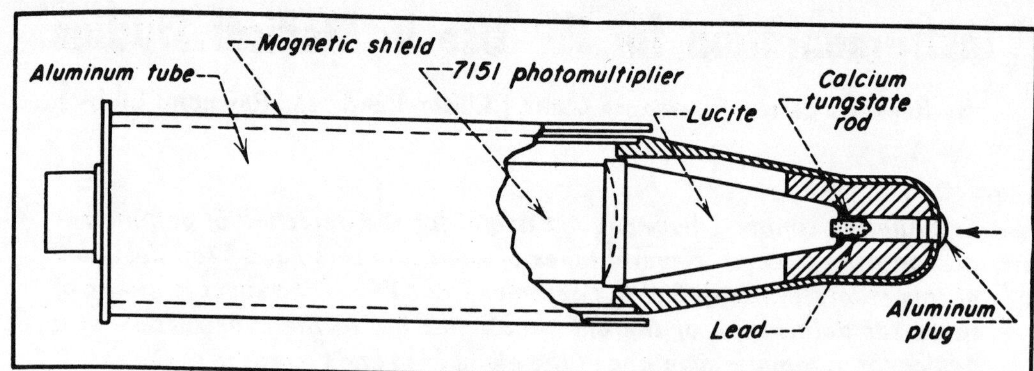

FIG. 1. Hand-held counter for tissue-boundary determination

Figure 1 shows this counter. An RCA 7151 photomultiplier tube is used. The scintillator is a single rod of clear calcium tungstate. The light produced is guided to the photosensitive surface by a conical Lucite light pipe that is cemented to the face of the phototube with Hyrax cement. This cement is also used to hold the calcium tungstate rod in place.

To obtain a sharp localizing effect with this arrangement, it is necessary to surround the calcium tungstate rod with a lead annulus of sufficient thickness and depth to shield most of the crystal from radiation coming in from outside a small angle. It is also necessary to surround the phototube with a mu-metal shield so the counting rate is not affected by the earth's or stray magnetic fields.

As a localizing detector, this counter is much more sensitive than the previous type. The over-all optical efficiency of the instrument is greater because the light can get to the photosensitive surface without reflections at air or vacuum interfaces. Also, the calcium tungstate rod is much closer to the layer of radioactive material. But the collimation of the gamma radiation is not as good and the spatial resolution suffers somewhat. If bias and amplification are set so that the background is about 4 cps, this counter, with a ¼-in. diameter circular aperture, is 3 to 4 times as sensitive as the earlier type with the same aperture.

Earlier, a modification of this type of detector was constructed using the larger 5819 photomultiplier tube and a much longer Lucite light pipe. The possibility was suggested of making radioactive the pontamine sky blue dye that Dr. Weinberg of the Long Beach Veterans Hospital injects into the mediastinal lymph plexus when making a radical removal of a lung. Usually the dye diffuses to the lymph nodes and makes those near enough to the surface visible so they can be excised in case of suspected lung cancer. Mixing radioactive di-iodofluorescein with the blue dye was suggested since with a gamma locater it would seem possible to locate more lymph nodes for excision, even if they were somewhat below the surface. Preliminary tests on rabbits have shown that the radioactivity of the di-iodofluorescein follows along with the visible dye.

For this application, the counter was made with a long light pipe so that the crystal and aperture could be introduced into a deep operation cavity. As yet it has not been used in a human operation.

3. *Sensitive Wide-Angle Counter*

Since a relatively small volume of calcium tungstate will absorb a high percentage of the incident 0.37-Mev gammas from radioiodine, a scintillation counter can be built with an overall sensitivity from 30 to 100 times greater than that of an ordinary G-M tube. Specially designed G-M tubes can do better than the usually available types. However, it was thought worth while to investigate scintillation counters for use in thyroid-gland uptake and biological half-life studies with radioiodine.

By removing the lead shield from the counter discussed in Section 1 of this article, it was found that the thyroid-uptake studies could be made with an administered dosage of only 1–5 μc of radioiodine. The calcium tungstate crystals which were cemented to the face of the 1P21 tube were placed close to the patient's thyroid gland and a series of cases were followed.

Somewhat later calcium tungstate crystals were cemented to the face of a 5819 tube. The arrangement is shown in Fig. 2. Tests showed that 0.002 μc of radioiodine placed 1 in. from the face of the crystal assembly could easily be detected at about twice a background of 4 cps. Thyroid uptake and biological half-life studies could easily be made with 1 μc, or less, administered dose.

It appears likely that this tube is sensitive enough to make a direct measurement of radioiodine in tissue by placing the counter over a part of the body. In such use the crystals would have to be particularly well shielded from the thyroid gland. Measurements along these lines are in progress.

4. Counter Characteristics

In Fig. 3 performance characteristics of the wide-angle counter tube discussed in Section 3 are given. The data plotted are from a 0.62-μc I^{131} source at a distance of 40.5 cm from the face of the crystals.

It was found that, over a limited range of photomultiplier plate voltage, the net counts of a sample at a fixed distance from the counter are approximately the same for the same background count. To get the same background count when the plate voltage is raised, the bias must be raised. If the plate voltage is raised too much, the sensitivity to the sample will decrease somewhat, even though the bias is adjusted to give the same background.

The three sets of points in Fig. 3 are for three different fixed bias settings, the plate voltage being varied to obtain various background levels. Background counts is chosen for the abscissa because the sample count is relatively independent of the physical factors, as long as the background is set at the same value.

The net counts increase rapidly with low background and then flatten out. The ratio of gross to background counts reaches a maximum value and then slowly decreases.

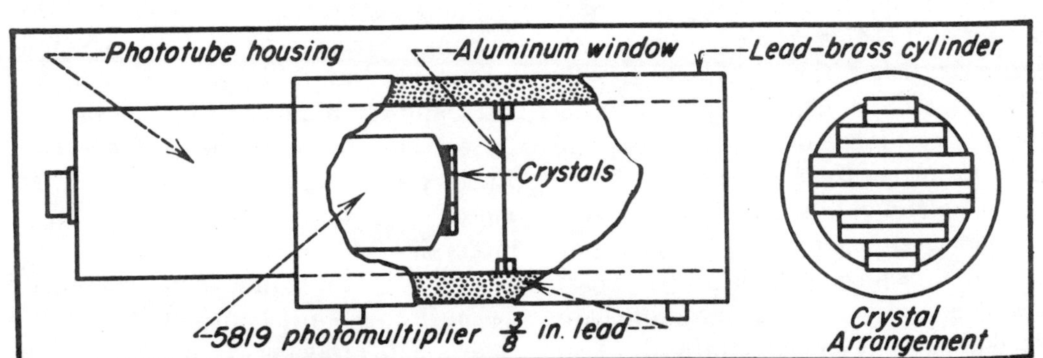

FIG. 2. Wide-angle scintillation counter designed for high sensitivity. The calcium tungstate crystals are cemented to the face of the photomultiplier

As is well known, the ratio of the standard deviation of the net counts, σ_{g-b}, to the net counts, $g - b$, is

$$\frac{\sigma_{g-b}}{g - b} = \frac{1}{\sqrt{g}} \frac{\sqrt{r^2 + r}}{r - 1}$$

where g = gross counts, b = background counts, and $r = g/b$.

The number of counts, C_p, required for a predetermined fractional accuracy, $p = \sigma_{g-b}/(g - b)$, is

$$C_p = \frac{1}{p^2} \frac{r^2 + r}{(r - 1)^2}$$

The time, t_p, required for C_p counts is

$$t_p = \frac{C_p}{g} = \frac{1}{gp^2} \frac{r^2 + r}{(r - 1)^2}$$

The third curve in Fig. 3 is $p^2 t_p$ plotted from this equation, with values of g taken from the experimental curve.

Counting with this particular counter is most accurate, then, if the background is about 8 cps, although the accuracy does not suffer too much over quite a range of background settings. In some applications a high gross-to-background ratio would be more useful than maximum accuracy. For this counter the maximum ratio is at about 6 cps, which is practically the same setting that gives maximum accuracy. The stability of the counting rate with respect to plate voltage fluctuations is at its best at higher backgrounds, say from 10 cps up.

5. *Automatic Scanner and Recorder*

The scintillation counter described in Section 1 of this article has been used for *in vivo* delineation of thyroid glands. The procedure requires taking individual readings over a rectangular network of positions and then estimating the gland outline by drawing a line through positions of a given reading or range of readings. With a little practice it is possible to get extraordinarily good agreement between the outlines so obtained and the actual outline of the glands as found either post operatively

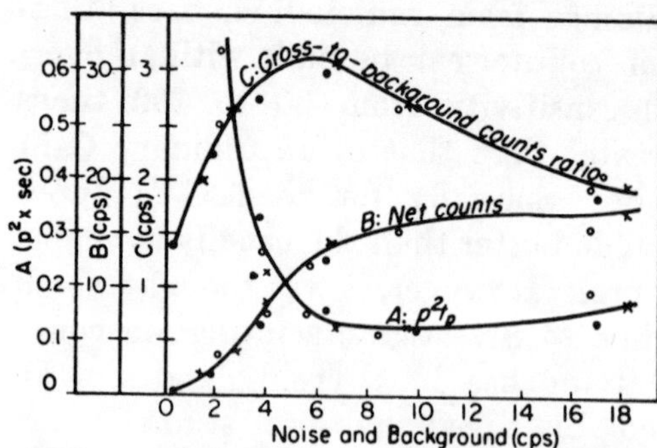

FIG. 3. Performance characteristics of a calcium tungstate scintillation counter

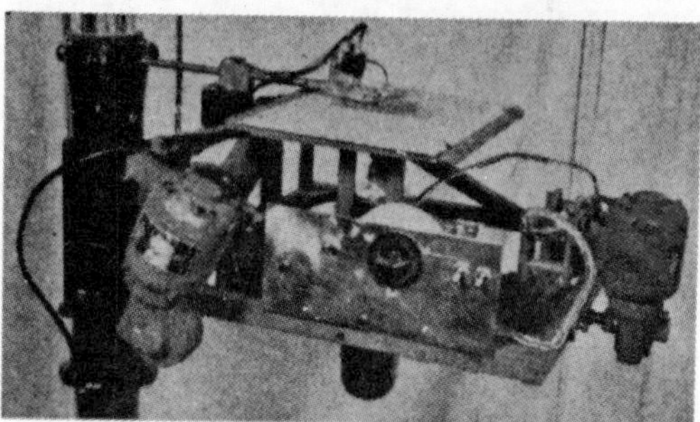

FIG. 4. Automatic scanner and recorder

or post mortemly. This procedure, however, is tedious and time consuming. An automatic scanner and recorder which would give a crude picture of the distribution of gland activity would obviously serve a very useful purpose.

The automatic scanner and recorder is shown in Fig. 4. The localizing scintillation counter is mounted on a carriage that is driven back and forth by a lead screw which in turn is driven by a reversing series motor operating through a reduction gear. The electrical reversing is accomplished by tripping a switch that is attached to the moving carriage, by a stationary but adjustable stop. The amplitude of back and forth motion can be adjusted by setting the positions of the stops. Each time reversal occurs the other motor is actuated for a small time interval. This interval is usually adjusted so that a scan is displaced about ⅛ in. from the previous one.

A small drawing board is rigidly mounted on the carriage that holds the counter. This drawing board is

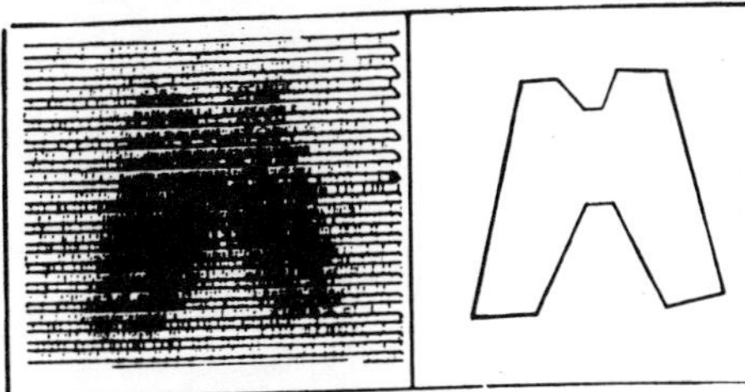

FIG. 5. Record of automatic scanning of filter paper soaked with 200 μc of I^{131} (left) and actual shape of the filter paper

scanned under an ink writing pen held rigidly on an arm attached to the main frame. The pen is attached to the arm of an electromagnet so that a short duration actuation of the magnet causes the pen to make a ⅛-in. pip in a direction at right angles to the direction of motion of the scanning table. The pen and relay assembly was adapted from one used on Esterline-Angus time-marking recorders.

The amplified pulses from the photomultiplier tube are fed into a multivibrator regularizer and scaler. The scaler can be set to feed a pulse to the pen for any power of 2 up to 256 counts. Obviously, when the ¼-in. aperture of the detector moves over an active area the pips will be closer together. The higher the signal-to-noise count ratio the higher will be the visual contrast in the scanning record. If the contrast is sufficient the effect of a picture of the gland will be obtained. However, even when the contrast is low, a sensation of a picture can often be obtained.

The first tests of the scanner were made with filter paper wetted with a solution containing radioiodine. Figure 5 shows such a record and the corresponding outline of the filter paper which had been wetted with 200 μc of I^{131}. On this record, one pip corresponds to four counts.

The next tests were made on a frozen trachea preparation with attached thyroid glands obtained from a terminal patient given 3 mc of I^{131} 14 hours before death. The gland uptake in this time was approximately 15%. A series of records were obtained from 11 to 29 days after death.

The relative success of these tests made it desirable to extend the trials to *in vivo* mapping of thyroid glands in actual patients. Tests were made and typical results are shown in Fig. 6.

* * *

The parts of this program of investigation requiring testing on patients at the Radioisotope Units of the Sawtelle and Long Beach Veterans Hospitals were authorized by the Division of Medicine and Biology of the Atomic Energy Commission, and by the Veterans Administration. At the Sawtelle Hospital the clinical programs were undertaken by Dr. Herbert Allen, Jr. and Dr. Raymond Libby. At the Long Beach Hospital some other types of testing were done under the direction of Dr. M. Morton. Much of the clinical findings reflected back on improved instrumentation development, and important suggestions were made by the clinicians concerned.

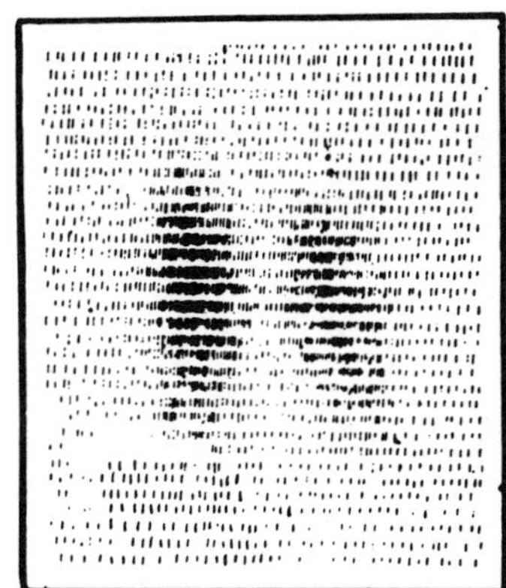

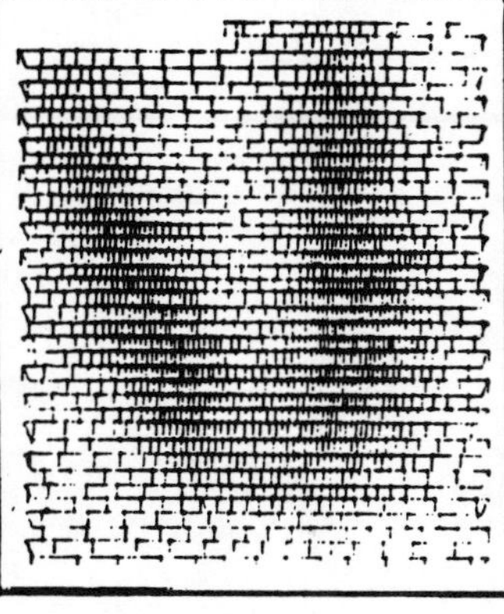

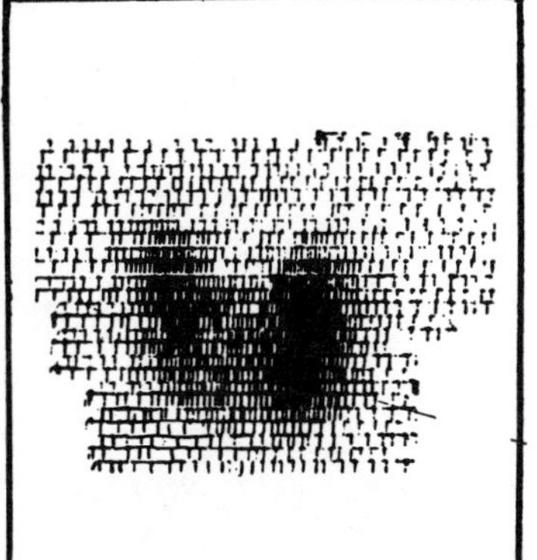

FIG. 6. Automatically recorded outlines of the thyroid glands of live patients

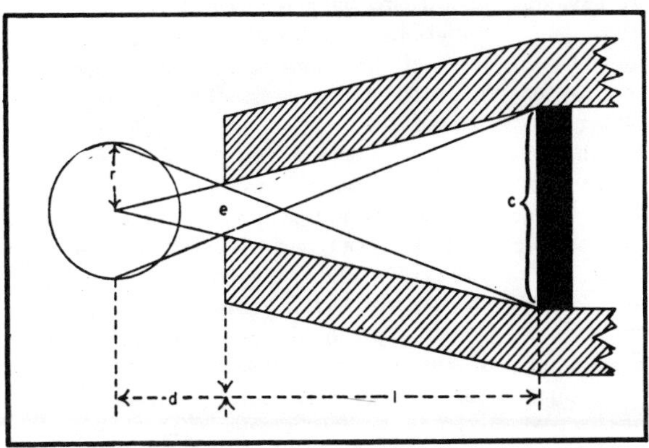

FIG. 1. Conical collimator that produces a scanning beam equal in diameter to a tumor at its focus

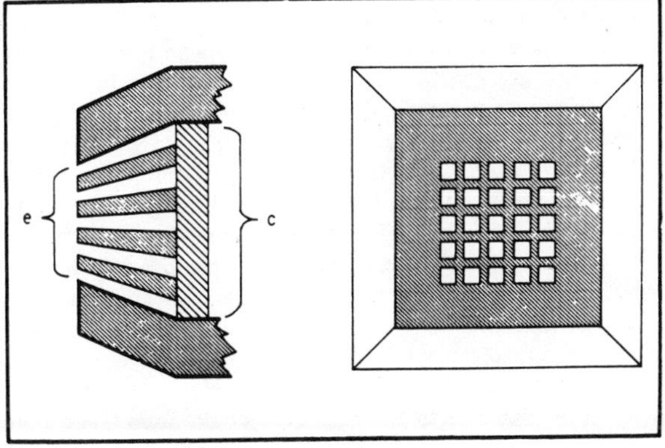

FIG. 2. Cross section and front view of a multichannel collimator used for gamma-ray scanning

Multichannel Collimators for Gamma-Ray Scanning with Scintillation Counters

To locate a tumor that has taken up radioiodine, the counter must look through a narrow collimator if the tumor is at the center of the brain. A multichannel collimator gives both a narrow scanning beam and a high counting rate

By R. R. NEWELL*
WILLIAM SAUNDERS†
and EARL MILLER‡

A BRAIN TUMOR that has taken up I^{131}-enriched diiodofluorescein can be detected with a counter by finding the point on the surface of the head where the counting rate is largest. This method, called the normal method by Moore (*1*), fails when the tumor lies at the center. Scanning must then be done with a counter which looks through a narrow collimator. Moore (*2*) thinks a conical collimator and a grid are both to be avoided. We believe this point needs further discussion.

Corbett and Honour (*3*) have designed a collimator for use with I^{131} gammas and a small cylindrical G-M tube. They mentioned the interesting possibilities of scintillation counters, but did not pursue this further and so had no call to study the adaptation of a collimator to a large frontal area of detector. They were interested in mapping the margins of the thyroid and were preoccupied with avoiding subsidiary peaks of response on the wings. They were little concerned with attaining a maximum signal, and readily accepted a very small aperture. Their analysis has, therefore, many differences from ours here.

To get a sufficient number of counts for statistical significance the counting rate must be high if the time available is limited. For example, the relatively high concentration of diiodofluorescein in a brain tumor persists for only an hour or two. The advantage of scintillation counters with their high efficiency for gamma rays becomes obvious. As much of the tumor radiation as possible should be caught by exposing a large area of crystal. The frontal area of the crystal is limited by

* Radiobiology Department, Stanford University School of Medicine, San Francisco, California.
† U. S. Veterans Hospital, San Francisco, California.
‡ University of California Medical School, San Francisco, California.

the ability of the light flashes to escape into the window of the photomultiplier.

The advantages of a collimator for these purposes are great. The problem is to design an optimum collimator. For a cylindrical collimator, however long, the crystal cannot be larger than the scanning beam (we call this a beam, although it is a limited bundle of rays coming in instead of going out). A conical collimator can be made to cover a large crystal.

Figure 1 shows a conical collimator that produces, at its focus, a scanning beam equal in diameter to the tumor. The collimator length, l, equals the tumor distance, d, multiplied by the ratio of crystal diameter, c, to tumor radius, r,

$$l = d\frac{c}{r}$$

The size of the entrance throat, e, equals the tumor radius multiplied by the ratio of collimator length to the sum of collimator length and tumor distance

$$e = r\frac{l}{l+d}$$

Thus, if the tumor is small and lies deep, the collimator has to be long, unless the crystal is small.

The larger the crystal, however, the longer the collimator, and the smaller the throat in relation to the crystal for a given narrow scanning beam. The ratio of throat area to crystal area is a measure of the efficiency of use of the crystal. It can be shown that

$$\text{efficiency} = \frac{d^2}{(d+l)^2}$$

The collimator should, therefore, be short. Since this means a narrow channel to get a narrow scanning beam, it uses only a small crystal.

To get a high counting rate, many of these narrow collimators are mounted abreast, all aimed at the same point. Such a multichannel collimator is shown in Fig. 2. The counting rate depends on how big the crystal is. The efficiency is measured by the ratio of areas of entrance throat and crystal, $(e/c)^2$, corrected for the area covered by the septa.

The optimum design of the multichannel collimator is not the same for all situations. Since large tumors close to the surface are easy diagnostic problems, they do not require optimum design. The optimum design pays off on the small deep-seated tumor.

As an example, take a 2-cm globular tumor (volume about 4 cm^3) in the middle of a 16-cm head (volume about 2,000 cm^3). Suppose that the specific uptake in the tumor is 4 times that in the brain generally. Let the total signal from the brain at a distance of 10 cm (2 cm from the surface) be 2,000 cps; this amounts to 1 cps/cm^3. Each cubic centimeter of tumor gives 4 cps, a total of 16 cps. The tumor displaces a volume of brain which would have given 4 cps. The effective tumor signal is the difference, 12 cps.

Noise-to-Signal Ratio

Without a collimator, the ratio of n, the total background including the brain, to s, the tumor signal, is 2,000/12 for the example above. But detection is hardly possible unless the tumor signal is at least three times the standard error of the measurement. To detect this tumor in the presence of such an overwhelming background without a collimator, even at the high counting rate of 2,000 cps, would require 10 min for each station, or setting, even if one had a dependable "normal" head for comparison.

In 300 sec the normal control head would give 600,000 counts. In another 300 sec one measures the patient's head and gets 603,600 counts. The difference, 3,600 counts, is due to the tumor. The standard error of the difference is $(600{,}000 + 603{,}600)^{1/2}$, which is about 1,100 counts. The difference, being more than three times the standard error, is taken as statistically significant.

The columnar signal. No matter how perfectly the scanning beam is adapted to the size of the tumor, the radiations from a column of brain in front of the tumor and behind it are accepted by the collimator and can't be stopped.

Figure 3 shows how a radioactive tumor is detected by scanning. The volume of brain enclosed in the scanning beam is a truncated pyramid. Its radiatively effective volume, for comparison with tumor volume, is equivalent to a prism with the cross section of the tumor. When the scanning beam moves "off tumor" a distance equal to ⅛ the diameter of the head, the length of path through the head is shortened by about 4%.

It will be shown later that the optimum scanning beam for a 2-cm tumor is about 3 cm square. For a beam of this size in a 16-cm head, the effective columnar volume of this beam that passes completely through the head is 144 cm^3. (The beam does actually expand toward the far side of the head, but the expansion is almost perfectly balanced by the reduction in effectiveness due to the distance.) This is 36 times the volume of the tumor, and even though the tumor has 4 times the concentration, the augmentation of the total column signal by the presence of the tumor is only 1 part in 9. About 1,500 counts are required for significant detection.

It is not apparent how this columnar radiation can be avoided, although some small amelioration becomes evident when the collimator's efficiencies for column and tumor are considered.

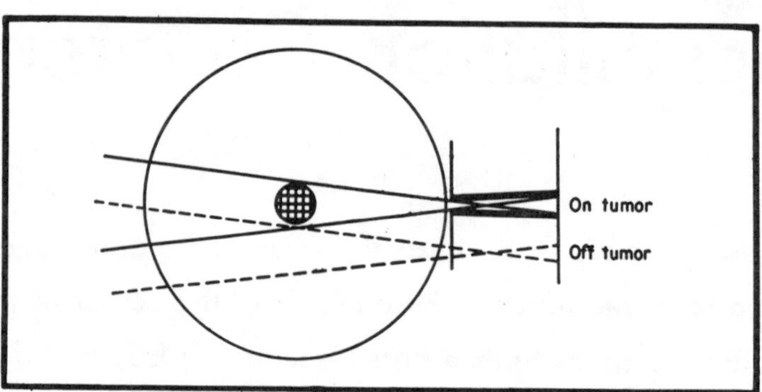

FIG. 3. Detection of a radioactive tumor in the center of the head

Length of Collimator

The mass of lead (or other material) in the collimator must be great enough to reduce to an acceptable level the radiation that comes from outside the scanning beam. Most of this radiation comes from the head.

One finds that one should not attempt to attenuate this to much less than $\frac{1}{4}$ of what comes (inescapably) from the column of brain lying along the scanning beam. The reason is that a longer collimator puts the crystal further away, and so reduces the counting rate, which results in an increase in the statistical error.

The collimator rejects most of the radiation coming from the lateral portions of the scanning beam. The average acceptance of the radiation coming from that portion of the brain enclosed within the scanning beam is $\frac{1}{4}$. When the tumor is at the focus of a collimator channel (Fig. 1) only the center of it sends radiation to the entire exposed crystal face. The radiation from all other source points is partly shielded, or occulted, by the collimator wall.

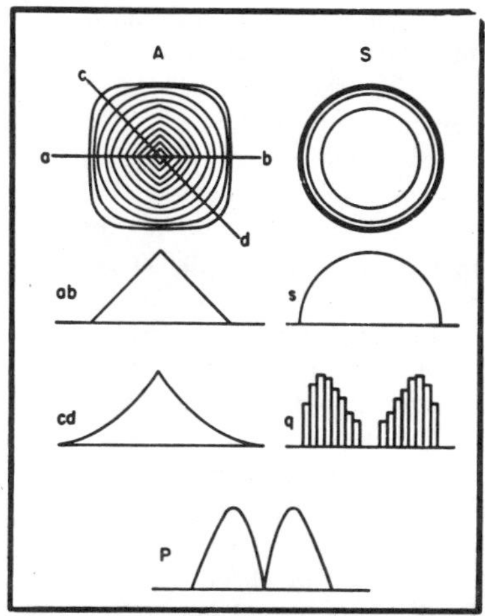

FIG. 4. Collimator acceptance contours (*A*), and tumor thickness contours (*S*)

Figure 4 illustrates the acceptance of the collimator. Diagram *A* shows, for a square scanning beam, the contours of equal percentage occultation over the face of the source of radiation, or what amounts to the inverse of the occultation, the acceptance, of the collimator for the radiation coming from the source. The contour lines are at intervals of 10%, from 100% at the center to essentially zero at the margins of the scanning beam. Section *ab* shows the profile square across, and *cd* shows the diagonal profile.

From a spherical tumor, more radiation per unit projected area comes from the thick center than from the edges. Diagram *S* in Fig. 4 shows contours of tumor thickness at intervals of 25%; *s* is the profile, and *q* is a histogram of the volumes in successive rings. The product of ring volume and percentage acceptance, when the tumor is exactly the size of the scanning beam, is shown at *P*. The area under *P* is a measure of the quantity of radiation that reaches the crystal. The shape of *P* changes when the ratio of scanning beam to tumor size changes.

In addition to reducing the beam to $\frac{1}{4}$ because of the average acceptance of the collimator, the septa of a multichannel collimator block off about half of the radiation within the beam (Fig. 2). This makes a total reduction to $\frac{1}{8}$. Consequently, the 144 cm^3 of a 3-cm-square beam column gives a signal only as large as 18 cm^3 would give without a collimator.

To reduce the radiation from the whole 2,000 cm^3 of head down to $\frac{1}{4}$ of what would come from 18 cm^3 means attenuation to $\frac{1}{440}$, which takes about 3.1 cm of lead, if the tracer is I^{131} (from our own absorption curve). If the collimator is half channels and half septa, its average density will be half as great as a block of solid metal, and its length will have to be twice as great, 6.2 cm, for the same attenuation.

Figure 5 summarizes the balance of effects between single and multichannel collimators. The curve labeled "inverse square" is calculated on the supposition that the channel of the collimator must limit the scanning beam to a 3-cm square at 8 cm from the face of the collimator. As the collimator is made longer, the crystal may be larger (Fig. 1), but the entrance aperture has a smaller ratio to the crystal size, cutting down the efficiency as shown. The points marked are where the exit aperture is large enough to expose crystals that are 0.5, 1.0, 1.55, 2.0, and 2.2 cm square.

When the channel is short and the efficiency high, a reduplication of the collimator multiplies the usable area of the crystal. If the sheaf of collimators is backed up by a single large crystal, the septa between channels shade part of the crystal face. The shorter the collimator the thicker these septa have to be to provide the necessary 3.1-cm lead-equivalent shielding.

The two "occultation by septa" curves show how this goes in terms of efficiency, which is the ratio of crystal face exposed to total crystal face. Obviously the efficiency goes to zero when a lead collimator is only 3.1 cm long, because then it has to be solid lead. But tungsten, being $\frac{3}{2}$ as dense, can be $\frac{1}{3}$ open channels and still give the necessary 3.1-cm lead-equivalent shielding when it is only 3.1 cm long.

The product of these two efficiency factors gives the resultant relative efficiency for every length of collimator. The highest efficiency for a multichannel tungsten collimator is the same as that of a single-channel collimator with a 1.55-cm-square exit aperture. To make use of a crystal larger than this, the multichannel collimator is better. For lead, the multichannel construction is better for crystals larger than 2.2-cm square. These critical sizes are shown by the horizontal dotted lines.

The vertical dotted lines in Fig. 5 show the required length of collimator for the optimum design in tungsten and lead. The optimum design for a 3-cm-square scanning beam focused at 8 cm from the face of the collimator gives an efficiency of 24% for gold or tungsten, and 16% for lead. For lead, a multichannel collimator is better than a single-channel one if the crystal is more than 5 cm^2 (2.2-cm square). For gold or tungsten, the balance tips at 2.4 cm^2. If one can use a 40-cm^2 crystal (a 6.3-cm square, or a 7-cm circle) we calculate that a multichannel collimator made of tungsten will prove 6.5 times as good as a single channel one. Made of lead, it would be only 4.3 times as good.

Optimum Size of Beam

For any single channel, either a pyramid or a truncated cone (Fig. 1), the rays from the center of the tumor reach, at the focus, the whole surface of the exposed crystal. They are 100% accepted. Rays from lateral portions are partly cut off, so that the acceptance gradually falls away to zero at the edges of the beam. Figure 4 shows the way the acceptance falls away from center to edge of the scanning beam. By arithmetic integration of the product of area and acceptance, we find that the acceptance for the total cross section of the beam (round or square) is about $\frac{1}{4}$.

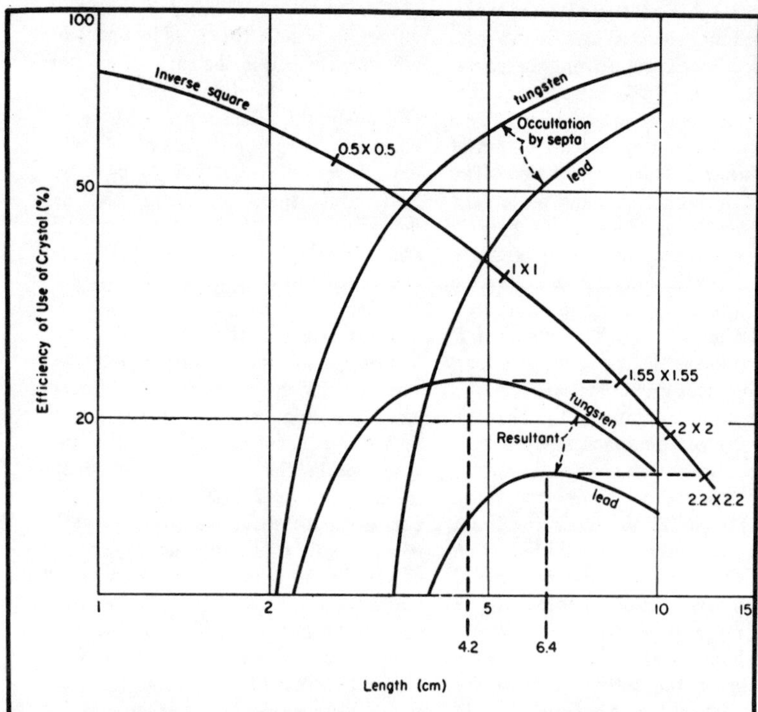

FIG. 5. Balance of effects between single and multichannel collimators

But the radiation from the tumor comes mostly from the middle, where the tumor is thickest. A similar arithmetic integration for a tumor of exactly the diameter of a round scanning beam focused at its center, results in an acceptance value of 0.38. If the beam is smaller than the tumor, the acceptance falls off markedly because the outer tumor rays are cut off completely. If the beam is larger than the tumor, the acceptance increases because the tumor is better limited to the center of the beam where collimator acceptance is high.

Figure 6 is a graph of collimator acceptance for various relative diameters of scanning beam. It is calculated for a 2-cm spherical tumor, at the focus of a conical collimator which is focused at a distance of 8 cm (Fig. 1).

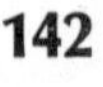

Figure 7 shows the optimum size of the scanning beam for a 2-cm tumor. As the scanning beam is made larger, the background increases because a larger column of brain is included. Tumor signal increases because more of it lies in the center of the larger beam, where collimator acceptance is higher, but this goes on more slowly.

The tumor signal keeps up with the background for a while because collimator acceptance is increasing for the tumor but remains constant at ¼ for the column through the head. With still larger beam, this effect can no longer overcome the fact that the volume of the tumor remains constant while the volume in the column increases with the beam cross section. As the tumor signal falls away, the ratio of background to signal grows larger, and the counts required increases as the square of this ratio.

The upper curve shows the time required (at that counting rate) to attain a tumor signal three times its standard error. The time can obviously be shortened by giving a larger dose of tracer isotope.

The necessary total number of counts to reduce the statistical error to the required degree goes up as the square of the ratio of background to tumor signal. But the increase in counting rate shortens the time required for a given number of counts. The result is that time is best conserved, not by choosing a maximum ratio of signal to noise (minimum ratio of background to tumor signal), but by choosing a somewhat larger beam.

The difference between a square beam and a round one is negligible (less than 10% in required time). The optimum is fairly broad, and any beam size between 0.9 and 2 times the diameter of the tumor will be within 20% of the optimum.

Detecting a Small Tumor

There might be hope of detecting a 2-cm tumor (4 cm^3) in a 16-cm head (2,000 cm^3). A multichannel lead collimator built for a 3-cm-square scanning beam at a distance of 8 cm, is 6.5 cm long, which puts the crystal 14.5 cm from the center of the head. The septa shade 48% of the surface of the crystal. The collimator blocks off radiation coming from all parts of the head that are not within the scanning beam. The equivalent volume of head within the scanning beam is that of a square prism 3 × 3 × 16 cm, which is about 7% of the volume of the head. The average acceptance for radiation from this column is 25%. The product of these factors is 0.0091.

If the patient has received a dose of I^{131}-enriched diiodofluorescein that makes the average activity in the head high enough to give 10,000 cps on a large crystal 14.5 cm from the center of the head, then the interposition of a perfect collimator of the above dimensions would reduce the columnar signal to 91 cps. But the collimator is not perfect. Its thickness is equivalent to only 3.1 cm of lead, and it attenuates the gamma rays by a factor of 1/440. Thus the radiation from the whole head adds only 23 cps to the signal, and the total signal is, 114 cps.

On this total background is superimposed the extra radiation from the tumor. We suppose the tumor to have a volume of 4 cm^3 and a specific activity four times that of its surroundings. It displaces 4 cm^3 of brain and substitutes 300% more radiation for this fraction (4/44) of the beam column. However, the acceptance of

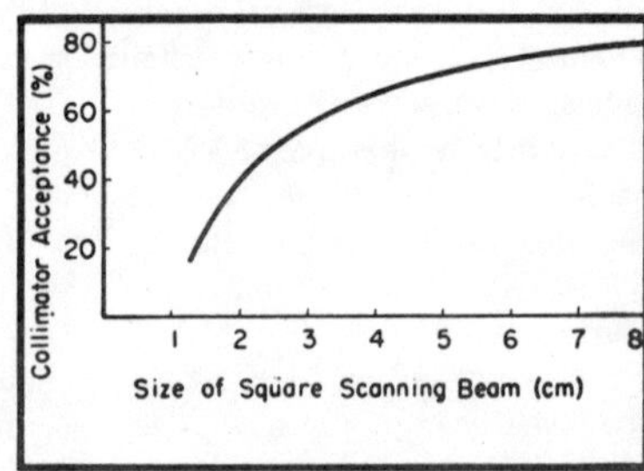

FIG. 6. Acceptance of collimator for radiations from tumors of different sizes

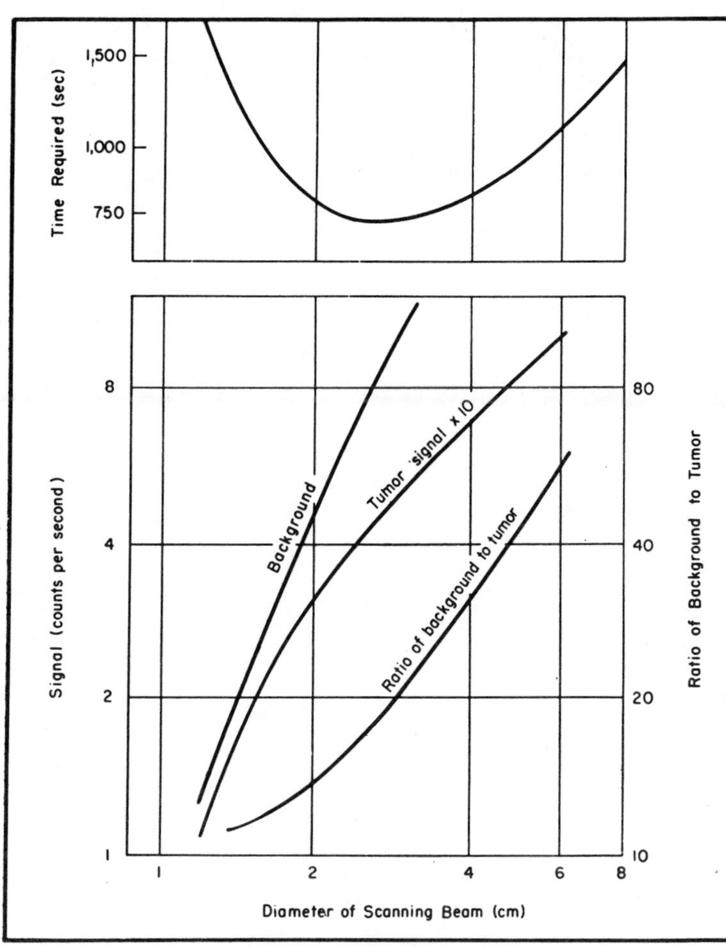

FIG. 7. Optimum size of scanning beam for a 2-cm tumor

this radiation is 56% instead of 25% (Figs. 5 and 6), so that the actual increment of signal is 18% of the column signal, or 16 cps. The background plus tumor is 130 cps.

Now displace the scanning beam laterally 2 cm (Fig. 3). The edge of the beam still cuts through 0.5 cm of the side of the tumor (15% of its volume), but collimator acceptance is so low at the edge of the beam that the tumor signal is reduced to about 5%, or 0.8 cps. The beam column is shortened about 6 mm, which reduces the column signal to 87.4 cps. The 23 cps from the whole head remains the same. The counting rate "off tumor" is the sum of all these, or 111.2 cps. The difference between this and 130 cps, the counting rate "on tumor," is 18.8 cps, of which 3.6 cps is attributable to the change in length of column path through the head, and only 15.2 cps is significant of the presence of tumor, i.e., a change of 11.7% from the "on tumor" signal.

Statistical error. If the "on tumor" and "off tumor" positions are each run to 2,000 counts, the standard error of each run is 2.5%. The standard error of the difference is $2.5\% \times \sqrt{2}$, which is 3.5%. The change in signal is more than three times its standard error, and can be taken as statistically significant.

Each station should be run to 2,000 counts, which takes about 18 sec. It should be possible to make enough such readings to survey the whole head in a reasonable total time.

If the isotope dose is smaller, so as to diminish the hazard to the patient, the time required for the measurements is correspondingly lengthened.

If the tumor is smaller it will be much more difficult to detect, unless its specific uptake is greater. If a 1-cm tumor is to be detected, it seems likely that it will require a collimator designed especially for it. Such a collimator made of lead would be 10 cm long, the time required would be increased 8 times, and the job of surveying the head would take half a day. It might be worth while to make a collimator for a 1-cm tumor, and hope for a higher specific uptake. For a tumor so very small, if a 25-cm² crystal is used, the multichannel collimator is 10 times as good as a single-channel collimator.

Collimator Construction

Our first collimators were made by casting lead around a number of smooth rods and driving out the rods.

We also made a collimator of sheet lead cut in the shape of a circular skirt. Several layers of masking tape were cemented along the greater and lesser curved edges, the greater being thicker. When rolled on itself, this sheet made a truncated cone. When the small end was pressed onto a spherical surface of proper size, this structure took a nearly perfect form, with the slit well focused on a point.

Since the parameters for good efficiency are moderately critical, it pays to calculate and make the collimator with more precision. We found that an easy way to do this is to make saw cuts in a block of light wood and cast a heavy alloy into this form. Wood's metal is convenient because it does not char the wood, although it is less dense than lead. The wood core is left in place. We hope to incorporate tungsten sheet, or tungsten powder to increase density and efficiency.

The saw cuts have parallel sides, instead of the theoretically correct wedge shape. This makes the bundle of channels point to a focus further away than the focus of the individual channel. The effect is a small one, and unimportant. With simple saw cuts, the density of the collimator is a little less than it ought to be for the chosen ratio of channel area. The collimator should, therefore, be a little longer, but this is also a small effect.

* * *

The opinions expressed here are those of the authors, and are not to be taken as reflecting any official views of the Veterans Administration.

BIBLIOGRAPHY

1. G. E. Moore, D. A. Kohl, J. F. Marvin, J. C. Wang, C. M. Caudill, *Radiology* **55**, 344 (1950)
2. G. Boyack, G. E. Moore, D. F. Clausen, NUCLEONICS **3**, No. 4, 62 (1948)
3. B. D. Corbett, A. J. Honour, NUCLEONICS **9**, No. 5, 43 (1951)

Cardiac Output of Men and Dogs Measured by in vivo Analysis of Iodinated (I^{131}) Human Serum Albumin

By REX L. HUFF, M.D., DAVID D. FELLER, PH.D., OLIVER J. JUDD, M.SC. AND GEORGE M. BOGARDUS, M.D.

A time-intensity analysis of I^{131} was carried out with a highly shielded well-collimated scintillation detector placed over the chest of normal men and women, patients and dogs. I^{131} human serum albumin solution was injected intravenously. The curves thus obtained when analyzed for cardiac output gave values not significantly different from simultaneously obtained direct Fick values.

THE first published effort to record the intensity of radioactivity as a function of time over the heart following a single intravenous injection was by Prinzmetal and associates.[1] They used a relatively unshielded Geiger tube and Na^{24}. Despite relative insensitivity of Geiger tubes to hard gamma rays, they were able to detect (by in vivo analysis) two peaks of radioactivity representing the entry of Na^{24} to the right and left heart. Work of a very similar nature was published shortly after by Waser and Hunzinger.[2] Their work also includes simultaneous measurements of the peripheral circulation.

This type of study has recently been made by Shipley and co-workers[3] with modern scintillation equipment and wide angle counting of I^{131}. A more extensive analysis of the data was made from the standpoint of the possibility of computing cardiac output, but the authors concluded that the method gave results roughly twice greater than those of conventional methods. They justify the use of a modified Hamilton equation with curves having the double rise on the basis that the equilibrium value truly represents the sum of the equilibrium values of the two components causing the double rise, that is, the radioactivity in the right and left sides of the heart. This leads to the assumption that the radioactivity of either of the waves does not reinforce the other. But this would tend to make the values for cardiac output too low and, therefore, is perhaps of little significance since their values were twice too high rather than too low. The major cause of the lack of correlation between their data with that of conventional methods for cardiac output is thought to be due to the inordinately high equilibrium value occurring due to the use of a wide angle counter. They discuss this possibility.[3]

Perfect simulation of the conditions for use of the Hamilton equation[4, 5, 6] for cardiac output on data obtained by external detection of gamma rays probably can never be achieved; however, the results of our studies correlate so well with the conventional direct Fick method that we think them worth reporting. The major modifications we have made from the preceding method,[3] and which we feel contribute to the success of the technic, are (1) collimation with a $\frac{3}{4}$ inch $\times$ 2 inch orifice[7]; (2) positioning of the counter on an area of the body where there is a relatively small or insignificant amount of intervening musculoskeletal blood; and (3) location near the aorta. The effects of these modifications in technic are discussed.

METHODS

Isotope. Human serum albumin tagged with I^{131} was used routinely in amounts varying from 100 to 200 μc. When it was necessary to repeat the test immediately, 300 μc. were given as the second injection. In such instances, Lugols solution was administered during the subsequent week.

From the Radioisotope Unit, and Divisions of Medicine and Surgery, Veterans Administration Hospital, Seattle, Washington, and the University of Washington Medical School Departments of Medicine and Surgery, Seattle, Wash.

This work was aided by a grant from the Life Insurance Medical Research Fund.

Received for publication June 8, 1955.

Apparatus. The scintillation detector consisted of a thalliated sodium iodide cylindrical crystal 3/4 inch high and 3/4 inch in diameter optically coupled to a photomultiplier tube. The detector was shielded by two inches of lead on all sides except for the 3/4 inch diameter cylindrical hole used to collimate the radiation. A cathode follower coupled the signal to either a scaler with a plug-in ratemeter or a ratemeter and/or scaler.

The method whereby the data were recorded depended on the driving units used. The output of the ratemeter registered on a potentiometer recorder and the output from the scaler was taken from the register driving impulse through a suitable voltage pulse shaping network and recorded on one channel of a galvanometer type recorder. The latter recorder gave a clear record of the register impulses when the paper speed was 2.5 cm. per second and the scaler was set to scale by 64. The potentiometer recorder had a paper speed of 180 inches per hour and its associated ratemeter had an integration time constant of 2.5 seconds. Both methods of recording could be used simultaneously. In order to evaluate the time constant of the ratemeter integration circuit and response of the recorder, a hand plotted histogram of the recorded register impulses of the scaler was prepared and compared to the pen written record. When a three second interval histogram was plotted, the integral under the primary circulation peak was not measurably different.

Evaluation of detector field. Positioning a point source showed that an angle of 30 degrees encompassed all of the high counting rates and that the rates fell off sharply; i.e., within 1 inch of the 30 degree solid angle. At three to four inches from the outer plane of the aperture, the diameter of the field is three and one-half inches.

Since the count rate of a point source falls off as the reciprocal of the distance squared while the "counted volume" increases with distance, an experiment was performed to evaluate the relative counting efficiencies of segments of a half-inch thickness and about 16 inches in diameter when present at different distances from the aperture. In this way it was possible to show that the layer of I^{131} solution nearest the counter contributed about twice as much as the layers between three and four inches away. The reduction in count rate with distance was roughly exponential with a half value of three inches.

Procedure of Injection. The human subject, seated and at rest for ten minutes prior to injection, had the detector placed on the skin between the first and second ribs or at the second rib at the left parasternal line and with the axis of the collimator forming an angle of approximately 10 degrees to the left side, posteriorly. The venopuncture was made using a 21 gage needle mounted on an empty syringe. This syringe was removed and after a free flow of blood was assured, the syringe containing the I^{131} human serum albumin (in a volume of 0.1 to 1.0 ml.) was attached; injection was made in a single continuous motion and required about 1 second. In 8 to 10 minutes, two venous blood samples were taken for blood volume determination.

Direct Fick cardiac outputs. Fick methods were carried out in the usual manner on unanesthetized patients. Mongrel dogs in a healthy state were anesthetized with pentobarbital (30 mg. per Kg.). In some cases, the catheter was placed in the pulmonary artery while in others it was placed in the right ventricle. The cardiac output determinations by Fick and dilution technics were carried out simultaneously.

Calculation of flow rate. The initial fall in intensity of radioactivity following the first rise was extrapolated in the manner of other investigators.[8] Extrapolation was done in the early studies on a hand plotted histogram from the data of the galvanometer type recorder, but in most of the studies the curves of the automatic pen writer were extrapolated directly on the recorder paper. The area under the primary extrapolated curve was measured with a planimeter in square inches. The area was divided by the length in inches which represented one minute since recorder speed was expressed in inches per minute. This quotient was then divided into the height in inches of the equilibrium value. Thus

$$\text{Blood volumes per minute} = \frac{\text{Ht. (inches) of equilibrium value}}{\text{Area (inches)}^2 \text{ of extrapolated curve / recorder paper speed in inches per min.}}$$

The dimension of blood volumes per minute is valid if it is assumed that the ordinate values of the curve can be reliably related to the equilibrium value where all the injected dose I, is diluted in the entire blood volume. This equation for computation of output differs from the formulation of Kinsman and associates,[4] only in the fact that concentration $C(t)$ is presented as $C(t) = \frac{I}{BV(t)}$, and the equation for flow F:

$$F = \frac{I}{\int_{t_1}^{t_2} C(t)\,dt} = \frac{I}{\int_{t_1}^{t_2} \frac{I}{BV(t)}\,dt} = \frac{1}{\int_{t_1}^{t_2} \frac{1}{BV(t)}\,dt}$$

where $BV(t)$ is the time varying fraction of blood in which the injected dose I is apparently diluted, and the time limit t_2 is the apparent termination of the extrapolated curve. Shipley and associates[3] discuss this derivation in a slightly different form.

Results and Discussion

The majority of the curves show only one major rise and fall in counting rate with time (fig. 1). These eight graphs are smoothed curves made from the three second interval histograms of eight normal subjects. The equilibrium value obtained after 3 to 10 minutes is also shown. The curves are similar to those obtained by direct arterial sampling.[8, 9, 10] About 20 per cent of these curves exhibited a double rise when one second interval histograms were plotted. They have some resemblance to the doubly peaked in vivo curves published by others;[1, 2] however, the decrease in counting rates between the two peaks was less. Cardiac output calculated with either the one second interval curve or the three second curve was the same.

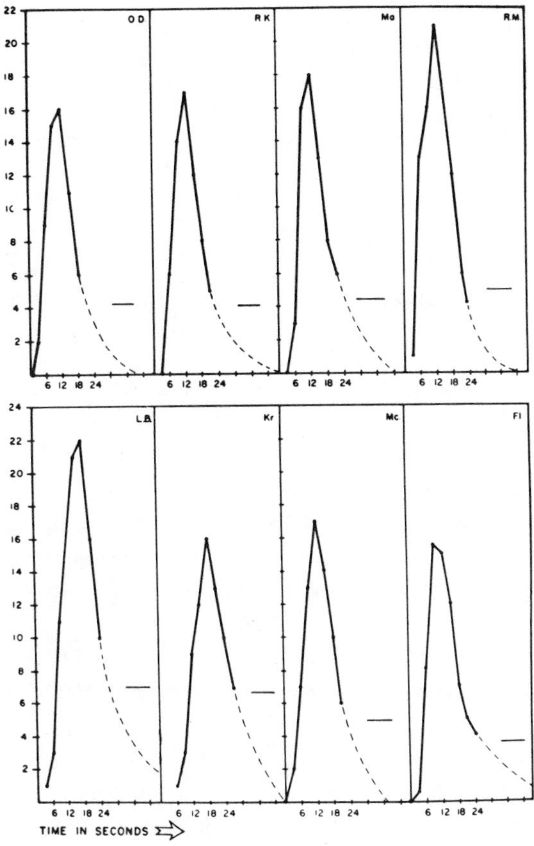

Fig. 1. Data from eight normal subjects, obtained by a crystal detector well-collimated and shielded, placed at the level of the second rib at the left parasternal border. Ordinates show the count rate divided by 64 at successive three-second intervals. Short horizontal line is the equilibrium level obtained after several minutes of measurement. Dashed line is the extrapolation used for measurement of the area under the curve, abscissae, time in seconds.

Table 1.—*Cardiac Output Values*

	No. of Subjs.	Blood Vol. L.	Cardiac Output	
			Blood Vol./min.	L./min./M²
Normal Women	28	4.1* ± 0.7†	1.3 ± 0.3	3.3 ± 0.8
Normal Men	36	5.5 ± 0.8	1.3 ± 0.2	3.6 ± 0.8

Patients	Fick L/min./M²	I^{131} HSA in vivo L/min./M²
1. RIT	2.05	2.04
	2.11	2.14
2. SHI	2.69	2.80
	2.75	2.66
3. HAN	1.60	1.53
4. MAC	4.03	4.15
5. SAN	1.77	1.34

* Mean.
† Standard deviation.

Table 1 gives the data of 28 normal women and 36 normal men. The age range was 17 to 57 years but most subjects are between 20 and 40 years. The mean cardiac index for the women was 3.3 L. per minute per square meter of body surface area with a standard deviation of 0.8; while the mean and standard deviation for the 36 men were 3.6 and 0.8 L. per minute per square meter of body surface area respectively.

The range of the average of Fick cardiac indices reported by various investigators is from 3.27 to 3.79,[11, 12, 13, 14, 15, 16] and the range for the direct dye method is 2.85 to 4.19 L. per minute per square meter of body surface area.[16, 17, 18] The mean cardiac index for the men and women by the in vivo method is 3.5 with a standard deviation of 0.8.

Table 1 also shows the calculated blood volumes of the subjects as well as the cardiac output in terms of blood volumes per minute. It is thought important, that these values are obtained as part of this method, since the former is useful information in the case of many cardiacs and the latter is a parameter of *blood turnover rate*. The parameter of blood turnover rate, although not a true representation of all segments of blood in the body, is a general indication of blood mixing efficiency. Inspection and analysis of the individual curves demonstrate the approximate volumes and rates of slowly mixing components. This type of analysis constitutes the subject of another study.

TABLE 2.—*Dog Data: Simultaneous Cardiac Output Determinations by the Direct Fick and in vivo I^{131} HSA Method*

Dog	Trial	Wt. Kg.	A-V Diff. O_2%	O_2 Consum. cc.	BV (cc.)	Cardiac Output		
						Fick cc./min.	In Vivo I^{131}	
							BV/min.	cc./min.
1	1	10.0	6.68	57	650	853	1.72	1120
2	2	16.5	2.55	138	1250	5400	4.46	5570
	3		2.04	115	1250	5640	4.17	5210
3	4	13.6	2.21	70	935	3180	3.04	2840
4	5	12.1	3.22	82	697	2540	3.51	2440
	6		3.63	78	712	2150	3.29	2340
5	7	17.6	2.61	120	1480	4510	2.54	3760
	8		2.78	123	1480	4430	2.39	3540
6	9	10.4	4.52	73	713	1630	2.32	1655
	10		4.39	81	713	1850	2.34	1680
	11		5.19	98	763	1900	1.87	1430
7	12	10.4	4.40	80	885	1819	1.93	1710
	13		3.54	94	815	2660	2.45	2000
8	14	19.8	5.00	94	1080	1880	2.47	2670
	15		3.32	92	1080	2770	2.52	2720
9	16	16.5	1.36	53	1545	3900	2.22	3430
	17		3.56	122	1545	3430	2.00	3080
10	18	11.0	2.00	62	1200	3100	2.50	3000
	19		2.20	64	1200	2950	3.00	3600
11	20	19.0	5.65	93	1092	1640	1.92	2100
	21		5.51	142	1335	2575	3.02	4030
12	22	10.0	2.00	59	934	2950	3.02	2820

Table 1 allows comparison of seven simultaneous Fick and in vivo isotope determinations (5 patients). These paired data with the exception of one (patient with very low output) are almost identical. The mean of the differences of the paired data is 0.072 L. per minute per square meter; while the standard deviation is 0.19 and the standard error of the mean 0.095. The "t" value is thus 0.762 and the corresponding "p" is equal to or greater than 0.5.

The accuracy of detector positioning on the chest is limited in several ways. The contour of the chest may have an irregular outward convexity in the region of the first and second ribs so that placing the axis of the collimator normal to the skin surface, while directing the axis perpendicular to the anterior topographic projection of the arch of the aorta, is impossible. In such an instance the detector was always placed with respect to the expected aortic projection based on location of bone prominences.

Although efforts were made to effectively isolate a segment of the vasculature so it alone would be in the radiation detector field, it is not thought that this is mandatory to the success of the method. That it is not necessary to "effectively isolate" certain volumes is true for the chambers of the heart and great vessels, but not for the various distal vascular beds. This fact was realized by Shipley and co-workers[3] and pointed out as justification for examination of their doubly humped curves by the Hamilton equation. Veall and associates,[19] have presented a mathematic proof for this contention. As pointed out above, such an application cannot be made to in vivo data which represent a large portion of some distal segment of the circulation, for example, musculoskeletal circulation. Thus the tissue nearest the detector, the intervening body wall, falls into this category. Thoroughgoing consideration of the effect of coronary blood flow on these measurements cannot be made at this time because of lack of data.

Table 2 presents data of simultaneous Fick and in vivo I^{131} cardiac output in dogs. The average absolute difference of the two methods of 22 trials in 12 dogs was 12 per cent. The mean of the differences of the paired data is 46 ml. per minute; while the standard deviation is 531 and the standard error of the mean is 116 ml. per minute. The "t" value is thus 0.397 and the corresponding "p" is equal to 0.7. The correlation coefficient was .90 with a high degree of significance. Although the animals were under deep anesthesia, their blood turnover rate was several blood volumes per minute, in contrast to slightly over one blood volume per minute in man.

That the I^{131} data of the dog studies differed so slightly from the Fick dog data was surprising in view of the difficulty of accurate counter localization and the use of a counter having the same collimation as in the human studies.

The similarity of the data gathered by these two methods leads us to conclude that for men and dogs the body surface measurements of I^{131} are a good approximation for a real arterial curve. We believe the chief reasons that the in vivo method described here gives values similar to the direct Fick method and the direct arterial sampling are:

(1) The early and main portion of the curve is produced by tagged blood in the major fixed vessels. The isotope in pulmonary artery and veins, as well as their branches and tributaries probably contributes slightly to the initial curve. The position used (second rib at the left parasternal line) assures us that in most individuals studied, the major "sampled" vessel is the aortic arch. The theory, developed and mentioned above,[3, 19] suggests that pure single vessel sampling is not required.

(2) The equilibrium value is measured over a very small portion of a relatively avascular bony area. The results of the two experiments described under "Methods" indicate the relative efficiency of counting tagged material at different distances from the outer plane of the orifice. The detected field in the mediastinum is nearly 100 per cent blood while that of the thoracic wall is only about 2 per cent blood.[20] Thus if one considers a core of musculoskeletal system 2 cm. $\times$ 3 cm. or about 10 $cm.^3$, there is not likely to be more than 0.6 $cm.^3$ of blood present or about 1/100,000 of the total radioactivity in the body. The value 0.6 $cm.^3$ is high; it is more likely in the order of 0.2 to 0.4 $cm.^3$ since musculoskeletal parts containing large quantities of fat or bone contain a lesser amount of blood.[20, 21] The position at the second rib near the midline has the advantage that it rarely, if ever, has a large thickness of fat or musculoskeletal tissue.

Almost simultaneously with our first presentation of the results of this method,[22] Veall and co-workers[19] reported a nearly identical method with comparable results. Through a personal communication from N. Veall, we learned that other investigators have obtained additional data confirming the reported similarity of the results of the in vivo isotope and direct Fick methods.

This in vivo method has several advantages, chiefly its simplicity. The subject may be readily studied in recumbent, erect or sitting positions. Except for marked uncontrollable chest movements, there are few abnormalities of the subjects which interfere with this procedure; it also gives additional useful information on blood volume and cardiac output in terms of blood volume per minute.

The test may be repeated as indicated without exceeding the tolerance dose if no more than 0.3 μc. is present in the body and Lugols solution is given to block the uptake of I^{131} by the thyroid. The 300 μc. value is calculated for total body distribution of I^{131}. It is somewhat less than the value of 8.3 μc. per Kg. given by Marinelli and co-workers,[23] which results in 0.1 Roentgen equivalent physical representation during the first day following the deposition.

Summary

A method for estimating cardiac output by external body counting of I^{131} following a single injection of I^{131} is described. A well-collimated and shielded scintillation detector was placed at the left parasternal line between the first and second ribs for recording a time concentration curve. Calculation of cardiac output was by a modification of the Hamilton dye method. Seven patient and 22 dog studies, carried out simultaneously by this method and the direct Fick method, when subjected to the "t" test, showed the means not to be significantly different. Sixty-four normal subjects studied by the external counting technic had a mean cardiac index very similar to published values obtained by conventional methods for normal subjects. This method has the advantage of simplicity in application. Serial arterial blood sampling is not required.

Acknowledgment

We are indebted to Doctors J. Michel, Belding H. Scribner and J. Thomas Payne for their assistance in cardiac catheterization. The constant encouragement and assistance of Dr. Robert S. Evans was of great value.

REFERENCES

[1] PRINZMETAL, M., CORDAY, E., SPRITZLER, R. J. AND FLIEG, W.: Radiocardiography and its clinical application. J.A.M.A., **139:** 617, 1949.

[2] WASER, VON P. AND HUNZINGER, W.: Bestimmung von Kreislaufgrössen mit radioaktiven Kochsalz Cardiologia **15:** 219, 1950.

[3] SHIPLEY, R. A., CLARK, R. E., LIEBOWITZ, D. AND KROHMER, J. S.: Analysis of the radiocardiogram in heart failure. Circulation Research **1:** 5, 428, 1953.

[4] KINSMAN, J. M., MOORE, J. W. AND HAMILTON, W. F.: Studies on the circulation. I. Injection method: Physical and mathematical considerations. Am. J. Physiol. **89:** 322, 1929.

[5] MOORE, J. W., KINSMAN, J. M., HAMILTON, W. F. AND SPURLING, R. G.: Studies on the circulation. II. Cardiac output determinations: Comparison of the injection method with the direct Fick procedure. Am. J. Physiol. **89:** 331, 1929.

[6] HAMILTON, W. F., RILEY, R. L., ATTYAH, A. M., COURNAND, A., FOWELL, D. M., HIMMELSTEIN, A., NOBLE, R. P., REMINGTON, J. W., RICHARDS, D. W., JR., WHEELER, N. C. AND WITHAM, A. C.: Comparison of Fick and dye injection methods of measuring cardiac output in man. Am. J. Physiol., **153:** 309, 1948.

[7] HUFF, R. L., ELMLINGER, P., GARCIA, J. F., ODA, J., COCKRELL, M. S., AND LAWRENCE, J. H.: Ferrokinetics in normal subjects and in patients having various hematopoietic diseases. J. Clin. Invest., **30:** 1512, 1951.

[8] MACINTYRE, W. J., STORAASLI, J. P., KRIEGER, H., PRITCHARD, W. AND FRIEDELL, H.: I^{131}-Labeled serum albumin: Its use in the study of cardiac output and peripheral vascular flow. Radiology, **59:** 849, 1952.

[9] PRITCHARD, W. H., MACINTYRE, W. J., SCHMIDT, W. C., BROFMAN, B. AND MOORE, D. J.: The determination of cardiac output by a continuous recording system utilizing iodinated (I^{131}) human serum albumin. II. Clinical Studies. Circulation, **6:** 572, 1952.

[10] NYLIN, G. AND CELANDER, H.: Determination of blood volume in the heart and lungs and the cardiac output through the injection of radiophosphorus. Circulation, **1:** 76, 1950.

[11] COURNAND, A., RILEY, R. L., BREED, E. S., BALDWIN, E. DEF., AND RICHARDS, D. W., JR.: Measurement of cardiac output in man using the technique of catheterifation of the right auricle or ventricle. J. Clin. Invest., **24:** 106, 1945.

[12] STEAD, E. A., JR., WARREN, J. F., MERRILL, A. J. AND BRANNON, E. S., The cardiac output in male subjects as measured by the technique of right atrial catheterization. Normal values with observations on the effect of anxiety and tilting. J. Clin. Invest., **24:** 326, 1945.

[13] EBERT, R. V., BORDEN, C. W., WELLS, H. S. AND WILSON, R. H.: Studies of the pulmonary circulation. I. The circulation time from the pulmonary artery to the femoral artery and the quantity of blood in the lungs in normal individuals. J. Clin. Invest., **24:** 326, 1945.

[14] CHAPMAN, C. B., TAYLOR, H. L., BORDEN, C., EBERT, R. V. KEYS, A.: Simultaneous determinations of the resting arteriovenous oxygen difference by the acetylene and direct Fick Methods. J. Clin. Invest., **29:** 651, 1950.

[15] DEXTER, L., WHITTENBERGER, J. L., HAYNES, F. W., GOODALE, W. T., GORLIN, R. AND SAWYER, C. G.: Effect of exercise on circulatory dynamics of normal individuals. J. Appl. Physiol., **3:** 439, 1951.

[16] DOYLE, J. T., WILSON, J. S., ESTES, E. H. AND WARREN, J. V.: The effect of intravenous infusions of physiologic saline solution on the pulmonary arterial and pulmonary capillary pressure in man. J. Clin. Invest., **30:** 345, 1951.

[17] FREIS, E. D., SCHNAPER, H. W., JOHNSON, R. L. AND SCHREINER, G. E.: Hemodynamic alterations in acute myocardial infarction. I. Cardiac output, mean arterial pressure, total peripheral resistance, "central" and total blood volumes, venous pressure and average circulation time. J. Clin. Invest., **31:** 131, 1952.

[18] KOWALSKI, H. J. AND ABELMANN, W. H.: The cardiac output at rest in Laennec's cirrhosis. J. Clin. Invest., **32:** 1025, 1953.

[19] VEALL, N., PEARSON, J. D., HANLEY, T. AND LOWE, A. E.: A method for the determination of cardiac output (Preliminary Report). Proc. Second Radioisotope Conference Oxford, July 19–23, 1954. London, Butterworths Scientific Publications, 1954, p. 183–192.

[20] HUFF, R. L., BOGARDUS, G., BROADBOOKS, H., AND FELLER, D.: Musculoskeletal circulatory rates determined with I^{131} human serum albumin. Am. J. Med. **17:** 111, 1954. Abstract.

[21] —, AND FELLER, D. D.: Circulating red cell volume and corporeal specific gravity. Federation Proc., **13:** 73, 1954.

[22] HUFF, R. L., FELLER, D. D. AND BOGARDUS, G.: Cardiac output by body surface counting of I^{131} human serum albumin. J. Clin. Invest., **33:** 944, 1954 (Abstract).

[3] MARINELLI, L. D., QUIMBY, E. H. AND HINE, G. J.: Dosage determination with radioactive isotopes. II. Practical considerations in therapy and protection. Am. J. Roentgenol. **59:** 260, 1948.

Medical Scintillation Spectrometry

This article tells how a simple new single-channel scintillation spectrometer makes isotope-uptake measurements more accurate by counting only in photopeak. Two new collimators, flat-field and focusing, are also described. Taken altogether this provides a new philosophy of how medical isotope measurements should be made

By J. E. FRANCIS, P. R. BELL, and C. C. HARRIS
Oak Ridge National Laboratory
Oak Ridge, Tennessee

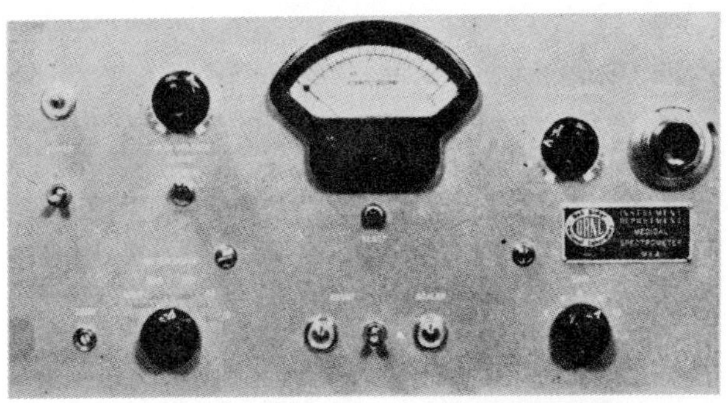

FIG. 1. Single-channel scintillation spectrometer panel

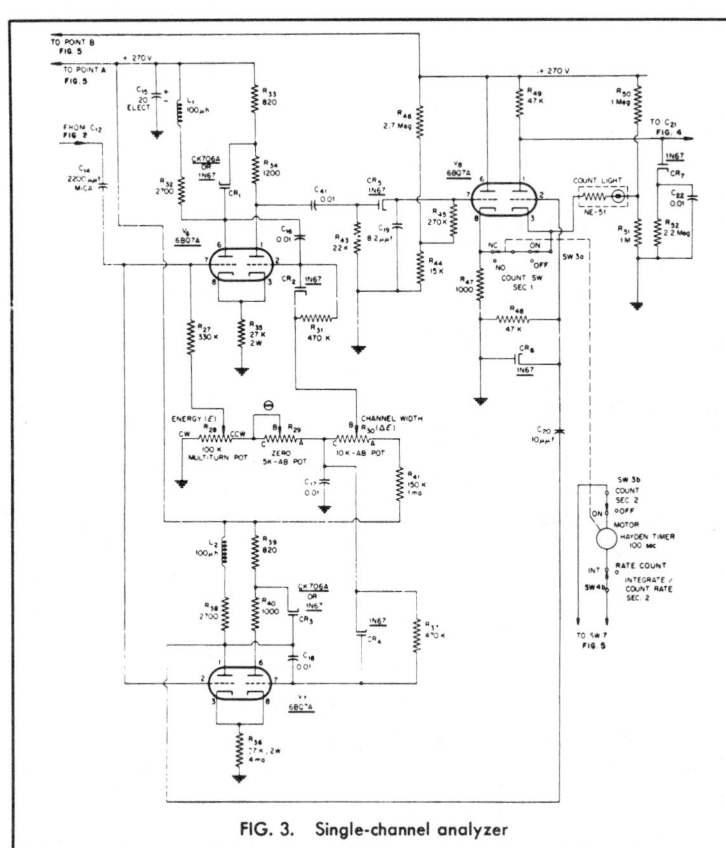

FIG. 3. Single-channel analyzer

ACCURATE SCINTILLATION COUNTING of radioiodine and other gamma-emitters in biological work has always been extremely difficult with equipment that includes scattered radiation in the measurements. The inclusion of scattered radiation can easily lead to an error of a factor of two or greater, making precision dosimetry very difficult.

We believe the spectrometer method is far superior to the integral method for measurement of iodine uptake. A scintillation spectrometer can measure the spectrum of gamma radiation falling on it. By selecting the full-energy peak, scattered radiation will not be detected. Counting rates are reduced, but usually less than in the integral method when shielding against scattered radiation. Background counting rates with the spectrometer are also much lower because only background pulses that occur within the channel being counted enter.

In addition to accurate thyroid-uptake measurements, this unit permits assay of material to be used, detection of radioactive impurities, measurement of samples for tracer chemistry, and high-contrast scanning.

1. TUBE SHIELD NEEDED FOR TUBE V_2 BECAUSE OF HUM PICKUP TO PLATE FROM HV AC. SHIELD ALSO V_{11}, V_{12}.
2. DELAY LINE (DISTANT END) MUST NOT GROUND TO CHASSIS DUE TO HUM PICKUP THROUGH GROUND CURRENTS.
3. DUE TO MAGNETIC PICKUP DELAY LINE MUST RETURN ON ITSELF
4. INPUT TIME CONSTANT MUST BE LONG (CRITICAL FOR OVERLOAD SIGNALS).
5. ALL RESISTORS ½ WATT ± 10% ALLEN BRADLEY UNLESS OTHERWISE SHOWN. * R_3, R_5, R_8, SHOULD BE STABILIZED BY BAKING AT 150°F FOR 24 hr BEFORE SELECTION.
6. CAPACITANCES ARE IN MICROFARADS UNLESS OTHERWISE SPECIFIED.
7. ALL CAPACITORS TO BE CERAMIC UNLESS OTHERWISE SPECIFIED.
8. POWER CABLE TO PREAMP IS MADE BY PULLING CENTER CONDUCTOR AND INSULATOR FROM RG 62/u AND INSERTING TEFLON COVERED NO. 22 AWG INTO THE COVERED BRAID REMAINING.

FIG. 2. Photomultiplier, preamplifier, and linear amplifier

Two special collimators designed for use with the spectrometer are described on p. 87. The first accepts radiation only from an arc of 30 deg in front of the scintillation crystal and very little in the back direction. The second is a new focusing collimator designed for measuring the distribution of activity in body organs.* This focusing collimator will be of great assistance in locating abnormalities, especially those that tend to absorb greater amounts of radioactive material than neighboring tissues.

Spectrometer Circuitry

The spectrometer is a new design developed at these laboratories and proven by actual laboratory use. It combines a linear amplifier, a single-channel analyzer, a count integrator together with preset timer, and a high-voltage supply for the photomultiplier in one relatively inexpensive 13- × 17-in. chassis. See Figs. 1, 2–5, and 6.

The main spectrometer schematics are shown in Figs. 2–4; the power

* Although developed independently, this collimator resembles that of Newell, et al. (*1*).

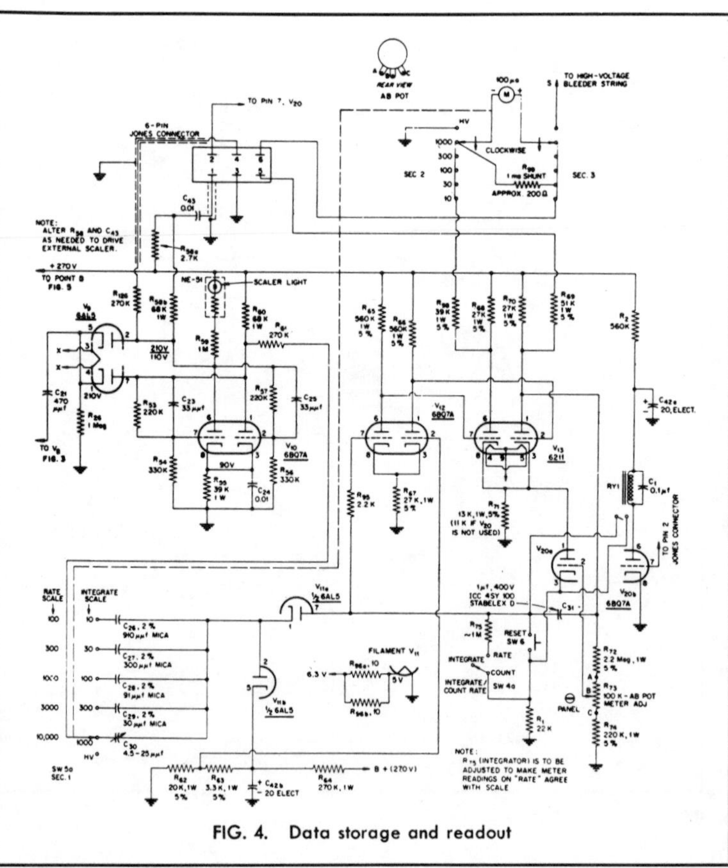

FIG. 4. Data storage and readout

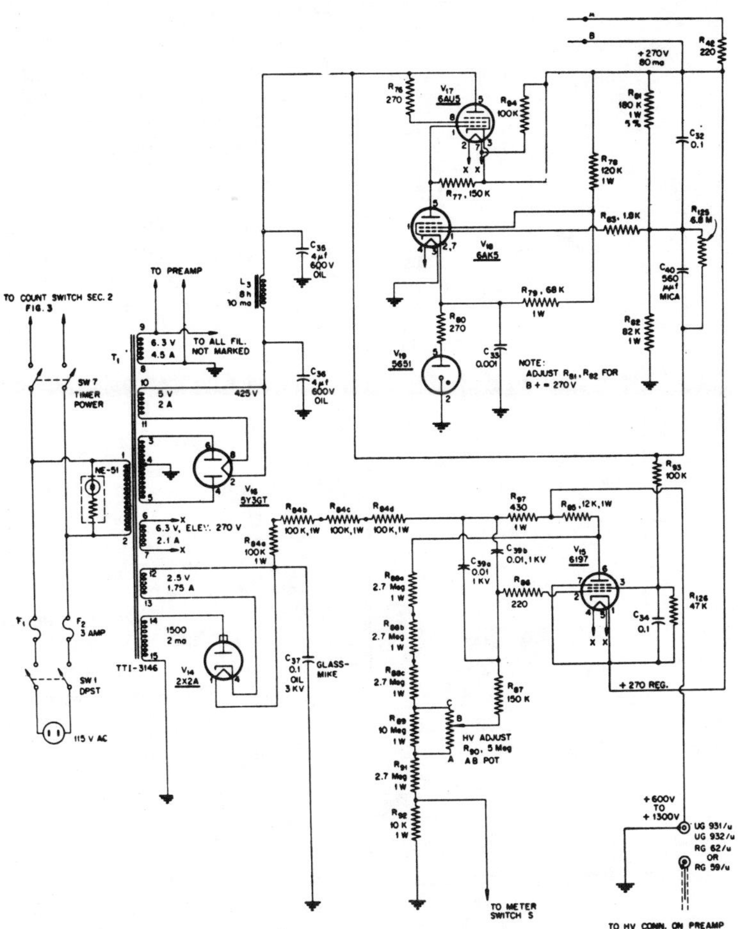

FIG. 5. Spectrometer power supply

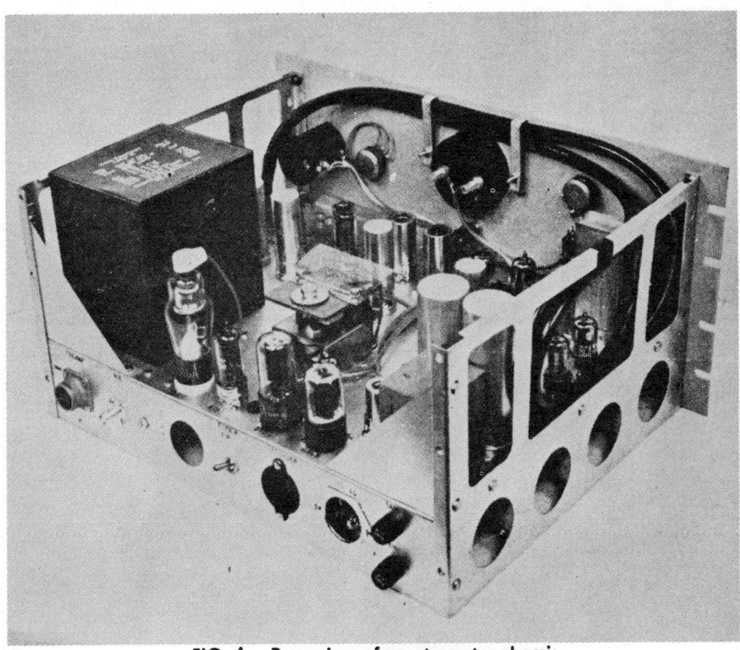

FIG. 6. Rear view of spectrometer chassis

supply is diagrammed in Fig. 5

By taking the signal from the last dynode of the photomultiplier a positive step pulse is obtained. This positive pulse is placed on the grid of a cathode follower (*V-1*), which drives a cable carrying the signal to the amplifier input, Fig. 2. The step pulse from the cathode of *V-1* is fed into a 1,500-ohm delay line through its characteristic impedance to obtain a 1-μsec pulse. The differentiated signal is placed on the input grid of the first feedback loop (*V-2*, *V-3*) of the linear amplifier, which has a gain of ~70. A step potentiometer provides gain control over a range of 16:1.

V-4 and *V-5* comprise the output group, which has a gain of 120; the output pulses vary from 0 to 100 volts.

Pulses from the amplifier are fed to the single-channel analyzer, Fig. 3. The analyzer contains two discriminators (*V-6*, *V-7*) whose discrimination level can be varied from a few volts to ninety volts by means of a multiturn potentiometer labeled E. The two discriminators are biased a fixed distance apart determined by the setting of a second potentiometer labeled ΔE.

For a small signal lying below the value determined by the setting E neither discriminator is triggered, and there is no output pulse. When an input signal is large enough to trigger only the lower discriminator, the plate of *V-7A* goes negative and charges the 10-$\mu\mu$f coupling condenser (*C-20*), which goes to the second grid of the anticoincidence tube *V-8*. When the input signal goes down below the trigger level, the plate of *V-7A* returns to its original voltage, and a positive signal is produced at the second grid of the anticoincidence tube *V-8*, which decays away with the time constant determined by the total shunt capacity and the 47-k grid resistor (*R-48*). This transfers the current from the first half of *V-8*, which is normally "on," to the second half giving a negative output from the second plate of *V-8*. If, however, the input signal from the amplifier is large enough to trigger both discriminators, a positive signal is obtained from the second plate of the upper discriminator (*V-6*) in addition to the signal from the lower discriminator. The signal from the upper discriminator is lengthened by a 1N67 diode (*CR-5*) and placed on the first grid of *V-8*. This keeps the first half of *V-8* "on" even when the signal from the lower discriminator appears at the second grid. By this means no output signal is obtained.

It should be noted that the signal from the lower discriminator does not appear on the grid of *V-8* until after the input pulse is no longer large enough to trigger the lower discriminator. This is necessary because of the finite rise and fall time of the pulses.

On-off operation for counting is obtained by means of two switches in series connecting the cathodes of *V-8* together. The switch operated by the timer is normally closed. Counting is started by closing the count switch. At the end of 100 sec the switch operated by the timer opens causing the counting operation to cease because the cathode of *V-8B* is now open.

The output pulse from *V-8* is fed into a scale-of-2 scaler (*V-10*) in the data-storage section, Fig. 4. When the plate changes from one stable-state voltage to the other, the coupling condenser (*C-26* to *C-29*) in use is charged or discharged through *V-11*. So for each two pulses into the scaling circuit a charge $q = VC$ is placed on the grid

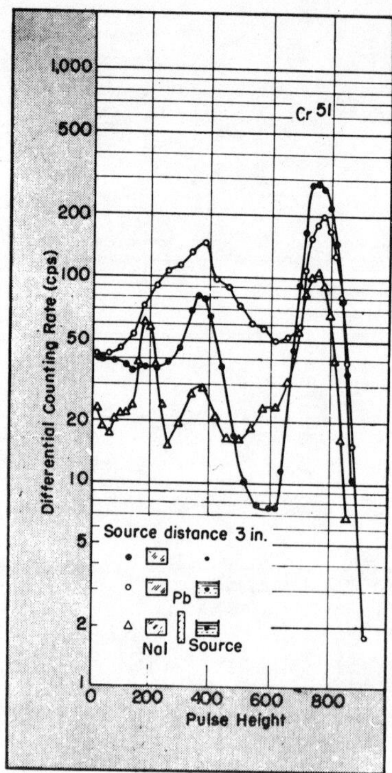

FIG. 7. Pulse height spectrum of Cr^{51} under three different conditions

of *V-12A*, where *V* is the difference in voltage of the two stable states of *V-10B* and *C* is the coupling capacity.

V-12 and *V-13* is a two-stage d-c amplifier with a 1-μf feedback condenser from the plate of *V-13B* to the grid of *V-12A*. The plate of *V-13B* has to go up 45 volts and the plate of *V-13A* down 45 volts to obtain 1 milliamp current in the cross resistor (*R-69*) and meter between the two plates. By using a 100-sec predetermined time, the current in the meter is calibrated in counts per second.

The value for the coupling condenser C_c is obtained from the relation

$$q = NE_1C_c/2 = E_2C_F$$

where E_2 is the change in voltage across C_F, E_1 is the voltage change of the scaler plate, and N is the count.

The meter can also be used to read count rate by connecting in resistor *R-75* to leak the charge continuously.

The positive high-voltage supply for the phototube is an ordinary shunt-regulated voltage supply except that the positive voltage supply at 270 volts is used for the reference voltage (Fig. 5).

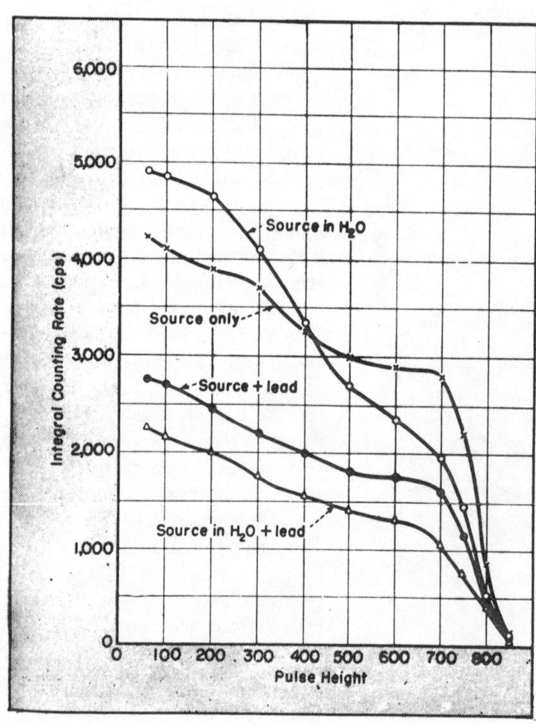

FIG. 8. Integral pulse height spectrum of Cr^{51}, showing scattering effects

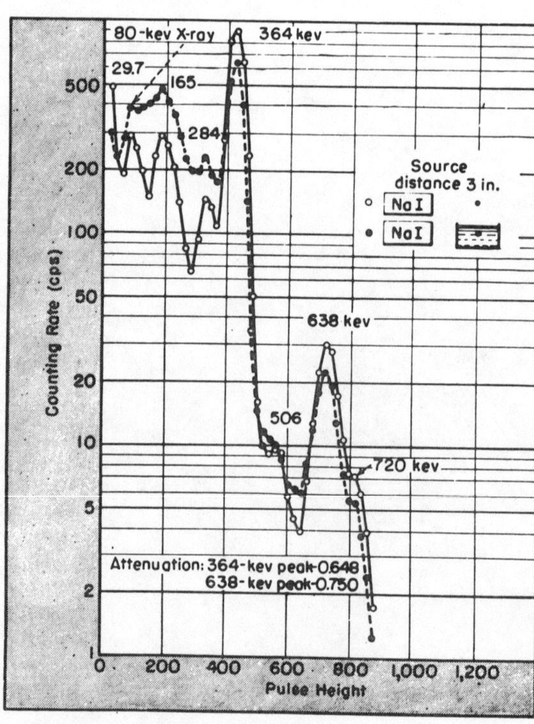

FIG. 9. Pulse height spectrum of I^{131} bare and in water bath. Window = 10 pulse-height units

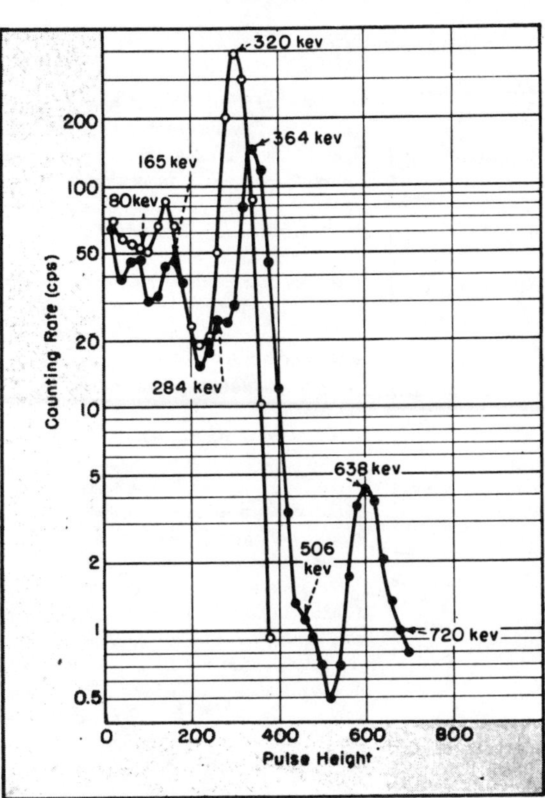

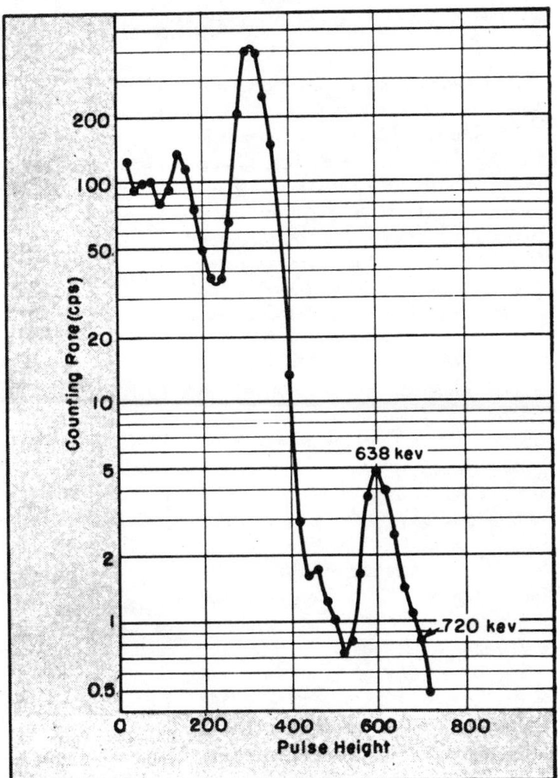

FIG. 10. Spectrum of 0.1 μc of I^{131} and of 1.6 μc of Cr^{51} under identical conditions—window = 200 pulse-height units, 1½- × 1-in. NaI crystal

FIG. 11. Spectrum of a mixture of 0.1 μc of I^{131} and 1.6 μc of Cr^{51}; window = 20 pulse-height units, 1½- × 1-in. NaI crystal

Spectrometer Performance

Spectra of I^{131}, Cr^{51}, and Cs^{137} were measured to check the operation of the spectrometer and also to show the effects of scattered radiation on measurements like thyroid uptake.

Chromium and cesium were chosen for these measurements, because each has a single gamma ray like one of the two main I^{131} gamma rays.

Figure 7 shows the spectrum obtained under three different conditions from Cr^{51}, which has a single 320-kev gamma ray. First, the solid dots represent the spectrum obtained with the source at three inches from the crystal. The main peak at 780 pulse-height units is the photoelectric peak, while the counts in the region 0 to 400 pulse-height units are produced largely by Compton-scattering events in the crystal, although a few of them are due to detection of scattered radiation from the source and the crystal container. The source was then immersed in an 800-cm^3 beaker of water to give a rough approximation of the conditions encountered in actual thyroid measurements. The spectrum shown by the circles was obtained under the above conditions. The main peak at 780 pulse-height units is attenuated by absorption of the gamma rays in the water. It should be noted that the number of counts in the entire region from 0 to 600 pulse-height units is increased due to the scattered radiation rather than reduced, as it should be.

The triangles show the spectrum obtained when a $\frac{1}{16}$-in. lead shield is placed between the source in water and the crystal. The entire spectrum is attenuated with the exception of the valley before the peak at 780 pulse-height units; also a peak appears at 180 pulse-height units due to lead X-rays.

Figure 8 shows the spectra obtained with integral counting, that is, recording all pulses whose amplitude is greater than a given pulse height. Note that when the source is immersed in water, there is an apparent increase in the source strength for low pulse-height settings. This is due to the scattered radiation. Even when a lead shield is used to minimize the effects of the scattered radiation, the attenuation measured varies greatly with different integral settings.

Using a wide channel width (ΔE setting) arranged to accept the photopeak one obtains the same counting rate from Cr^{51} with a source alone as is obtained with the integral method using a lead shield. The differential method of counting gives the correct value for the attenuation of the gamma ray. In addition to obtaining the same counting rate using a wide channel width and the right answer for the attenuation, the background will be cut down as much as a factor of ten using the differential method of counting. Integral and differential backgrounds are included in the calculation on p. 88 to demonstrate this point.

Figure 9 shows spectra of I^{131} under two different conditions. The circles show the spectrum for the bare source and the solid dots were obtained when the source was immersed in water. The detail of the spectrum for the bare source is good enough to permit detec-

Two collimators have been developed for use with the spectrometer.

The first is a flat-field collimator to be used for thyroid-uptake studies. It accepts radiation only from a 30-deg arc. The response of this collimator, as a source is moved in a circle around the collimator, is shown in Fig. 12 for a source of Cr^{51} *(320-kev gamma ray) and (where different) for a source of* Cs^{137} *(661-kev gamma ray).*

The unique feature of this collimator is that while the transmission of the gamma rays from the back direction is low, it was not necessary to extend the lead portion of the shield around the back of the photomultiplier tube. Instead a light pipe made from a NaI crystal that was not activated with thallium was used to obtain the necessary shielding for the back direction. This reduces the weight considerably while still giving the same shielding characteristics.

The second type of collimator is intended for scanning body organs to map the radioisotope distributions within them. This collimator (Fig. 13) is called a focusing collimator and has nineteen tapering hexagonal holes in a 2-in. lead shield. The axes of the holes meet at a point 2 in. from the face of the collimator. The transmission of the collimator is high—at 2 in. the counting rate obtained is about 58% of that obtained without the collimator.

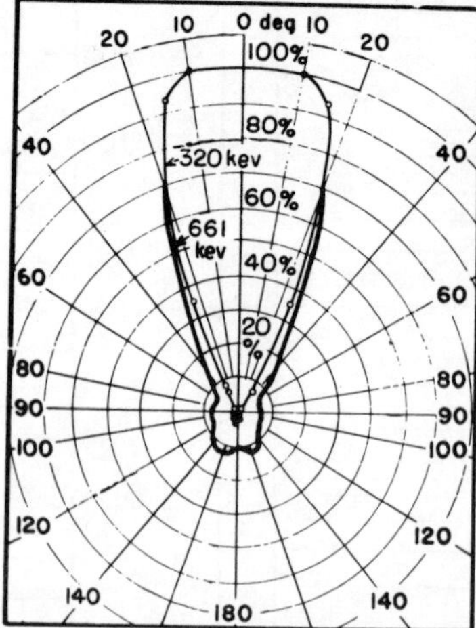

FIG. 12. Polar diagram showing response of flat-field collimator to 320-kev gamma ray of Cr and to the 661-kev gamma ray of Cs, where it differs substantially from the former

Figure 9 shows a contour map of the response of this collimator to a point source of 320-kev gamma rays. Note that a source on the axis gives a lower counting rate when in contact with the front face of the collimator than it does when 1.5 in. away, the point of maximum sensitivity.

Using this focusing collimator it was possible to detect a 1-cm-diameter void at a depth of 0.75 in. in a solution tank 5 in. in diameter and 1.5 in. deep. The solution contained 0.07 μc/ml of I equivalent.

To demonstrate the value of this collimator with the spectrometer, a mock thyroid gland was measured. This gland contained 0.6 μc I/cm³ with an additional source 1 mm in diameter in one lobe containing 0.67 μc of I and two voids in the other lobe of 0.5-cm and 1.0-cm diameter. A map of the counting rate from the 364-kev gamma ray in iodine was made. This map (Figure 14) definitely shows the location of the hot spot and the 1-cm void. The location of the 0.5-cm void, while visible, would not be definite enough to be used for a diagnosis without experience based on the shape of the contour to be expected from normal thyroid measurements.

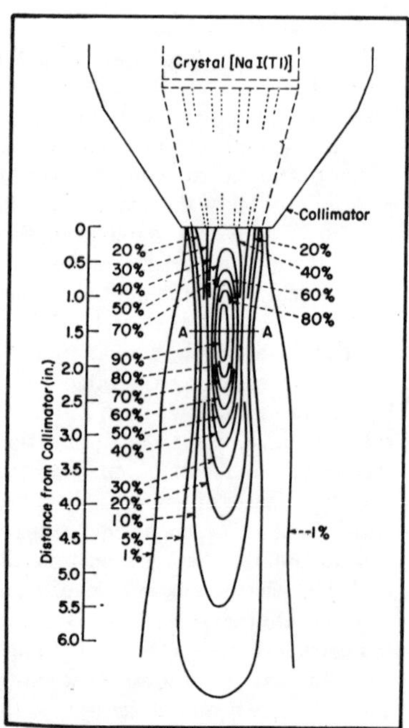

FIG. 13. Response for Cr^{51} gamma rays; 50% width at AA is 0.38 in.

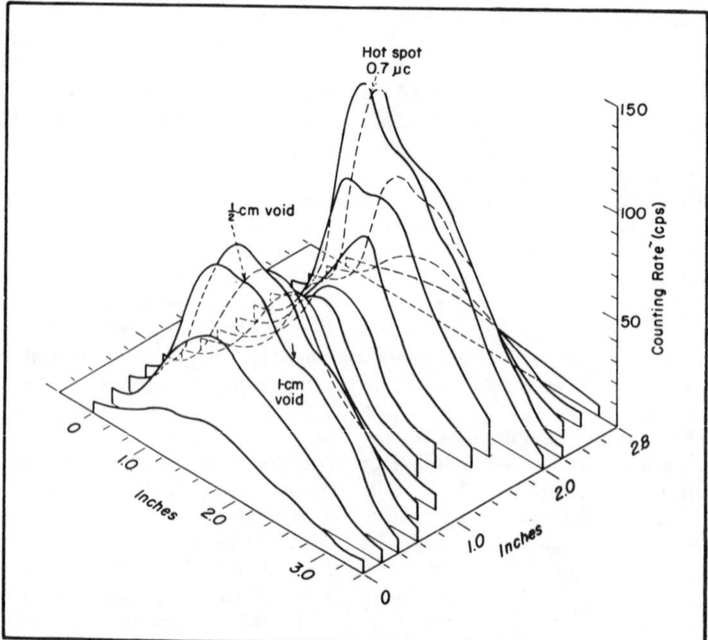

FIG. 14. Isometric drawing of distribution of I^{131} in mock thyroid as measured with focusing collimator

156

Calculated Peak Counting Rates per Microcurie

Isotope and gamma-ray energy (kev)	Efficiency	Percent gamma	Geometry	Specific counting rate (cps/μc)
	1- × 1½-in. crystal			
Cr(320-kev)	0.33	0.1	.5	610
I(364)	0.27	0.84	.5	4,190
(638)	0.13	0.078	.5	188
	3- × 3-in. crystal, source in well			
Cr(320)	0.747	0.1	1.0	2,765
I(364)	0.642	0.84	1.0	19,950
(638)	0.381	0.078	1.0	1,110

Determining Source Strengths in a Cr + I Mixture

Calibration numbers*

Source	Pulse height	cps per μc
I^{131}(364)	220	16,900
(638)	500	882
Cr (320)	220	2,300

Weak source determination

Source	Pulse height	Counts	Time (sec)	cps − bg = true cps
I alone	220	4,096	291	14.05 − 1.915 = 12.13
Cr alone	220	4,096	752	5.44 − 1.915 = 3.52
I + Cr	220	4,096	238.9	17.15 − 1.915 = 15.23
I + Cr	500	4,096	3,085	1.328 − 0.705 = 0.623
Background	220	2,816	1,471	1.915
Background	500	512	714	avg. 0.705
			718	
			738	
			735	
Integral	40 (60 kev)	4,096	230	17.8
background	220 (270 kev)	4,096	500	8.2

Source strength

$$\text{Assay of Cr alone by 320-kev peak} = \frac{3.52}{2{,}300} = 1.53 \times 10^{-3}\ \mu c$$

$$\text{Assay of I alone by 364-kev peak} = \frac{12.13}{16{,}900} = 0.78 \times 10^{-3}\ \mu c$$

Calculating Cr and I from mixture

$$\text{Assay of I by 638-kev peak} = \frac{0.625}{882} = 0.71 \times 10^{-3}\ \mu c$$

(0.71×10^{-3}) 16,900 = 12 cps calculated counts expected for I at 220 pulse height from 638-kev measurement.

17.15 − 12 = 5.15 cps due to Cr and background at 220 pulse height.

5.15 − 1.92 (background) = 3.23 cps due to Cr.

$\frac{3.23}{2{,}300} = 1.41 \times 10^{-3}$ μc Cr is the calculated value. This value is to be compared to the assay value of 1.53×10^{-3} μc.

---

* Assume 3 × 3-in. NaI crystal, source in ½ × 1½-in. well, ΔE = 100 pulse-ht units.

tion of radioactive contaminants if any were present.

Multiple Tracers

This instrument is also useful for the simultaneous determination of I and Cr in a blood sample as demonstrated by the following curves.

Figure 10 shows the spectrum of Cr and I separately, taken under the same conditions. Figure 11 shows the spectrum obtained when both sources are measured simultaneously. Although the 320-kev peak from Cr and the 364-kev peak from I are not resolved, it is possible by matching the 638-kev peak of Fig. 11 with the 638-kev peak of Fig. 10 to obtain the Cr spectrum in Fig. 10 by point-by-point subtraction.

Using a narrow channel width and running a complete spectrum shows in detail the physics of the situation, and source strengths can then be computed by measuring the area under the curve. But this is a time-consuming process. For routine tests where the physics is understood and the sources known, the concentration of the two substances can be measured much more rapidly by using a wide channel width and appropriate calibration.

As an example the relative amounts of Cr and I in the same sample were determined by taking a measurement at only two points.

The table on this page gives intrinsic peak efficiencies for two crystal sizes and the counting rates expected in the peaks of the spectrum for a 1-μc source.

Experimental calibration numbers used and data obtained when measuring a weak source containing 1.5×10^{-3} μc of Cr^{51} and 0.7×10^{-3} μc of I^{131} are shown in the calculation below the table. The calibration numbers listed are experimental determinations where the window did not cover the entire peak. These were used to determine the source strength of an iodine sample and a chromium sample separately. Then these same two sources were counted simultaneously using two pulse height settings, namely 220 and 500. From the data obtained at these two settings the source strengths of the iodine and the chromium were again calculated. The value obtained for each isotope is found to be comparable when measured separately or in the presence of the other.

BIBLIOGRAPHY

1. R. R. Newell, William Saunders, Earl Miller, NUCLEONICS 10, No. 7, July 1952.

Scintillation Camera

HAL O. ANGER
Donner Laboratory of Biophysics and Medical Physics and Radiation Laboratory, University of California, Berkeley, California

(Received August 19, 1957; and in final form, October 21, 1957)

A new and more sensitive gamma-ray camera for visualizing sources of radioactivity is described. It consists of a lead shield with a pinhole aperture, a scintillating crystal within the shield viewed by a bank of seven photomultiplier tubes, a signal matrix circuit, a pulse-height selector, and a cathode-ray oscilloscope. Scintillations that fall in a certain range of brightness, such as the photopeak scintillations from a gamma-ray-emitting isotope, are reproduced as point flashes of light on the cathode-ray tube screen in approximately the same relative positions as the original scintillations in the crystal. A time exposure of the screen is taken with an oscilloscope camera, during which time a gamma-ray image of the subject is formed from the flashes that occur. One of many medical and industrial uses is described, namely the visualization of the thyroid gland with I^{131}.

AN important problem in the use of radioisotopes is determining the distribution of an isotope contained in a given subject. It is often desirable to produce a gamma-ray image or map that shows the exact areas where a gamma-ray-emitting isotope is located. The image will then show, for example, the size, shape, and location of the functioning parts of the thyroid gland in a human subject, or an area of radioactive contamination in an industrial device.

The conventional method of producing a gamma-ray image is to scan the subject with a directional counter or counters. An image of the subject is produced by a printing device which moves in synchronism with the counter and displays the counts as dots or lines on paper or photographic film.[1–6] Another method is to take a picture of the subject with a gamma-ray camera. The camera consists of a stationary lead shield with a pinhole aperture and a gamma-ray sensitive film, perhaps with an intensifying screen.

This paper describes an improved gamma-ray camera, previously described briefly,[7] which is much more sensitive than others that have been reported.[8,9] In addition to the lead shield with pinhole aperture, it employs a large flat scintillating crystal within the shield viewed by a bank of

[1] Mayneord, Turner, Newberry, and Hodt, Nature **168**, 762 (1951).
[2] Cassin, Curtis, Reed, and Libby, Nucleonics **9**, No. 2, 46 (1951).
[3] H. C. Allen, Jr., and J. R. Risser, Nucleonics **13**, No. 1, 28 (1955).
[4] Francis, Bell, and Harris, Nucleonics **13**, No. 11, 82 (1955).
[5] Gorden L. Brownell and William H. Sweet, Nucleonics **11**, No. 11, 40 (1953).
[6] H. O. Anger, Am. J. Roentgenol. Radium Therapy Nuclear Med. **70**, 605 (1953).
[7] Hal O. Anger, "A New Instrument for Mapping Gamma-Ray Emitters, in Biology and Medicine Quarterly Report," UCRL-3653, January 1957, p. 38.
[8] H. O. Anger, Nature **170**, 200 (1952).
[9] Mortimer, Anger, and Tobias, "The Gamma-Ray Pinhole Camera with Image Amplifier," UCRL-2524, March 1954.

seven photomultiplier tubes, a signal matrix circuit, a pulse-height selector, a cathode-ray oscilloscope, and a conventional camera to photograph the oscilloscope screen.

Briefly, the operation of the scintillation camera is as follows. Gamma rays are emitted from the subject, some of which travel through the aperture in the lead shield and continue traveling in straight lines until they impinge on the scintillating crystal. The light that is produced in any given scintillation is emitted isotropically and divides between all the phototubes, with those closest to a given scintillation receiving the most light. The duration of each scintillation is short compared to the average time interval between them.

The pulses obtained from the phototubes are applied to the signal matrix circuit which adds and subtracts the amplitudes in such a way that three output signals are obtained. Two of the signals are positioning signals, which are applied to the X and Y input terminals of the oscilloscope. The third, or Z signal, is obtained by adding together the pulses from all of the seven phototubes, with equal value being given to each. Then a scintillation of a given magnitude produces a Z signal of substantially the same magnitude regardless of where it originated in the crystal. This signal is applied to the input of the pulse-height selector and then to the intensity-input terminal of the oscilloscope.

When a scintillation occurs, the oscilloscope beam, which is normally in a blanked or extinguished state, is deflected by the X and Y signals to a point corresponding to the location of the original scintillation in the crystal. Then the beam is unblanked or turned on momentarily, provided the Z signal passes the pulse-height selector. The result is that scintillations in the crystal are reproduced as flashes on the oscilloscope screen at greatly increased brightness, with the provision that only scintillations falling within a narrow range of brightness are reproduced. In normal operation the pulse-height selector is adjusted to accept the photopeak pulses from a given gamma-ray-emitting isotope.

The flashes on the oscilloscope screen are photographed, usually by a Polaroid-Land camera which develops the picture within the camera in one minute. The exposure time may last from a few seconds to an hour or more. During this time an image is built up from the flashes that occur. If only a few flashes are recorded, they appear as separate dots which are more numerous in the places of maximum activity. If many are photographed in one exposure and the camera lens is suitably adjusted, the dots
160 merge together and show a gamma-ray image of the subject in shades of gray and white against a black background.

Although seven phototubes are employed, the number of picture elements which can be resolved is not limited to this number because scintillations which occur at intermediate points between the phototubes are reproduced approximately in that position. The actual limitations on resolution are discussed later in the paper.

Among the advantages of the scintillation camera are the following. It is concurrently sensitive to all parts of its field of view, an advantage when rapidly changing activity patterns are studied. There is no line structure to the image, since scanning is not employed. An area of any size may be examined by moving the camera closer or further away. It can be oriented readily in any direction so that horizontal, vertical, and oblique views can be taken; remote viewing and recording are quite feasible. It can be adjusted to be sensitive only to photopeak scintillations of the isotope being studied, thus rejecting radiation scattered by adjacent objects or tissue.

DETAILED DESCRIPTION

A sectional view of the camera is shown in Fig. 1. The camera housing is made of lead, and it shields the scintillating crystal on all sides except for the pinhole aperture through which the gamma rays enter. Above the aperture is the thallium-activated sodium iodide crystal, which is 4 in. in diameter and $\frac{1}{4}$ in. thick. It is backed with magnesium oxide to reflect maximum light. A short distance above the crystal is the bank of seven 1.5-in.-diameter photomultiplier tubes. The tubes are spaced a minimum distance apart and the spaces between the photocathodes are covered by light reflecting surfaces. Some of the light-reflecting surfaces are painted white, and others are mirror surfaces. The space between the crystal and the phototubes is filled with a transparent optical fluid.

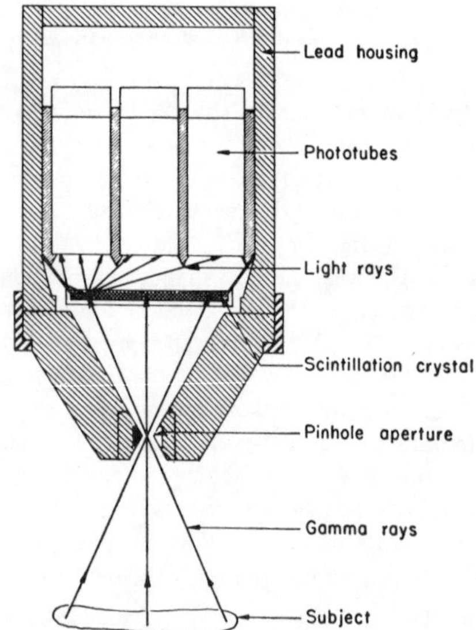

FIG. 1. Sectional drawing of scintillation camera.

A diagram showing the paths of the signals after they leave the phototubes is in Fig. 2. The signal matrix circuit is shown with a block diagram of the other main parts of the electronic circuit.

The Y-axis positioning signal is obtained in the following way. The outputs from Phototubes 2 and 3 are fed through resistances R_{12} and R_{13} to one terminal of the Y-axis difference circuit, and the outputs from Phototubes 5 and 6 are fed through resistances R_{15} and R_{16} to the other terminal of the difference circuit. The four resistances are equal in value. The amplitudes of the two signals are then subtracted one from another to obtain the Y signal, which has an amplitude and polarity dependent upon the location along the Y axis of the scintillation in the crystal. The signal is amplified and is then shaped by means of a shorted delay line. The resulting pulse is about 1 μsec long, and is rectangular in shape with a flat top. It is applied to the Y-axis input of the oscilloscope.

The X-axis signal is obtained in almost the same way as the Y signal. The outputs from Phototubes 1, 2, and 6 are added through resistances R_{21}, R_{22}, and R_{26}. Here R_{22} and R_{26} are of equal value but R_{21} is one-half the value of the others. This is necessary because Phototube 1 has twice the linear displacement along the X axis of the other two phototubes. The outputs of Phototubes 3, 4, and 5 are also added through resistances R_{23}, R_{24}, and R_{25}. The value of R_{24} is half the value of the others. The signals are applied to the two terminals of the X-axis difference circuit, and the resulting output signal is amplified and shaped in the same way as the Y signal. The amplitude and polarity of this signal depend on the location of the scintillation along the X axis. It is applied to the X input of the oscilloscope.

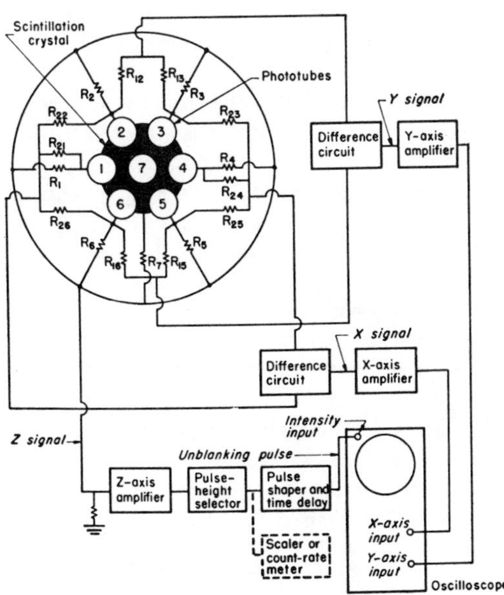

FIG. 2. Block diagram of electronic circuit.

The Z signal is obtained by adding the outputs of all the phototubes through resistances R_1–R_7, all of which are of equal value. The resulting signal is amplified and fed to the input of the pulse-height selector. The output signal goes to a pulse shaper and delay circuit, which shortens the pulses and delays them so that the oscilloscope beam is unblanked only at the peak of the excursion caused by the X and Y positioning signals. This signal, called the unblanking pulse, is applied to the intensity input of the cathode-ray oscilloscope.

ADJUSTMENT AND OPERATION

The operation of the camera depends upon the phototubes all being equally sensitive to light. They can be adjusted to meet this condition quite easily in the following way. A sample of the gamma-emitting isotope to be used is first placed inside the camera near the pinhole aperture so that the entire scintillating crystal is irradiated with gamma rays. The pulse-height selection window is set to a fixed height and the width is set to about 10% of the height. Then the phototube supply voltage is increased from below the threshold voltage until a maximum number of flashes appears on the screen. Then, by adjustment of the individual phototube voltages, the pattern on the screen is made symmetrical about the origin and evenly illuminated. The voltages on phototubes 1–6 are adjusted for equal maximum deflection from the origin, and the voltage on the center phototube is adjusted for the most even distribution of the flashes radially over the screen.

After the pattern has been made symmetrical, the supply voltage is usually readjusted for maximum counting rate from the photopeak portion of the pulse-height spectrum. The pulse-height selector will then be accepting pulses from photopeak scintillations that occur anywhere in the crystal. The window width is set to the minimum value at which most of the pulses within the photopeak are passed. This results in the clearest picture and the lowest background.

Normally, the camera is set to the photopeak, as described above, because the counting efficiency is then relatively high and scattered radiation is rejected. However, it is also possible to set it to a portion of the Compton spectrum. This may be necessary when viewing a source containing a mixture of isotopes of different energy.

FACTORS AFFECTING RESOLUTION

The resolution obtained with four different aperture sizes is shown in Fig. 3. The test pattern consisted of 12 small sources of I^{131} arranged in a square array with two sources each in the top and bottom rows and four each in the others. The exposure time was varied so that an

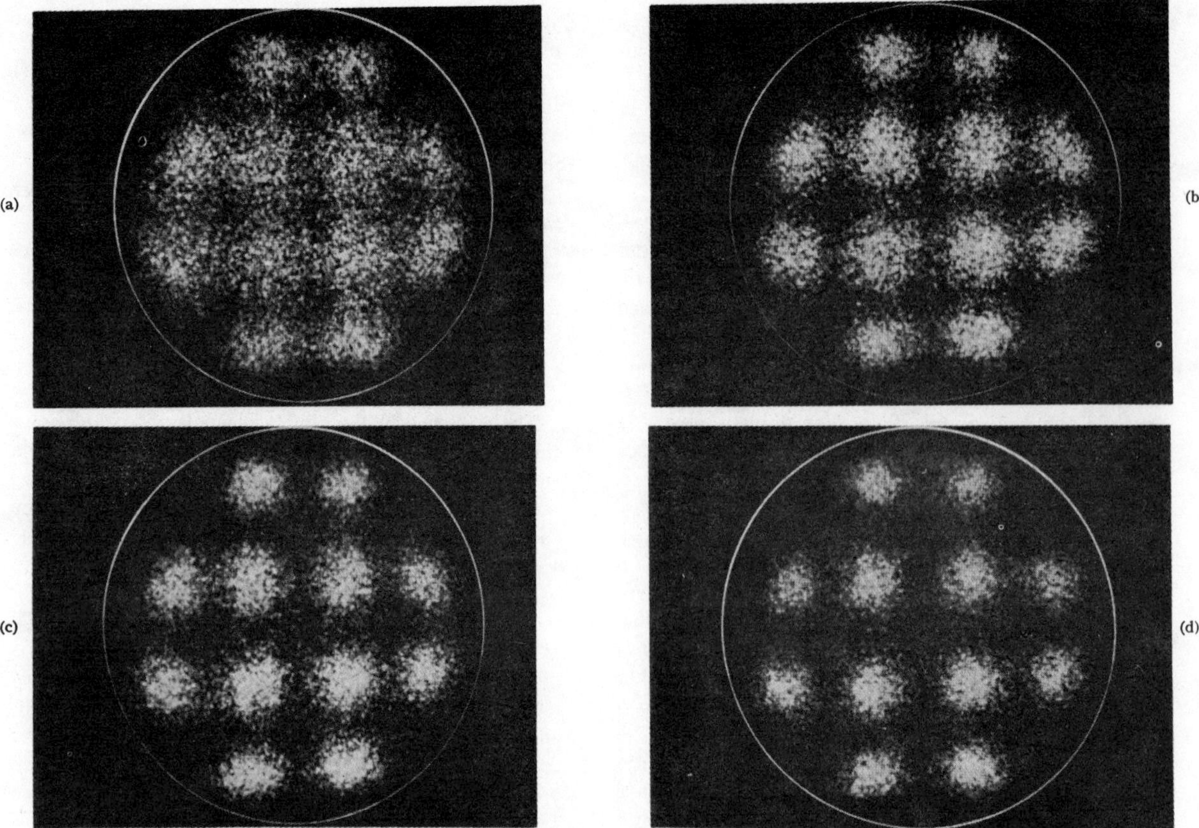

FIG. 3. Scintillation pictures taken with apertures of $\frac{5}{16}$-, $\frac{1}{4}$-, $\frac{3}{16}$-, and $\frac{1}{8}$-in. diam. The test pattern consisted of 12 small sources of I^{131}.

equal number of counts was recorded with each aperture. The $\frac{1}{8}$-, $\frac{3}{16}$-, and $\frac{1}{4}$-in. apertures are made of platinum, because of its relatively high stopping power for gamma rays, although tungsten would have been almost as good. The $\frac{5}{16}$-in. aperture was made of lead. The definition is shown to be progressively better as the aperture size is decreased.

A list of the major factors affecting definition include: The pinhole aperture size and the distances between the aperture, subject and scintillator; statistical variations in the distribution of the scintillation photons among the phototubes, the production of electrons at the photocathodes, and their subsequent multiplication; the width of the pulse-height selector window; and mislocation of the flash on the oscilloscope screen when a single gamma ray produces first a Compton recoil and then a photoelectric recoil in the scintillating crystal. In addition, the definition of any given picture depends on the number of counts or dots contained in it. This is a function of subject activity and exposure time as well as of the aperture size and the distances involved.

The geometric factors affecting definition are relatively straightforward, but they are complicated by the fact that the effective aperture size is somewhat larger than the actual size because some of the gamma rays go through the edge of the aperture. This effect is reduced by the use of a very dense material for the aperture, such as platinum or tungsten. When the camera is adjusted to the photopeak, gamma rays that are scattered through a wide angle by the aperture are eliminated by the pulse-height selector, since they have been degraded in energy. However, the few gamma rays that happen to be scattered through only a small angle are not rejected if the change in their energy is very small.

Regarding the statistics of photon distribution and of photoelectron production, a photoelectric recoil of the 0.36-Mev gamma ray of I^{131} occurring at the center of the crystal in the present instrument results in the production of about 40 photoelectrons[10] at the photocathode of each of the six phototubes located near the circumference of the crystal. The number of photoelectrons released by any given scintillation is, of course, subject to statistical variations. This in turn produces a statistical variation in the amplitudes of the positioning signals from one scintil-

[10] G. J. Hine and G. L. Brownell, Eds., *Radiation, Dosimetry* (Academic Press, Inc., New York, 1956), p. 252.

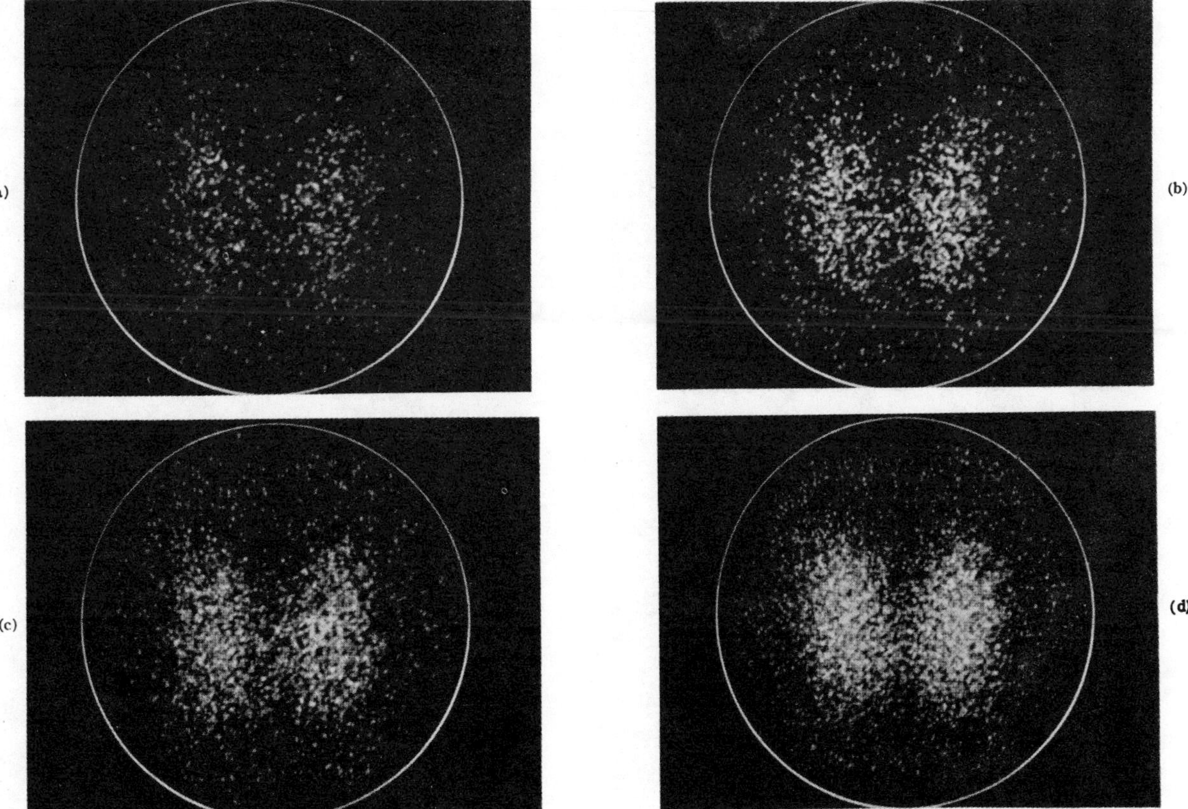

Fig. 4. Scintillation camera pictures taken of a thyroid phantom containing 5 microcuries of I^{131}.

lation to the next and a loss in definition of the picture. This places a limit on the improvement in resolution that can be obtained by decreasing the size of the pinhole aperture. The loss is such that there is very little advantage to be obtained by decreasing the pinhole size to less than $\frac{1}{8}$ in. in the present instrument. Actually a $\frac{1}{4}$-in. aperture is usually used in medical tracer applications to obtain higher sensitivity, and the maximum resolution capability is not realized because of the geometry.

The pulse-height selector window width should not be greater than necessary to pass most of the photopeak pulses, for the background due to stray gamma rays and cosmic rays would then be larger than necessary. Also, scintillations of greater or less energy than those desired could appear on the oscilloscope screen and the X- and Y-positioning signal magnitudes would not be correct for them. The effect would be similar to superimposing images of varying magnification, one upon the other, producing an astigmatic blurring at the edge of the picture.

When a gamma ray produces a scintillation by the Compton process and the secondary gamma ray reacts again with the crystal to produce another scintillation by the photoelectric process, the light from the two scintillations, when added together, is the same as that which would be produced if the original gamma ray had produced a photoelectric recoil. Therefore, the signal produced will pass the pulse-height selector but the positioning signals will place the flash at some point intermediate between the two scintillations. Since only the original scintillation is at the correct site, the flash is misplaced. Fortunately this is a fairly rare occurrence, since most secondary gamma rays produced in Compton interactions escape from the scintillator without producing a second reaction. When they do undergo a secondary photoelectric reaction, the second recoil is usually a considerable distance from the first, and the net effect is only to produce a slight increase in background over a large area around the subject. Furthermore, if the second reaction is another Compton recoil, and the gamma ray then escapes, the signal will not pass the pulse-height selector, provided the escaping gamma ray carries off sufficient energy. Multiple scintillations such as these are probably a limiting factor on the thickness of crystal that can be employed.

In Fig. 4 is shown the effect of the number of counts or dots on the appearance of the image. The number of

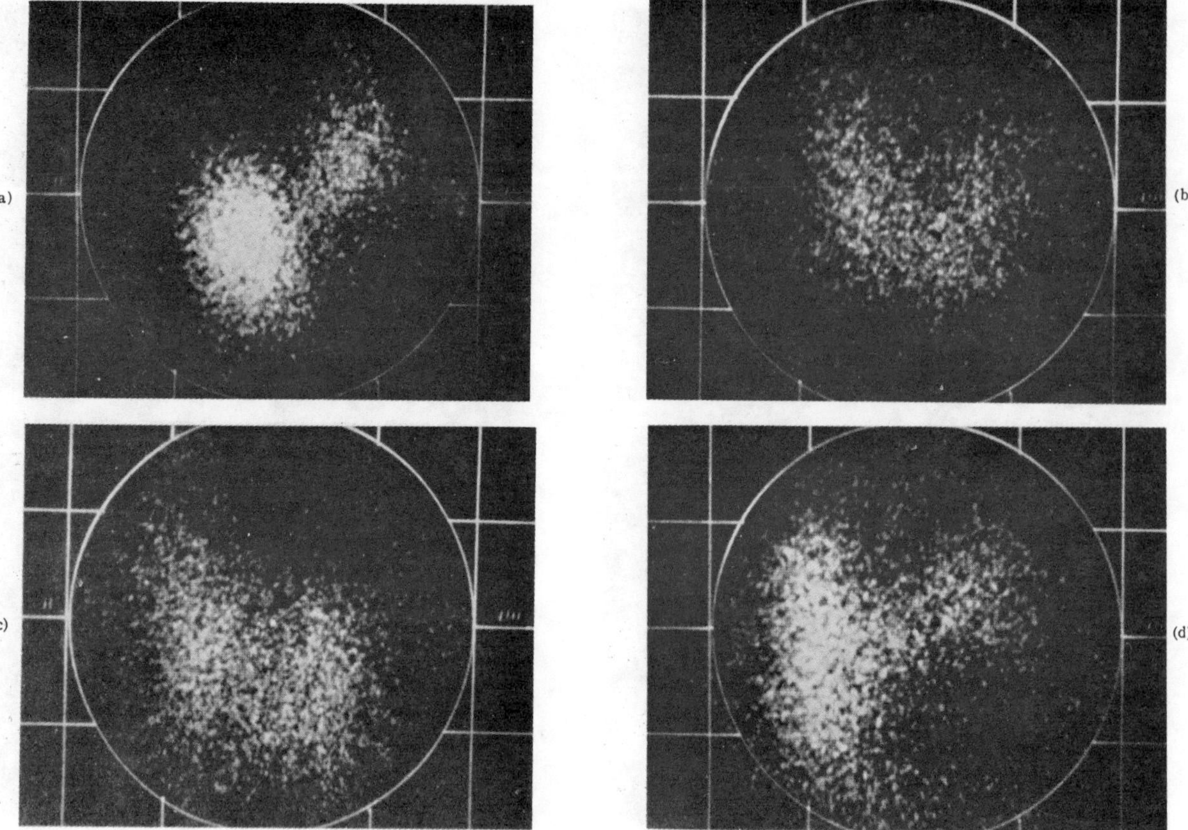

FIG. 5. *In vivo* pictures of the human thyroid.

counts is, of course, a function of subject activity, exposure time, and aperture size. The same test pattern is shown with 800, 1600, 3200 and 6400 counts comprising the image. The increase in clarity of the image with an increasing number of counts is apparent. The subject in this case is a phantom thyroid consisting of a radioactive solution contained in a Lucite form. Each lobe was elliptical in shape and of constant activity per unit area. The phantom contained 5 μC of I^{131} and was covered with $\frac{3}{4}$ in. of Lucite to represent overlying tissue. The exposure times for the four pictures were 5, 10, 20, and 40 min, respectively. The aperture size was $\frac{1}{4}$ in., and the distance between the aperture and the phantom was 5 in.

SENSITIVITY AND DISTORTION

The sensitivity of the present camera is such that about 10% of the 0.365-Mev gamma rays of I^{131} that impinge on the scintillating crystal produce a photoelectric recoil. The background is about 30 counts per minute. Of the remainder of the gamma rays, 75% pass through the crystal without producing any scintillation at all, and 15% produce Compton recoils,[11] which are not normally reproduced on the oscilloscope screen. The sensitivity can probably be increased by the use of a thicker crystal, or by revising the electronic circuit so that scintillations caused by Compton recoils are shown as well as those caused by photoelectric recoils. However, this would have the disadvantage that radiation scattered in the subject and the aperture would no longer be rejected.

If a small radioactive source is placed at the geometric center of the pinhole aperture, and a picture is taken with the entire scintillating crystal evenly illuminated by I^{131} gamma rays, some distortion of the pattern is evident. Ideally the image should be a round, evenly illuminated disk, since the scintillating crystal is round. Instead the pattern is a rounded hexagon, with the six points on the circumference corresponding to the six radial phototubes. Also, a few more of the counts are concentrated near the border of the pattern than over the remainder of the area. The distortion can be decreased if the distance between the scintillator and phototubes is increased, but the definition decreases at the same time owing to the change in the distribution of light among the phototubes. Therefore, a compromise must be made between definition and distortion. With the configuration chosen, the distortion

[11] C. M. Davissen and R. D. Evans, Revs. Modern Phys. 24, 99 (1952).

is negligible for most purposes, as shown by the approximately regular spacing of the test pattern image in Fig. 3. The distortion is confined almost entirely to the edges of the picture and is absent for all practical purposes from the central area.

It is possible to obtain an image by employing a multi-aperture collimator plate between the subject and the scintillating crystal instead of the pinhole aperture. The collimator consists of a plate made of lead or other dense material with many regularly spaced parallel holes. The area covered by the holes corresponds to the area of the crystal. For best definition and sensitivity, the subject should be as close to the multi-aperture plate as possible.

It has been found, however, that when the plate is made of lead, and the hole sizes and spacing are optimum for I^{131} gamma rays, the hole structure is so coarse that the shape of the image is appreciably distorted by the collimator structure. The distortion could, of course, be eliminated if the collimator plate were continually moved in relation to the scintillator and the subject during the exposure time. If the plate were made of tungsten or some other very dense material, the hole structure might be refined to the point where movement of the plate during exposure would not be necessary. Somewhat higher sensitivity might be obtained in this way. The holes in the plate could be angled inward or outward to view subjects smaller or larger than the scintillating crystal.

THYROID MAPPING

In Fig. 5 are shown a few examples of *in vivo* pictures of the human thyroid gland taken with the scintillation camera.[12] The amount of I^{131} in the gland varied from 7.5 to 12.5 μC, and the exposure times varied from 12 to 15 min. In all cases a $\frac{1}{4}$-in.-diameter platinum pinhole aperture was used, and the distance from the aperture to the thyroid gland was about 5 in. It is evident that the definition is adequate at the present time for thyroid mapping, and the amount of I^{131} required in the gland is quite low. Pictures could be taken with half the amount of I^{131} if the exposure time were doubled, or conversely pictures could be taken in half the time if the I^{131} dose were doubled. However, no fixed relation between activity and exposure time must be maintained, because the picture quality improves with increasing activity in the gland and increasing exposure time.

[12] The author is indebted to Dr. John C. Weaver and Dr. Donald J. Rosenthal for referring the subjects of these pictures.

If any abnormal uptake of I^{131} is suspected in a patient, a picture is usually taken with the scintillation camera at an increased distance from the subject. Then, the field of view is quite large, and if there is any substernal or upper cervical uptake, or any active nodule at some distance from the thyroid, it will be shown. A relatively large aperture and short exposure are used for this view, since the object is not to show detail, but to show the location of any abnormal uptake. Then the large aperture is replaced with a smaller one and the camera is moved closer to take longer, more detailed exposures of the thyroid and other points of uptake.

The amount of I^{131} present in the thyroid can be determined at the same time a picture is taken by recording the number of pulses per unit time that pass the pulse-height selector. This can be done with a scaler or count-rate meter connected as shown in Fig. 2. The counting efficiency can be determined in the usual way by counting a known amount of I^{131} in a thyroid phantom. These measurements will be more accurate if they are made with the camera at an increased distance to minimize the error due to variation in depth of the thyroid under the skin.

FUTURE DEVELOPMENT

Further development of the scintillation camera should improve the definition and sensitivity. The sensitivity may be increased by use of a thicker scintillator, or perhaps for some applications by displaying Compton, as well as photoelectric, recoils. Work is proceeding along these lines at the present time. The background, although it is not high, can probably be reduced by use of a thicker camera housing. The definition may be improved if phototubes of increased sensitivity become available, by using an increased number of phototubes, or perhaps by improvement of the optical coupling between the scintillator and the phototubes.

An image storage tube might be used in the oscilloscope to integrate and retain the image. This would have the advantage that the image could be seen without delay as it was building up. The controlled persistence of the tube could be used to advantage when watching changing patterns of activity. When the activity pattern is changing very slowly, time-lapse motion picture techniques might be used to visualize the action. The motion of tracers in plants and animals, as well as industrial processes, could be studied this way.

RADIOBIOLOGY

Assay of Plasma Insulin in Human Subjects by Immunological Methods

WE have previously reported on the immuno-assay of beef insulin and certain other animal insulins, employing antiserums from human subjects treated with commercial mixtures of beef and pork insulin[1]. The insulin-binding antibodies present in these antiserums do not form precipitable complexes with insulin, but with the use of insulin labelled with iodine-131 the complexes are readily demonstrable by paper chromatography and electrophoresis[2]. Beef, pork, sheep and horse insulins can be assayed quantitatively by measurement of the degree of competitive inhibition of binding of any insulin labelled with iodine-131[1–3]. As might have been anticipated, however, human insulin competes too weakly in systems employing human antiserum to be measurable at concentrations which obtain *in vivo*. Furthermore, the lack of availability of significant quantities of pure human insulin precludes its use as an antigen for animal immunization. However, in the present work, it has been found that human insulin cross-reacts strongly with insulin-binding antibodies in guinea pigs immunized with crystalline beef insulin, and that guinea pig anti-beef insulin serum has characteristics suitable for the detection and measurement of human insulin at concentrations which exist in the plasma of normal fasting subjects.

The methods employed and results obtained in this work will be described in detail elsewhere. It is sufficient to note here that, following incubation of antiserum with tracer quantities of crystalline beef insulin-^{131}I of high specific activity (40–100 mc. iodine-131/mgm. insulin) radio-active insulin bound to antibody is readily distinguished from unbound ('free') insulin-^{131}I by paper chromato-electrophoresis[2] (Fig. 1) and that the ratio of bound to free insulin at trace concentrations of insulin-^{131}I can be lowered to any desired level by appropriate dilution of the antiserum. Dilutions yielding ratios of bound to free insulin between 1 and 3 at trace insulin-^{131}I concentrations are most satisfactory for precise work. At any fixed dilution of antiserum, the ratio of bound to free insulin decreases progressively with increments in the concentration of added human insulin. The precision of the technique and the sensitivity for detection of insulin are greater according as the slope of bound to free insulin concentration is sharper. The minimum amount of tracer beef insulin-^{131}I which can be used is limited by the sensitivity of the counting system employed but must be low enough to avoid saturating the initial portion of the curve where the slope is sharpest. Best results are therefore obtained with preparations of the highest specific activity. Fig. 1 shows some representative radio-chromato-electrophoretograms. From such results a curve for bound to free insulin versus concentration of human insulin in known standards can be obtained. Table 1 gives the concentrations of human insulin in plasma samples of subjects W. and B. before and after administration of glucose.

Table 1

Subject	Endogenous insulin concentration (micro-units/ml. plasma): fasting	½ hr. after 100 gm. glucose *per os*	1 hr. after 100 gm. glucose *per os*	2 hr. after 100 gm. glucose *per os*
W	98	145	302	302
B	64	145	236	

Known standards of human insulin

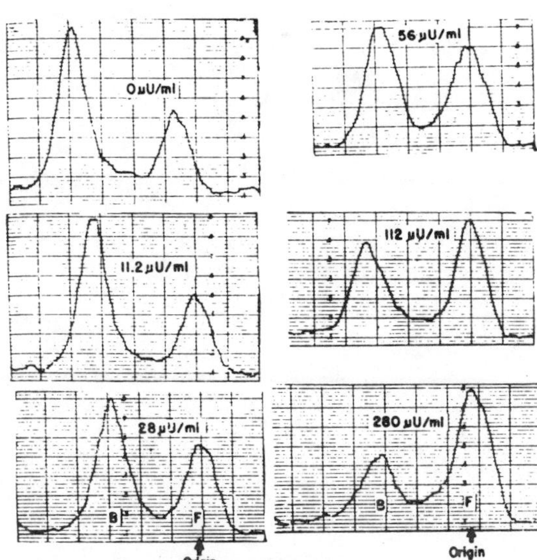

Plasma-subject W. 1 : 4 dilution

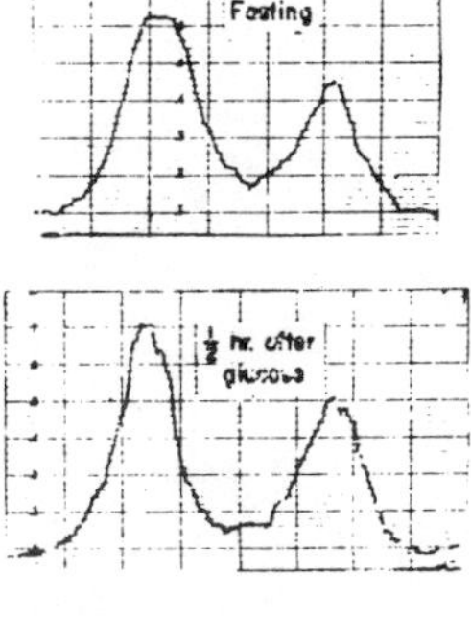

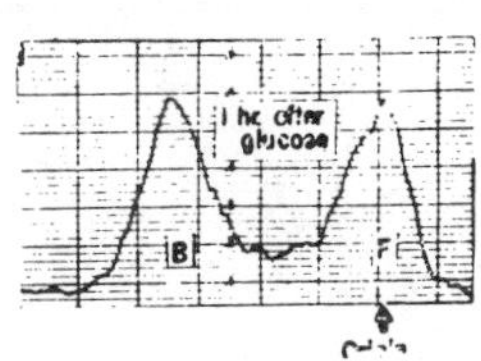

Fig. 1. Radio-chromato-electrophoretograms of mixtures containing the same concentrations of tracer crystalline beef insulin-^{131}I and guinea pig anti-beef insulin serum but varying concentrations of human insulin from known standards (left), or 1 : 4 dilutions of plasma from a human subject before and after administration of glucose (right). Two-tenths ml. of mixtures was applied to paper strips along line marked 'origin'; veronal buffer, ionic strength 0·1, *p*H 8·6 ; 15 V./cm. Free insulin (*F*) is adsorbed to paper at origin ; antibody,bound insulin (*B*) migrates with serum proteins towards left under influence of water-flow chromatography and electrophoresis

Two to three micro-units of human insulin were detectable in the experiment depicted, but in other experiments employing beef insulin-^{131}I preparations of higher specific activity and more sensitive anti-serums, amounts of human insulin in the range 0·25–1·0 micro- units (1·25–5·0 micro-units/ml.) have been measured.

We are indebted to Drs. F. Tietze and J. Field for the human insulin employed as standard in this work.

ROSALYN S. YALOW
SOLOMON A. BERSON

Radioisotope Service,
Veterans Administration Hospital,
Bronx 68, New York.

1 Berson, S. A., and Yalow, R. S., "Adv. in Biol. and Med. Physics", 6, 350 (1958).
2 Berson, S. A., Yalow, R. S., Bauman, A., Rothschild, M. A., and Newerly, K., *J. Clin. Invest.*, 35, 170 (1956).
3 Berson, S. A., and Yalow, R. S., *Fed. Proc.*, 18, 11 (1959).